Manual of Cardiac Intensive Care

Manual of Cardiac Intensive Care

DAVID L. BROWN, MD

Professor, Cardiovascular Medicine (retired)
Washington University School of Medicine
St. Louis, Missouri

DAVID WARRINER, MD, PhD

Consultant Cardiologist
Department of Cardiology
Doncaster Royal Infirmary
Doncaster and Bassetlaw Teaching Hospitals NHS Foundation
Doncaster, United Kingdom;
Consultant Cardiologist
Department of Adult Congenital Cardiology
Leeds General Infirmary
Leeds Teaching Hospital NHS Trust
Leeds, United Kingdom;
Honorary Senior Lecturer Department of Infection, Immunity and Cardiovascular Disease
Faculty of Medicine, Dentistry and Health
The University of Sheffield
Sheffield, United Kingdom

ELSEVIER

Elsevier
1600 John F. Kennedy Blvd.
Ste 1800
Philadelphia, PA 19103-2899

MANUAL OF CARDIAC INTENSIVE CARE   ISBN: 9780323825528

ISBN: 9780323825528

Content Strategist: Robin Carter
Content Development Specialist: Akanksha Marwah
Publishing Services Manager: Shereen Jameel
Project Manager: Nadhiya Sekar
Design Direction: Margaret Reid

Printed in India

Last digit is the print number: 9   8   7   6   5   4   3

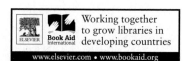

Dedicated to my children and life force, Noah and Erin.

David L. Brown, MD

Dedicated to Beth, Agnes, Bob and my parents.

David Warriner, MD, PhD

ACKNOWLEDGMENTS

Special thanks to Robin Carter who first proposed the idea of this handbook in a succinct e-mail sent on February 25, 2020, and the many other outstanding professionals at Elsevier who helped bring this book to fruition. Responsibility for any mistakes that find their way into the finished book falls solely on the authors' shoulders. We also owe a great deal of gratitude to the authors of the original chapters in *Cardiac Intensive Care* textbook, which we condensed to form this handbook.

David L. Brown, MD

Thank you to all the inspiring colleagues, teachers, mentors, peers, juniors, seniors and everyone in between who encouraged me to keep doing what I love doing; reading, writing and teaching.

David Warriner, MD, PhD

This handbook is a distillation of the most important concepts presented in the textbook *Cardiac Intensive Care*, now in its third edition. It was compiled by two co-authors who are at opposite ends of the career spectrum. Hopefully, that combination of vitality and experience results in a unique contribution to the cardiology literature. Our goal was to create a portable, easy-to-read, pocket-sized compendium of cardiac intensive care medicine that could be quickly referenced while in the midst of caring for these very ill patients. Our hope is that this handbook will translate into better understanding of the diagnosis and treatment of patients with severe cardiac diseases by learners at all levels and, most importantly, improved outcomes for patients.

David L. Brown, MD
David Warriner, MD, PhD

We would like to acknowledge the following for their contributions to *Cardiac Intensive Care*, the book from which this manual was derived:

Masood Akhtar, MD, FHRS, MACP, FACC, FAHA
Richard G. Bach, MD
Eric R. Bates, MD
Brigitte M. Baumann, MD, MSCE
Dmitri Belov, MD
Andreia Biolo, MD, ScD
Daniel Blanchard, MD
Matthew J. Chung, MD
Wilson S. Colucci, MD
Leslie T. Cooper Jr, MD
Mark Gdowski, MD
Michael M. Givertz, MD
Barry Greenberg, MD
George Gubernikoff, MD
Colleen Harrington, MD
Alan C. Heffner, MD
Bettina Heidecker, MD
Brian D. Hoit, MD
Ruth Hsiao, MD
Ulrich Jorde, MD
Mark S. Link, MD
Jacob Luthman, MD
Rohit Malhotra, MD
Pamela K. Mason, MD
Theo E. Meyer, MD, DPhil
Joshua D. Mitchell, MD
Jonathan D. Moreno, MD, PhD
Marlies Ostermann, PhD, MD, FICM
Nimesh Patel, MD
Richard M. Pescatore II, DO

Abhiram Prasad, MD, FRCP, FESC, FACC
Thomas M. Przybysz, MD
Claudio Ronco, MD
Michael Shehata, MD
Jeffrey A. Shih, MD
Adam Shpigel, MD
Daniel B. Sims, MD
Hal A. Skopicki, MD, PhD
Ali A. Sovari, MD, FACC, FHRS
Peter C. Spittell, MD
Jonathan D. Wolfe, MD
Paria Zarghamravanbakhsh, MD
Jodi Zilinski, MD

TABLE OF CONTENTS

CHAPTER 1

Cardiac Physical Examination in the Cardiac Intensive Care Unit

Common Misconceptions

- The physical examination in the Cardiac Intensive Care Unit (CICU) no longer contributes to achieving optimal patient outcomes in the era of ubiquitous laboratory testing and imaging.
- There is a single normal value for blood pressure.
- *Elevated jugular venous pressure* and *jugular venous distention* are synonymous terms.

Vital Signs

RESPIRATION

- The respiratory effort, rate, and pattern should be assessed in both ventilated and nonventilated patients.
- Accessory muscle use is common with pulmonary edema, chronic obstructive pulmonary disease (COPD), asthma exacerbations, and pneumonia.
- With acute tachypnea (a respiratory rate > 25 breaths/min), an immediate assessment should be performed to distinguish peripheral cyanosis (dusky or bluish tinge to the fingers and toes without mucosal or buccal changes) from central cyanosis (associated with a bluish tinge to the lips or mucosa under the tongue) (see below).
- Tachypnea, when secondary to hypoxia, should nearly always be associated with a reflex tachycardia.
- When tachypnea is present with a history of orthopnea, it suggests pulmonary edema, pleural effusion, or both.
- Hypopnea is defined as less than 10 shallow or slow breaths per minute. It may be caused by severe cardiopulmonary failure, sepsis, central nervous system (CNS) depressants (e.g., sedative-hypnotics, narcotics, and alcohol), or CNS disease (e.g., cerebrovascular accident, meningitis).

Breathing patterns can reveal underlying pathology (Table 1.1).

PULSE

The pulse should be assessed bilaterally for presence, rate, volume, contour, and regularity. An initial examination should always contain a description of the radial and carotid arteries, in addition to the brachial, femoral, popliteal, and pedal pulses.

- A discrepancy in bilateral upper extremity pulses (especially with decreases in rate or volume on the left side) raises the possibility of aortic dissection, subclavian narrowing secondary to atherosclerosis, or congenital webs.
- Aortic dissection is suggested by a pulse deficit, focal neurologic signs, and mediastinal widening on the chest radiograph.

TABLE 1.1 ▪ **Breathing Patterns**

Respiratory Pattern	Consider	Eponym/ Classification
Deep and rapid	Diabetic ketoacidosis	Kussmaul respiration
Snoring with episodic apnea	Obstructive sleep apnea	
Waxing and waning tachypnea/hypopnea alternating with apnea	Oversedation	Cheyne-Stokes breathing
	Heart failure	
	Severe CNS process	
	Respiratory failure	
	Renal disease (uremia)	
Irregularly irregular (yet equal) breaths alternating with periods of apnea	Damage to the medulla oblongata (intracranial disease)	Biot breathing
Completely irregular breaths (pauses with escalating periods of apnea)	Severe damage to the medulla oblongata	Ataxic respiration
No breaths or occasional gasps	Severe cardiovascular or neurologic disease	Agonal breathing

CNS, Central nervous system.

- Diminished lower extremity pulses are consistent with coarctation of the aorta or atherosclerotic disease of the abdominal aorta and/or the arterial supply of the lower extremities.
- Pulsus alternans is a pulse with alternately strong and weak beats.
- In patients with normal heart rates, pulsus alternans indicates severe left ventricular (LV) dysfunction.

When tachycardia (heart rate > 100 beats/min) is present, the regularity of the rhythm offers important diagnostic clues.

- Regular rhythm rates between 125 beats/min and 160 beats/min suggest sinus tachycardia, the presence of atrial flutter with 2:1 block, or ventricular tachycardia.
- Intermittent cannon A waves in the neck veins are highly sensitive, whereas a changing intensity of the first heart sound (S_1) is highly specific for the detection of ventricular tachycardia.
- Atrial flutter may be accompanied by rapid undulations in the jugular venous pulse (flutter waves or F waves).
- Detection of an irregular tachycardia suggests atrial fibrillation, atrial premature beats, or ventricular premature contractions.
- In atrial fibrillation, assessment of the apical rate (counting heartbeats via auscultation) is more accurate than counting the radial pulse, accounting for a "pulse deficit."
- Bradycardia (heart rate < 50 beats/min) in a patient with fatigue, mental status changes, or evidence of impaired peripheral perfusion or pulmonary congestion raises the possibility of pharmacologic toxicity (i.e., digoxin, β-blockers, or calcium channel blockers), hypothermia (owing to hypothyroidism or exposure), or an atrioventricular nodal or ventricular escape rhythm that occurs with complete heart block or sick sinus syndrome.

Appreciation of the pulse volume and contour is also informative (Table 1.2). Irregular rhythms are classified as either *regularly irregular,* in which the irregular beat can be anticipated at a fixed interval, or *irregularly irregular,* in which the irregular beat occurs without predictability.

- A regularly irregular pulse commonly occurs with second-degree atrioventricular block (either Mobitz I or II, depending on whether the PR interval is constant or lengthening before the dropped beat) or with interpolated ventricular premature beats.

TABLE 1.2 ■ **Pulse Characteristics**

Pulse Description	Consider
Bounding	Septic shock, hyperthyroidism, chronic AR
Weak and thready	Severe LV dysfunction, hypovolemia, severe MR, complete heart block, pericardial effusion
Slow rising and weak	Severe AS
Alternating between strong and weak	LV dysfunction, pericardial tamponade
Double tap (pulsus bisferiens)	Hypertrophic cardiomyopathy, AS with AR

AR, Aortic regurgitation; *AS*, aortic stenosis; *LV*, left ventricular; *MR*, mitral regurgitation.

- On the physical examination, the PR interval can be visualized as the distance between the *a* wave and *c* wave on the jugular venous pulse.
- This distance, before and after the dropped beat, can be diagnostic when the electrocardiogram is unable to differentiate between Mobitz type I and Mobitz type II second-degree block.
- When an interpolated ventricular premature beat is present, it may be accompanied by a weakened pulse (owing to inadequate ventricular filling) that occurs at a fixed interval from the regular pulse.
- An irregularly irregular pulse implies that the examiner cannot anticipate when the next beat will occur; it may be caused by ventricular premature beats, atrial premature beats, multifocal atrial tachycardia, or atrial fibrillation.
- Although ventricular premature beats and atrial fibrillation are associated with a pulse deficit (in which the auscultated apical rate is greater than the palpable radial pulse), the impulse that follows a ventricular premature beat should be stronger.
- If the beat following a ventricular premature beat is diminished (Brockenbrough sign), hypertrophic cardiomyopathy or severe LV dysfunction should be considered.
- No pulse deficit (or compensatory pause) should be present with atrial premature beats or multifocal atrial tachycardia.

Blood Pressure

There is no rigid definition of "normal" blood pressure. *Adequate* blood pressure varies by patient and clinical status, but is generally believed to consist of a mean perfusion pressure of at least 60 mm Hg and the absence of end-organ hypoperfusion.

In patients with LV systolic dysfunction, hypotension may be caused by volume depletion from overly aggressive diuresis or because of volume overload.

- The presence of tachycardia with orthostatic hypotension (a blood pressure decrease of > 20 mm Hg systolic or > 10 mm Hg diastolic when the patient is assessed first in the supine position and then again after 2 minutes with the patient standing or sitting with legs dangling) is consistent with volume depletion.
- The differential diagnosis of hypotension includes factors that reduce systemic vascular resistance (e.g., infection, inflammation, adrenal insufficiency, anesthetic agents, atrioventricular malformations, and vascular insufficiency), stroke volume (e.g., hypovolemia; aortic stenosis; severe mitral regurgitation; ventricular arrhythmias; and LV dysfunction owing to infarction, ischemia, or a cardiomyopathy), and heart rate (e.g., heart block or pharmacologic bradycardia).

- A pulsus paradoxus (a $> 10\,mm$ Hg decrease in systolic blood pressure occurring at end expiration with the patient breathing *normally*) can occur with cardiac tamponade (very sensitive when occurring with tachycardia, jugular venous distention, and an absent y descent), constrictive pericarditis (occurring with jugular venous distention that persistently augments with inspiration, a pericardial knock, hepatomegaly, and an exaggerated y descent), severe hypertension, pulmonary embolism, COPD, and severe obesity.

The pulse pressure (systolic blood pressure – diastolic blood pressure) may be normal, narrow, or wide.

- A narrow pulse pressure may be present with the decreased stroke volume of hypovolemia, tachycardia, severe aortic or mitral stenosis, pericardial constriction, or cardiac tamponade.
- With appropriate clinical suspicion, a narrow pulse pressure has high sensitivity and specificity to predict a cardiac index less than $2.2\,L/min/m^2$ when the pulse pressure divided by the systolic pressure is less than 0.25.
- A wide pulse pressure ($> 60\,mm$ Hg) can be seen with hyperthermia, but may also suggest severe chronic aortic regurgitation or highoutput heart failure from severe anemia, thyrotoxicosis, atrioventricular malformation, sepsis, vitamin B_1 deficiency, or Paget disease.

Jugular Venous Pressure

The jugular venous pressure (JVP) is a useful manometer for central venous or right atrial pressure.

- The JVP measured in centimeters of water (H_2O) is converted to mm Hg by multiplying by 0.735.
- Elevated JVP and jugular venous distention are not synonymous, and the latter term should be abandoned because jugular venous distention can occur in the supine position with normal JVP.
- JVP is accurate in indicating intravascular volume status and pulmonary capillary wedge pressure in the absence of tricuspid stenosis, right ventricular dysfunction, pulmonary hypertension, and a restrictive or constrictive cardiomyopathy.
- The JVP should be sought by asking the patient to lift the chin up and turn to the left against the resistance of the examiner's right hand. Within the triangle formed by the visible heads of the sternocleidomastoid muscle and the clavicle, the examiner should then search, with the neck muscles relaxed, for the weak impulses of the jugular vein along a line from the jaw to the clavicle.
- Simultaneous palpation of the radial pulse, assuming that the patient is in sinus rhythm, allows detection of a neck pulsation (a wave) immediately preceding the peripheral pulse (Fig. 1.1).
- Alternatively, one can visualize the x descent as an inward movement along the line of the jugular vein that occurs simultaneously with the peripheral pulse.
- In patients with volume overload, elevation of JVP may be best assessed with the patient sitting upright, a position in which the clavicle is approximately 7 to 8 cm above the right atrium (equivalent to the upper limit of normal for right atrial pressure, 5 to 7 mm Hg).
- The 7 to 8 cm is added to the maximal vertical distance at which any venous pulsations are seen above the clavicle to estimate the right atrial pressure.
- If the JVP cannot be appreciated in the upright position, an attempt can be made to visualize it by progressively reducing the angle of the upper body until pulsations become apparent.
- If venous pulsations are still difficult to discern, either of two extremes may be present: either there is no elevation of the JVP, or the JVP is so far above the angle of the jaw, even in the upright position, that it is lost in the hairline. The ear lobe should always be assessed for movement in these cases.
- A low JVP may be investigated further by increasing right atrial filling (i.e., with deep inspiration or passive leg elevation).

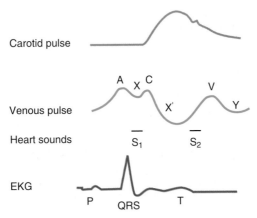

Fig. 1.1 Timing of jugular venous pressure. *ECG*, Electrocardiogram.

- When an increasing creatinine value is seen in the presence of an elevated JVP (with or without diuresis), the differential diagnosis includes refractory LV dysfunction requiring inotropic support, severe right ventricular (RV) dysfunction, restrictive or constrictive cardiomyopathy, RV failure, or secondary renal dysfunction (cardiorenal syndrome).
- With RV dysfunction, the assessment of JVP as a measure of pulmonary capillary wedge pressure (PCWP) becomes progressively less accurate.

Chest and Lung Examination
Different breath sounds provide important diagnostic clues regarding underlying lung pathology (Table 1.3).

Precordial inspection and palpation

Visible or palpable precordial pulsations may be a sign of cardiac disease.
- Pulsations in the second intercostal space to the left of the sternal border suggest an elevated pulmonary artery pressure.
- Pulsations seen in the fourth intercostal space at the left sternal border are consistent with RV dysfunction or an acute ventricular septal defect.

LV Apical Impulse
- The LV apical impulse is palpated by placing the right hand transversely across the precordium under the nipple and is perceived as an upward pulsation during systole against the examiner's hand.
- An LV apical impulse displaced to the left of the midclavicular line increases the probability that the heart is enlarged on chest radiograph, the ejection fraction is reduced, the LV end-diastolic pressure is increased, and the pulmonary capillary wedge pressure is increased.
- As measured in the left lateral decubitus position at 45 degrees, an apical impulse of 4 cm or more increases the probability that the patient has a dilated heart.
- LV enlargement is suggested by the presence of a sustained apical impulse (persisting more than halfway between S_1 and S_2 during simultaneous auscultation and palpation).
- If the LV apical impulse is detectable at end-systole, a dyskinetic apex is likely.
- If the apical impulse retracts during systole, constrictive pericarditis or tricuspid regurgitation should be considered.

TABLE 1.3 ■ Auscultation of the Lungs

Breath Sound	Consider
Rhonchi	
Diffuse	COPD
Localized	Pneumonia, tumor, foreign body
Stridorous	Large airway obstruction
Wheezes	
Expiratory	Reactive small airway obstruction (asthma, allergies, β-blockers)
De novo	Nonasthmatic causes (mass, pulmonary embolism, pulmonary edema, aspiration, foreign body)
Crackles or rales	Pulmonary edema, interstitial lung disease, COPD, amiodarone toxicity

COPD, Chronic obstructive pulmonary disease.

- All auscultatory fields should be palpated with the fingertips to detect a thrill (required for the diagnosis of a grade IV/VI murmur) or other abnormal pulsations.
- The presence of a palpable P_2 (an upward pulsation during diastole in the pulmonic position) suggests the presence of either secondary (acute pulmonary embolism, chronic mitral regurgitation, or stenosis) or primary pulmonary hypertension.
- A palpable pulsation in the aortic position during systole suggests hypertrophic cardiomyopathy or severe aortic stenosis.
- A thrill over the left sternal border in the fourth intercostal space, especially in the setting of an acute myocardial infarction (AMI), raises the possibility of a ventricular septal defect.
- A presystolic impulse (correlating with the *a* wave and equivalent to an audible S_4) suggests ventricular noncompliance and may be present with myocardial ischemia or infarction, with LV hypertrophy secondary to hypertension, aortic stenosis, acute mitral regurgitation, or hypertrophic cardiomyopathy.

AUSCULTATION OF THE HEART

- Cardiac auscultation allows for the detection of abnormal heart sounds (S_1, S_2, S_3, S_4) (Table 1.4) and common holosystolic (mitral regurgitation and ventricular septal defect), systolic ejection (aortic stenosis or hypertrophic cardiomyopathy), and diastolic (aortic regurgitation and mitral stenosis) murmurs.

HEART MURMURS: STATIC AND DYNAMIC AUSCULTATION

- Heart murmurs are categorized as systolic, diastolic, or continuous and should be further described according to their location, timing, duration, pitch, intensity, and response to dynamic maneuvers (Table 1.5).
- The optimal locations for detecting specific valvular pathology must be recognized.
- The aortic valve area is located right of the sternal border in the second intercostal space.
- The pulmonic valve area is to the left of the sternal border in the second intercostal space.
- The tricuspid valve area is found left of the sternal border in the fourth intercostal space.
- The mitral valve area is located midclavicular on the left side of the chest in the fifth intercostal space.
- The pathophysiology of murmurs may be divided into regurgitant and stenotic defects.

TABLE 1.4 ■ **Clinical Auscultation of S_1, S_2, S_3, and S_4**

Heart Sound	Consider
S_1	
Accentuated	Atrial fibrillation, mitral stenosis
Soft	Immobile mitral valves, MR, or severe AR
S_2	
Accentuated	(P_2) Pulmonary hypertension; (A_2) systemic hypertension; aortic dilation
Soft	(A_2) AR, sepsis, AV fistula
A_2-P^2 Splitting	
Wide	Severe MR, RBBB, atrial septal defect (secondary), pulmonary hypertension
Paradoxic	Severe TR, WPW, LBBB, severe hypertension, or AS
Fixed	Large atrial septal defect, severe RV failure
S_3	
Present	Heart failure, HOCM, thyrotoxicosis, AV fistula, sepsis, hyperthermia
S_4	
Present	Ischemic or infarcted LV, hypertrophic, dilated, or restrictive cardiomyopathy

AR, Aortic regurgitation; *AS*, aortic stenosis; *AV*, atrioventricular; *HOCM*, hypertrophic obstructive cardiomyopathy; *LBBB*, left bundle branch block; *MR*, mitral regurgitation; *RBBB*, right bundle branch block; *TR*, tricuspid regurgitation; *WPW*, Wolff-Parkinson-White.

- Although the gradations I to III are arbitrary (grade I, very faint, difficult to hear; grade II, faint, but readily identified; and grade III, moderately loud), the presence of a grade IV murmur always denotes the presence of an associated palpable thrill.
- Grade V is a louder murmur with a thrill.
- Grade VI occurs when the murmur is heard with the stethoscope physically off the chest wall.
- Holosystolic murmurs, with a soft or obliterated S_2, occur with tricuspid regurgitation, ventricular septal defects, and mitral regurgitation. Tricuspid regurgitation is suggested when the holosystolic murmur is best appreciated in the fourth intercostal space along the left sternal border and augments with inspiration, passive leg elevation, and isometric handgrip.
- In the setting of an acute inferior wall or extensive anterior wall MI, the presence of a new holosystolic murmur occurring with a palpable RV lift requires that an acute ventricular septal defect be excluded.
- The holosystolic murmur of mitral regurgitation is best appreciated at the apex during end expiration in the left lateral decubitus position and is associated with a soft S_1.
- With acute mitral regurgitation, the murmur may be absent or it may appear earlier or later in systole.
- When mitral regurgitation is severe, evidence of pulmonary hypertension may also be present.
- Posterior mitral leaflet involvement results in a murmur that radiates anteriorly, whereas posterior radiation into the axilla suggests anterior mitral valve leaflet dysfunction.
- Isometric handgrip results in a rapid increase in venous return and peripheral resistance that causes the murmur of mitral regurgitation (and aortic regurgitation) to grow louder.
- The harsh crescendo-decrescendo systolic ejection murmur of aortic stenosis begins shortly after S_1, peaks toward mid-systole, and ends before S_2.

TABLE 1.5 ▓ Dynamic Cardiac Auscultation

Maneuver	Physiology	TR	PS	VSD	MR	AS	HOCM	AR
Inspiration	Increased venous return and ventricular volume	↑	↑		nc/↑			
Expiration	Brings heart closer to the chest wall	↑			nc/↑			
Leg elevation	Increased SVR; increased venous return						↓	
Mueller maneuver	Decrease CVP/BP/SNA (10 sec), then increase in BP/SNA (5 sec) and surge in BP/decrease SNA with release	↑						
Valsalva maneuver	Decreased venous return and ventricular volumes (phase 2)		↓		↓	↓	↑	↓
Squatting to standing	Decreased venous return and volume	↓	↓	↓	↓	↓	↑	
Standing to squatting	Increased venous return; increased SVR			↑	↑	↑	↓	↑
Handgrip	Increased SVR; increased CO; increased LV filling pressures			↑	↑	↓	↓	↑

Inspiration also increases the murmur of tricuspid stenosis and pulmonary regurgitation. *AR*, Aortic regurgitation; *AS*, aortic stenosis; *BP*, blood pressure; *CO*, cardiac output; *CVP*, central venous pressure; *HOCM*, hypertrophic obstructive cardiomyopathy; *LV*, left ventricular; *MR*, mitral regurgitation; *PS*, pulmonary stenosis; *nc*, no changes; *TR*, tricuspid regurgitation; *SNA*, sympathetic nerve activity; *SVR*, systemic vascular resistance; *VSD*, ventricular septal defect.

- The aortic stenosis murmur is best appreciated in the second intercostal space to the right of the sternal border and radiates into the right side of the neck.
- A systolic thrill may be palpable at the base of the heart, in the jugular notch, and along the carotid arteries.
- Associated findings include an ejection click (occurring with a bicuspid valve, which disappears as the stenosis becomes more severe) and, with increasing severity, a slow increase and plateau of a weak carotid pulse (pulsus parvus et tardus).
- The severity of the obstruction is related to the duration of the murmur to its peak and not to its intensity.
- An early-peaking murmur is usually associated with a less stenotic valve; a late-peaking murmur, suggesting a longer time for the ventricular pressure to overcome the stenosis, suggests a more severe stenosis.
- A nearly immobile and stenotic aortic valve can result in a muted or absent S_2.
- The high-pitched, diastolic blowing murmur of aortic regurgitation frequently occurs with aortic stenosis.
- Hypertrophic cardiomyopathy is also associated with a crescendo-decrescendo systolic murmur.
- It is best appreciated *between* the apex and left sternal border, however, and although it radiates to the suprasternal notch, it does *not* radiate to the carotid arteries or neck.
- The murmur of hypertrophic cardiomyopathy can also be distinguished from aortic stenosis by an increase in murmur intensity (when the outflow tract gradient is increased) that occurs

during the active phase of the Valsalva maneuver, when changing from sitting to standing (the LV volume abruptly decreases), and with the use of vasodilators.

- Hypertrophic cardiomyopathy may also be accompanied by the holosystolic murmur of mitral regurgitation owing to the anterior motion of the mitral valve during systole.
- Additional findings include a laterally displaced double apical impulse (resulting from the forceful contraction of the left atrium against a noncompliant LV) or a triple apical impulse (resulting from the late systolic impulse that occurs when the nearly empty LV undergoes near-isometric contraction).
- Similarly, a double carotid arterial pulse (pulsus bisferiens) is common because of the initial rapid increase of blood flow through the LV outflow tract into the aorta, which declines in mid-systole as the gradient develops, only to manifest a secondary increase during end-systole.

  Diastolic murmurs are caused by regurgitation of the aortic or pulmonary valves or stenosis of the mitral or tricuspid valves.

- Chronic aortic regurgitation is heralded by a high-frequency, early diastolic decrescendo murmur, best appreciated in the second to fourth left intercostal space with the patient sitting up and leaning forward.
- As aortic regurgitation becomes more severe, the murmur takes up more of diastole.
- When LV dysfunction results in restrictive filling, the murmur of aortic regurgitation may shorten and become softer.
- Moderate to severe aortic regurgitation may also be accompanied by an Austin Flint murmur, a low-frequency, mid-diastolic to late-diastolic murmur best appreciated at the apex caused by left atrial flow into an "overexpanded" LV.
- Aortic regurgitation may be accompanied by a soft S_1, prominent S_3, and a diastolic rumble.
- Severe aortic regurgitation is associated with wide pulse pressure and a multitude of eponym-rich clinical findings including a
  - Corrigan or water-hammer pulse
  - De Musset sign (a head bob with each systole)
  - Müller sign (systolic pulsations of the uvula)
  - Traube sign ("pistol shot" systolic and diastolic sounds heard over the femoral artery)
  - Hill sign (when the popliteal cuff systolic pressure exceeds the brachial cuff pressure by more than 60 mm Hg)
  - Quincke sign (capillary pulsations seen when a light is transmitted through a patient's fingernail)
  - Duroziez sign (an audible systolic murmur heard over the femoral artery when the artery is compressed proximally along with a diastolic murmur when the femoral artery is compressed distally)

Other Diastolic Murmurs

- Pulmonary regurgitation is a diastolic decrescendo murmur that is localized over the second intercostal space. When it is caused by dilation of the pulmonary valve annulus, it produces the characteristic Graham-Steele murmur.
- Mitral stenosis is a mid-diastolic rumble that is appreciated with the bell as a low-pitched sound at the apex, immediately after an opening snap, which increases in intensity with exercise.
- Anatomic or functional tricuspid stenosis (the latter with the delayed opening of the tricuspid valve seen with large atrial or ventricular septal defects) is associated with a mid-diastolic rumble or with the aforementioned Austin Flint murmur of aortic regurgitation.
- Mitral stenosis can be differentiated from tricuspid stenosis by the localization of the latter to the left sternal border and its augmentation with inspiration.

Friction Rubs

- The superficial, high-pitched, or scratchy sound of a pericardial friction rub is best heard with the patient in the sitting position while leaning forward at end-expiration.
- This sound may be systolic, systolic and diastolic, or triphasic and should be suspected in the postinfarction or acute pericarditis setting in the presence of pleuritic chest pain and diffuse ST segment elevations on ECG.

Skin and Extremities Examination

- Detection of cool legs, mottling of the skin, and prolonged capillary refill time (see below) increases the probability of low cardiac output.
- Clubbing suggests central cyanosis, right-to-left shunting with or without congenital heart disease, or bacterial endocarditis.
- Arachnodactyly (long, spidery fingers) may be found in patients with Marfan syndrome.
- Capillary pulsations under the fingernails may be seen with aortic regurgitation, sepsis, or thyrotoxicosis.
- Splinter hemorrhages raise the possibility of bacterial endocarditis.
- Osler nodes (painful reddish papules approximately 1 cm on the fingertips, palms, toes, or soles of the feet) also suggest endocarditis.

Capillary Refill Time

- Capillary refill time (CRT) is defined as the time taken for color to return to an external capillary bed after pressure is applied to cause blanching.
- CRT has been shown to be influenced by ambient temperature, age, sex, and the anatomic testing and lighting conditions.
- The most reliable and applicable site for CRT testing is the finger pulp (not at the fingernail).
- The average value for CRT in healthy persons is 2 seconds.
- A prolonged CRT may be a sign of shock and can also indicate dehydration or peripheral arterial disease.

Cyanosis

- Cyanosis is an abnormal bluish discoloration of the skin and mucous membranes caused by blue-colored blood.
- In central cyanosis, the blood leaving the heart is blue. Typical causes are pulmonary edema, pneumonia, and intracardiac right-to-left shunts.
- In peripheral cyanosis, the blood leaving the heart is red, but it becomes blue in the peripheral circulation owing to increased extraction of oxygen by peripheral tissues. Typical causes are low cardiac output, arterial disease, and venous disease.
- Approximately 4 to 5 g/dL of unoxygenated hemoglobin in the capillaries generates the blue color appreciated clinically as central cyanosis.
- Central cyanosis often improves with supplemental oxygen.
- Cyanosis that does not improve with supplemental oxygen should suggest increased amounts of methemoglobin (e.g., with use of dapsone, nitroglycerin, or topical benzocaine) or sulfhemoglobin.
- If the lower limbs are cyanosed but the upper limbs are not, a patent ductus arteriosus should be expected.
- Pseudocyanosis, a blue color to the skin without deoxygenated hemoglobin, may occur with the use of amiodarone, phenothiazines, and some metals (especially silver and lead).

CHAPTER 2

Acute Myocardial Infarction

Common Misconceptions

- All patients suffering an acute myocardial infarction will complain of chest pain.
- In evaluating a patient with a suspected acute coronary syndrome, it is important to note the severity of chest pain on a scale of 1 to 10.
- The response of chest pain to nitroglycerin or antacids is useful in ruling in or ruling out an acute coronary syndrome as a cause of chest pain.
- A normal electrocardiogram (ECG) rules out an acute myocardial infarction.

Pathogenesis of Acute Myocardial Infarction (MI)

CORONARY THROMBOSIS AND THE PATHOGENESIS OF ACUTE MYOCARDIAL INFARCTION

- Although Herrick attributed fatal acute MI to a thrombotically occluded coronary artery in 1912, autopsy studies in the late 1970s did not demonstrate coronary thrombosis in patients who had died of an acute MI.
- Thus, coronary thrombosis was considered a consequence, rather than the underlying cause, of acute MI.
- In 1980, DeWood and colleagues reported the results of coronary angiography performed early after the onset of an acute transmural MI: within 4 hours of symptom onset, 87% of infarct-obstructed arteries were completely occluded. However, 12 to 24 hours after onset, the prevalence of coronary occlusion was only 65%.
- When patients with subtotal occlusion of the obstructed artery were included, the prevalence of angiographically demonstrable coronary thrombosis in the first 4 hours was 98%.
- Over the past decade, further understanding of the pathology underlying acute coronary occlusion has come from autopsy studies, angiography, and intracoronary imaging: underlying culprit soft lipid plaques, thin cap fibroatheromas, bulky plaques with characteristic erosion, and/or calcified nodules have all been found to predispose to plaque rupture and coronary occlusion (Fig. 2.1).

Diagnosis of Acute Myocardial Infarction

- Myocardial infarction describes the process of myocardial cell death caused by ischemia or the imbalance between myocardial oxygen supply via the coronary arteries and demand.
- In the United States each year, an estimated 1.1 million people experience an acute MI or die from coronary heart disease.
- In 2016, it was estimated that approximately every 34 seconds one American would have a coronary event and about every 1 minute 24 seconds an individual would die from a coronary event.

Thrombus-Predominant
STEMI Pathophysiology

Plaque-Predominant
STEMI Pathophysiology

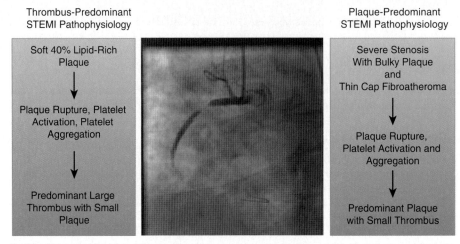

Soft 40% Lipid-Rich
Plaque

↓

Plaque Rupture, Platelet
Activation, Platelet
Aggregation

↓

Predominant Large
Thrombus with Small
Plaque

Severe Stenosis
With Bulky Plaque
and
Thin Cap Fibroatheroma

↓

Plaque Rupture,
Platelet Activation and
Aggregation

↓

Predominant Plaque
with Small Thrombus

Fig. 2.1 The pathophysiology of acute ST elevation myocardial infarction requires thrombosis and occlusion of a coronary artery. Thrombosis is mediated by plaque rupture related to lipid pools, thin cap fibroatheroma, calcific nodules, and plaque erosion.

- According to the most recent World Health Organization report in 2015, coronary heart disease is the leading cause of death worldwide.
- The early recognition and diagnosis of an acute MI are vital for the institution of therapy to limit myocardial damage, preserve cardiac function, and reduce mortality.
- Patients can be grouped into two major categories of acute MI:
  - 1. Patients with new ST segment elevation on the ECG that is diagnostic of acute ST segment elevation myocardial infarction (STEMI)
  - 2. Patients with non–ST segment elevation myocardial infarction (NSTEMI) who have elevated cardiac biomarkers in an appropriate clinical setting, with or without ischemic ECG changes
- Clinical trials have established the benefit of early reperfusion therapy in patients with STEMI and an early invasive strategy in patients with high-risk NSTEMI; thus a rapid and accurate assessment of patients with suspected acute MI is essential for optimal management.

Definition of Myocardial Infarction

- MI is defined as myocardial necrosis caused by prolonged myocardial ischemia.
- The diagnosis of an acute MI requires the rise and/or fall of cardiac biomarkers (preferably troponin) with at least one value exceeding the 99th percentile of a normal reference population (the upper reference limit) and at least one of the following:
  - Symptoms of ischemia
  - ECG changes indicative of active ischemia (new ST segment–T wave changes or new left bundle branch block [LBBB]) or infarction (new pathologic Q waves)
  - 3. Identification of an intracoronary thrombus by angiography or autopsy
  - 4. Imaging evidence of a new regional wall motion abnormality, or new loss of viable myocardium
- The type of acute MI can be classified further depending on the etiology of the infarct (Table 2.1).

TABLE 2.1 ■ Universal Classification of Myocardial Infarction (MI)

Type	Description
1	Spontaneous MI resulting from an atherosclerotic plaque rupture, ulceration, fissuring, erosion, or dissection with resulting intraluminal thrombus
2	MI associated with ischemia owing to an imbalance in myocardial oxygen supply and demand, such as in coronary endothelial dysfunction, coronary artery spasm, coronary embolism, anemia, arrhythmias, hypertension, or hypotension
3	MI resulting in cardiac death, with symptoms suggestive of myocardial ischemia, accompanied by new ischemic electrocardiogram changes, but death occurring before blood samples could be obtained, or at a time before the appearance of cardiac biomarkers in the blood
4a	MI associated with percutaneous coronary intervention
4b	MI associated with stent thrombosis as documented by angiography or autopsy
5	MI associated with coronary artery bypass graft surgery

Modified and adapted from Thygesen K, Alpert JS, Jaffe AS, et al. Third universal definition of myocardial infarction. *J Am Coll Cardiol.* 2012;60:1581–1598.

Biochemical Markers of Acute Myocardial Infarction

■ Cardiac biomarkers are an essential component of the criteria used to establish the diagnosis of acute MI (Table 2.2).

■ Cardiac troponins (I or T) have become the preferred biomarkers for the detection of myocardial necrosis; their use is a class I indication in the diagnosis of MI.

■ The improved sensitivity and tissue specificity of cardiac troponins compared with creatine kinase-myocardial band (CK-MB) and other conventional cardiac biochemical markers of acute MI has been well established.

■ Troponins are not only useful for diagnostic implications, but they also impart prognostic information and can assist in the risk stratification of patients presenting with suspected acute coronary syndromes (ACS).

■ Although detectable increases in cardiac biomarkers are indicative of myocardial injury, cardiac biomarker elevations are not synonymous with acute MI.

■ Many disease states, such as sepsis, congestive heart failure, pulmonary embolism, myocarditis, intracranial hemorrhage, stroke, and renal failure can be associated with an increase in cardiac biomarkers.

■ These elevations arise from mechanisms other than thrombotic coronary artery occlusion and require treatment of the underlying cause rather than the administration of antithrombotic and antiplatelet agents.

■ Acute MI should be diagnosed when cardiac biomarkers are abnormal, and the clinical setting is consistent with myocardial ischemia.

TROPONIN

■ Cardiac troponins are regulatory proteins that control the calcium-mediated interaction of actin and myosin, which results in contraction and relaxation in striated muscle.

■ The troponin complex is composed of three subunits: troponin C, which binds calcium; troponin I, which inhibits actin-myosin interactions; and troponin T, which attaches the troponin complex by binding to tropomyosin and facilitates contraction.

TABLE 2.2 ▦ Biochemical Markers of Myocardial Necrosis

Marker	Initial Appearance (h)	Mean Time to Peak	Return to Basal	Sampling Schedule
Myoglobin	1–4	6–7h	12–24h	Initially, then every 1–2h
CK–MB (tissue isoform)	2–6	18h	48–72h	Initially, then every 3–6h
Cardiac troponin I	3–6	24h	7–10 days	Initially, then every 3–6h
Cardiac troponin T	3–6	12–48h	10–14 days	Initially, then every 3–6h
CK	3–12	24h	72–96h	Initially, then every 8h
Lactate dehydrogenase (LDH)	10	48–72h	10–14 days	Once at least 24h after chest pain

Modified from Adams J, Abendschein DR, Jaffe AS. Biochemical markers of myocardial injury: is MB creatine kinase the choice for the 1990's? *Circulation*. 1993;88:750–763.
CK-MB, creatine kinase-myocardial band isoenzyme.

- Troponin C is expressed by cells in cardiac and skeletal muscle; in contrast, the amino acid sequences of troponins I and T are unique to cardiac muscle.
- This difference between troponin C vs troponin I and T, has allowed for the development of rapid, quantitative assays to detect elevations of cardiac troponins in the serum.
- Troponin is the preferred biomarker for use in the diagnosis of acute MI because of superior tissue specificity and sensitivity for MI and its usefulness as a prognostic indicator.

Diagnosis

- Troponin is released early in the course of an acute MI.
- An increased concentration of cardiac troponin is defined as exceeding the 99th percentile of a normal reference population.
- Troponin exceeding this limit on at least one occasion in the setting of clinical myocardial ischemia is indicative of an acute MI.
- Elevated troponin can be detected within 3 to 4 hours after the onset of myocardial injury.
- Serum levels can remain increased for 7 to 10 days for troponin I and 10 to 14 days for troponin T (Fig. 2.2).
- The initial release of troponin is from the cellular cytosol, whereas the persistent elevation is a result of the slower dispersion of troponin from degrading cardiac myofilaments.
- As a result of these kinetics, the sensitivity of troponin increases with time.
- At 60 minutes after the onset of an acute MI, the sensitivity is approximately 90%, but maximal sensitivity of troponin (≈ 99%) is not achieved until 6 or more hours after the initiation of myocardial necrosis.
- As a result of its high tissue specificity, cardiac troponin is associated with fewer false–positive results in the setting of concomitant skeletal muscle injury compared with CK-MB.
- This inherent characteristic of troponin is useful in the assessment of myocardial injury in patients with chronic muscle diseases, perioperative MIs, and after electrical cardioversion or blunt cardiac trauma.
- It is important to note that, although cardiac troponin is highly tissue specific, its elevation does not indicate the mechanism of myocardial injury; if elevated troponins are found in the

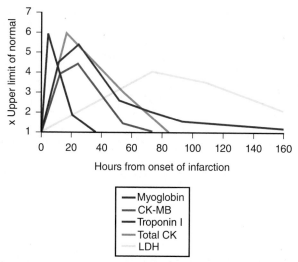

Fig. 2.2 Time course of biochemical marker levels during acute myocardial infarction. The relative timing and extent of the increase above normal values of the commonly used serum markers during acute myocardial infarction are shown. *CK*, creatine kinase; *CK-MB*, creatine kinase-myocardial band isoenzyme; *LDH*, lactate dehydrogenase.

absence of myocardial ischemia, an evaluation for alternative etiologies of myocardial injury should be pursued.

- Elevated troponins are not only vital to the diagnosis of NSTEMI, but also serve to direct treatment by identifying patients who would benefit from an early invasive management strategy.
- In the Treat Angina with Aggrastat and Determine Cost of Therapy with an Invasive or Conservative Strategy–Thrombolysis in Myocardial Infarction 18 (TACTICS–TIMI 18) study, patients with any increase in troponin who underwent early angiography (within 4 to 48 hours) and revascularization (if appropriate) achieved an approximately 55% reduction in the odds of death or MI compared with patients undergoing conservative treatment.

CREATINE KINASE MB

- Creatine kinase is a cytosolic carrier protein for high-energy phosphates.
- CK-MB is an isoenzyme of CK that is most abundant in the heart.
- However, CK-MB also constitutes 1% to 3% of the CK in skeletal muscle and is present in a small fraction in other organs, such as the small bowel, uterus, prostate, and diaphragm.
- The specificity of CK-MB may be impaired in the setting of major injury to these organs, especially skeletal muscle.
- Although cardiac troponin is the preferred marker of myocardial necrosis, CK-MB by mass assay is an acceptable alternative when cardiac troponin is unavailable.
- The diagnostic limit for CK-MB is defined as the 99th percentile in a sex-specific reference control group.
- All assays for CK-MB show a significant two-fold to three-fold higher 99th percentile limit for men compared with women.
- In addition, CK-MB can have two-fold to three-fold higher concentrations in African Americans than in caucasians.

- These discrepancies have been attributed to physiologic differences in muscle mass.
- It is recommended that two consecutive measurements of CK-MB above the diagnostic limit in a rise-and-fall pattern be required for sufficient evidence of myocardial necrosis because of the inherent lower tissue specificity of CK-MB compared with troponin.
- The temporal increase of CK-MB is similar to that of troponin in that it occurs within 3 to 4 hours after the onset of myocardial injury, but in contrast to troponin, CK-MB decreases to the normal range by 48 to 72 hours (see Fig. 2.2).
- The rapid decline of CK-MB to the reference interval by 48 to 72 hours allows for the discrimination of early reinfarction when ischemic symptoms recur between 72 hours and 2 weeks after the index acute MI; during this time, troponin may still be elevated from the original event.
- Similar to troponin, the amount of CK-MB released is useful for estimation of infarct size, which correlates with left ventricular function, incidence of ventricular arrhythmias, and prognosis.

Clinical Evaluation

- The evaluation of a patient presenting with acute MI should begin with a targeted history that ascertains the following:
  - Characterization and duration of chest discomfort and any associated symptoms
  - Prior episodes of myocardial ischemia, MI, percutaneous coronary intervention (PCI), or coronary artery bypass surgery
  - History of hypertension, hyperlipidemia, diabetes mellitus, tobacco use, cerebrovascular disease, and other cardiovascular risk factors
  - Assessment of bleeding risk and contraindications to anticoagulation
- The classic description of an acute MI consists of crushing, substernal chest pain or vice-like tightness with or without radiation to the left arm, neck, jaw, interscapular area, or epigastrium.
  - This presentation is associated with an estimated 24% probability of an acute MI; the probability decreases to about 1% if the pain is positional or pleuritic in a patient without a prior history of coronary artery disease.
  - Alternatively, the chest pain may be described as burning like indigestion, or sharp and stabbing, which are associated with a 23% and 5% probability of acute MI, respectively.
  - Patients may commonly deny pain, but describe a sensation of chest discomfort.
  - The duration of the discomfort is usually prolonged, lasting more than 30 minutes, but may wax and wane or even remit completely.
  - There may be associated vagal symptoms of nausea, vomiting, lightheadedness, and diaphoresis.
  - The severity of chest pain, commonly graded on a scale of 1 to 10, is not useful in discriminating ischemia or infarction from other causes of pain and should be abandoned.
  - The index of suspicion for different chest pain characteristics in diagnosing acute coronary ischemia is shown in (Fig. 2.3).
- Elderly patients and women more commonly have atypical presentations that mimic abdominal pathology or a neurologic event (Table 2.3).
- One third of all MIs are unrecognized, especially in patients without a prior history of MI, and about half of these unrecognized MIs are associated with atypical presentations.
- Response of chest pain to antacids, nitroglycerin, or analgesics can be misleading and should not be relied on.
- Nitroglycerin can reduce pain from esophageal spasm or pericarditis (by reducing heart size) and, conversely, pain from an acute MI may not always respond well to nitroglycerin because the pain is caused by infarction rather than ischemia.

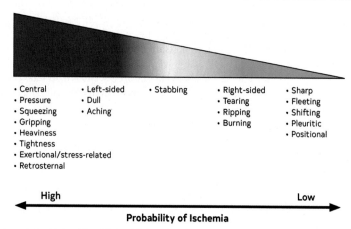

- Central
- Pressure
- Squeezing
- Gripping
- Heaviness
- Tightness
- Exertional/stress-related
- Retrosternal

- Left-sided
- Dull
- Aching

- Stabbing

- Right-sided
- Tearing
- Ripping
- Burning

- Sharp
- Fleeting
- Shifting
- Pleuritic
- Positional

High

Low

Probability of Ischemia

Fig. 2.3 Index of Suspicion That Chest "Pain" Is Ischemic in Origin on the Basis of Commonly Used Descriptors. From: Gulati M, Levy PD, Mukherjee D, et al. 2021 AHA/ACC/ASE/CHEST/SAEM/SCCT/SCMR guideline for the evaluation and diagnosis of chest pain: executive summary: a report of the American College of Cardiology/American Heart Association Joint Committee on Clinical Practice Guidelines. J Am Coll Cardiol. 2021;78(22):2218–2261.

TABLE 2.3 ■ **Atypical Symptoms of Myocardial Infarction in Elderly Patients**

Symptom	Percentage Of Patients With Symptoms		
	Age 65–74 y	Age 75–84 y	Age ≥ 85 y
Chest pain	77	60	37
Shortness of breath	40	43	43
Sweating	34	23	14
Syncope	3	18	18
Acute confusion	3	8	19
Stroke	2	7	7

Gulati M, Levy PD, Mukherjee D, et al. 2021 AHA/ACC/ASE/CHEST/SAEM/SCCT/SCMR guideline for the evaluation and diagnosis of chest pain: executive summary: a report of the American College of Cardiology/American Heart Association Joint Committee on Clinical Practice Guidelines. *J Am Coll Cardiol.* 2021;78(22):2218–2261.

Physical Examination

- Although an uncomplicated acute MI has no pathognomonic physical signs, the physical examination is crucial in the early assessment of the complications of acute MI and in establishing a differential diagnosis for the chest pain.
- The general assessment may reveal a restless and distressed patient with or without confusion owing to poor cerebral perfusion.
- A clenched fist across the chest, known as the Levine sign, may be observed.
- The patient may appear ashen, pale, or diaphoretic and may be cool and clammy to the touch.
- Tachycardia and hypertension indicate high sympathetic tone and they are usually consistent with an anterior MI.
- Bradycardia and hypotension signify high vagal tone and may be seen with inferior-posterior MI with or without right ventricular involvement.

- Hypotension could also be secondary to the development of cardiogenic shock or a result of medications, especially nitroglycerin, morphine sulfate, or beta-blockers.
- Visualization of elevated jugular venous pressure may indicate significant left or right ventricular dysfunction.
- Auscultation for additional heart sounds, cardiac murmurs, and friction rubs is mandatory.
- A soft S_1 is heard with decreased left ventricular contractility and an S_4 gallop indicates decreased left ventricular compliance.
- Killip and Kimball proposed a prognostic classification in 1967 that is still useful today for the evaluation of patients with acute MI.
- The classification scheme is based on the presence of a third heart sound (S_3) and rales on physical examination.
    - Class I patients are without S_3 or rales.
    - Class II patients have rales over less than 50% of the lung fields with or without S_3.
    - Class III patients have pulmonary edema with rales covering greater than 50% of the lung fields.
    - Class IV patients are in cardiogenic shock.
- Evidence of heart failure on physical examination correlates with greater than 25% of the myocardium being ischemic.
- A systolic murmur should prompt an evaluation for complications of MI, such as mitral regurgitation from papillary muscle rupture or the formation of a ventricular septal defect, which may also be accompanied by a palpable precordial thrill in half of cases.
- The chest wall should be palpated to assess for its effect on chest pain.
- Significant worsening of chest pain with palpation using moderate pressure is a clue that supports a musculoskeletal etiology.
- All peripheral pulses should be evaluated and documented.
- The finding of asymmetric or absent pulses, especially in the presence of tearing chest pain with radiation to the back, may indicate the presence of aortic dissection as an alternative diagnosis.

ELECTROCARDIOGRAM

- The ECG aids in the diagnosis of acute MI, suggests the distribution of the infarct-related artery, and estimates the amount of myocardium at risk.
- The presence of ST segment elevation in two contiguous leads or a new LBBB identifies patients who benefit from early reperfusion therapy.
- In the absence of a bundle branch block, the more abnormal the ECG leads, the greater the amount of ischemic myocardium.
- New LBBB or anterior infarction is an important predictor of mortality.
- In patients being evaluated for ACS, ST segment depression has a specificity of 95% and a sensitivity of 25% for diagnosing ACS.
- Conversely, the probability of an acute MI in patients with chest pain and an initially normal or nonspecific ECG is low, approximately 3%.
- Comparison with a previous ECG (if available) is indispensable and may help to avoid unnecessary treatment in patients with an abnormal baseline ECG.
- If the initial ECG is not diagnostic of STEMI, but the patient remains symptomatic, serial ECGs at 15- to 30-minute intervals should be performed to detect acute or evolving changes.
- The classic evolution of acute MI on ECG begins with an abnormal T wave that is often prolonged, peaked, or depressed.

- Most commonly, increased, hyperacute, symmetric T waves are seen in at least two contiguous leads during the early stages of ischemia followed by ST segment elevation in the leads facing the area of injury with ST segment depression in the reciprocal leads.
- Increased R wave amplitude and width in conjunction with S wave diminution are often seen in leads exhibiting ST segment elevation.
- This evolution may conclude with the formation of Q waves.
- The time course of development of these changes varies, but usually occurs in minutes to several hours.
- In patients with inferior STEMI, right-sided ECG leads should be obtained to screen for ST segment elevation suggestive of right ventricle infarction.
- Right ventricle infarction is likely when the ST segment is elevated 1 mm or more in the right precordial leads from rV_4 to rV_6.
- This finding has a sensitivity of about 90% and a specificity of 100% for proximal right coronary artery occlusion.
- Other changes reported to be associated with right ventricle infarction are (1) ST segment elevation isolated to lead V_1, (2) elevated ST segments in leads V_1 to V_4, and (3) T wave inversion isolated to lead V_2.
- The ECG changes of right ventricle infarction are usually transient, persist for hours, and then resolve within a day.
- A normal ECG can be seen in 10% of cases of acute MI owing to the infarction occurring in an electrocardiographically silent area, such as the posterior or lateral wall in the distribution of the left circumflex artery.
- Acute posterior injury is suggested by marked ST segment depression in leads V_1 to V_3 in combination with dominant R waves (R/S ratio > 1) and upright T waves.
- These ECG findings are neither sensitive nor specific for posterior infarction, however, and frequently are not evident on the initial ECG.
- In the case of patients who present with clinical evidence of an acute MI but have a non-diagnostic ECG, it is reasonable to obtain supplemental posterior ECG leads, V_7 through V_9, to assess for left circumflex occlusion.
- Several studies have shown that ST segment elevation in leads V_7 through V_9 assists in the early identification and treatment of patients who are having ischemic chest pain owing to acute posterior wall infarction, but do not display ST segment elevation on the standard 12-lead ECG.
- Several conditions can potentially confound the ECG diagnosis of an acute MI or cause a pseudoinfarct pattern with Q waves or QS complexes in the absence of MI, including preexcitation, obstructive or dilated cardiomyopathy, bundle branch block, left and right ventricular hypertrophy, myocarditis, cor pulmonale, and hyperkalemia.

Bundle Branch Block Patterns and Acute Myocardial Infarction

- The presence of an LBBB or ventricular pacing can mask the ECG changes of acute MI.
- In the Global Utilization of Streptokinase and Tissue Plasminogen Activator for Occluded Coronary Arteries (GUSTO)-1 trial, LBBB was seen in about 0.5% of patients with acute MI.
- Based on this finding, Sgarbossa developed criteria to evaluate for MI in the presence of left ventricular conduction abnormalities (Table 2.4).
- Because these changes in the ST segment or T waves, although very specific, are not seen in a significant proportion of patients, other modalities, such as biomarkers and adjunctive imaging, may be required for a diagnosis of acute MI.
- The same criteria used to assess for acute MI in the presence of LBBB are also applicable to patients with endocardial ventricular pacemakers, except for the T-wave criteria.

TABLE 2.4 ■ **Sensitivity and Specificity of Electrocardiogram (ECG) Changes in Left Bundle Branch Block for Diagnosis of Acute Myocardial Infarction**

ECG Changes	Sensitivity (%)	Specificity (%)
ST segment elevation ≥1 mm concordant with QRS polarity	73	92
ST segment depression ≥1 mm in leads V_1, V_2, V_3	25	96
ST segment elevation ≥5 mm discordant with QRS polarity	31	92
Positive T waves in leads V_5 and V_6	26	92

Modified from Sgarbossa EB. Recent advances in the electrocardiographic diagnosis of myocardial infarction: left bundle branch block and pacing. *Pacing Clin Electrophysiol*. 1996;19:1370–1379.

- The most indicative finding of acute MI in the presence of ventricular pacing is an ST segment elevation 5 mm or greater in the leads with predominantly negative QRS complexes.
- In right bundle branch block, the initial pattern of ventricular activation is normal, so the classic pattern of acute MI on ECG usually is not altered.

PRIMARY PERCUTANEOUS CORONARY INTERVENTION FOR STEMI

- Efforts to reduce mortality have focused on rapid restoration of blood flow in thrombotically occluded coronary arteries.
- First-line reperfusion therapy for STEMI in the late 1980s was coronary thrombolysis.
- Nevertheless, limitations of fibrinolysis alone were readily apparent: experience with fibrinolysis alone demonstrated that in approximately 15% of patients, recanalization failed completely and, for 50% of patients, restoration of flow in the infarct-related artery was suboptimal.
- Reinfarction occurs in 10% of patients in whom recanalization was initially successful.
- However, in influential early TIMI trials in which strategies of PCI were performed with balloon angioplasty after thrombolysis, no clinical benefit was observed with either immediate or delayed PCI compared with conservative therapy.
- In fact, immediate PCI led to a much higher incidence of bleeding and emergency coronary artery bypass graft surgery.
- Given the discouraging early results of combined balloon angioplasty and fibrinolysis, several investigators explored the possibility that stand-alone balloon angioplasty would be a safe and effective alternative to stand-alone fibrinolysis for patients with STEMI.
- Early results by O'Neill and coworkers in comparisons of angioplasty to intracoronary streptokinase demonstrated that balloon angioplasty was superior in improving ventricular function and reducing residual stenosis in the setting of acute MI.
- Over the next 15 years, multiple trials directly comparing stand-alone fibrinolysis with primary PCI were undertaken, eventually validating the utility of primary PCI and its superiority compared with thrombolysis in inducing more complete and more frequent recanalization of the infarct-related artery.
- In 2003, Keeley and colleagues reviewed 23 trials involving 7739 patients and found primary PCI (with adjunctive stenting in 12 trials) to be superior to thrombolytic therapy with respect to short-term mortality (7% compared with 9%; P = .0002), reinfarction (3% compared with 7%; P < .0001), and stroke (1% compared with 2%; P = .004).
- With long-term follow up, the benefits of primary PCI remained robust, with a substantial reduction in mortality (P = .0019), nonfatal reinfarction (P < .0001), and recurrent ischemia (P < .0001).

ADJUNCTIVE THERAPY

- Marked improvements in primary PCI over the past 2 decades have been a result of advancing technology (stents), pharmacology, and access approaches, as well as an emphasis on time to reperfusion (Fig. 2.4).
- Stents, both bare metal and later drug eluting, have improved short- and long-term outcomes after primary PCI.
- Effective adjunctive medical therapy inhibits both the plasma protein-based coagulation system and the activation and aggregation of platelets.
- Anticoagulation options for primary PCI are listed in Table 2.5.
- European and United States recommendations for anticoagulation are listed in Box 2.1.

ORAL ANTIPLATELET AGENTS: ASPIRIN, CLOPIDOGREL, PRASUGREL, AND TICAGRELOR

- Aspirin is routinely utilized in primary PCI—no randomized trials have compared aspirin with placebo in this setting and aspirin is considered *de facto* therapy in all patients with STEMI unless they are known to be allergic.
- Results in multiple trials have established that platelet adenosine diphosphate receptor antagonism with P2Y$_{12}$ receptor inhibitors is beneficial in the setting of PCI; thus, a second oral antiplatelet therapy agent is uniformly prescribed at the time of primary PCI.

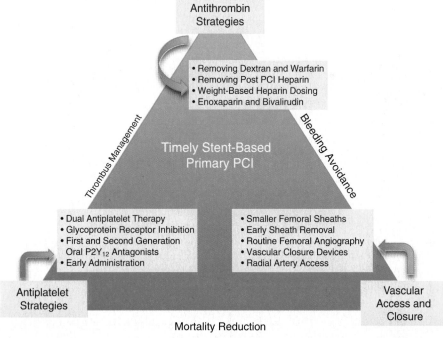

Fig. 2.4 Primary percutaneous coronary intervention has improved over the past two decades with active investigation in areas of stent technology, time to reperfusion, as well as adjunctive therapy and access methodology. (From Dauerman HL. Anticoagulation strategies for primary percutaneous coronary intervention: current controversies and recommendations. Circ Cardiovasc Interv. 2015;8.)

TABLE 2.5 ■ Anticoagulation Options for Primary PCI

Anticoagulant	Mechanism of Action	Pharmacokinetics	Advantages	Disadvantages	Key Primary PCI Clinical Trials
Unfractionated heparin	Activation of antithrombin: indirect antithrombin	Half-life of ~60 min but depends on bolus amount	Inexpensive and extensively studied Reversible Easily measurable anticoagulant effects	Heparin-induced thrombocytopenia (rare) Platelet activation Inactive against clot-bound thrombin Optimal dosing unclear	PAMI CADILLAC ADMIRAL HEAT ATOLL
Low-molecular-weight heparin: enoxaparin	Inhibition of Factor Xa and IIa 4:1 ratio of effect, predominantly acting on Factor Xa	Anti-Xa effects negligible after 8 hours	More reliable thrombin-inhibitory effect than heparin Partially reversible	Heparin-induced thrombocytopenia (rare) Difficult to measure anticoaguant effect	ATOLL
Fondaparinux	Indirect inhibitor of Factor Xa	Half-life of ~20 hours	Daily dosing	Heparin-induced thrombocytopenia (rare) Difficult to measure anticoaguant effect Catheter-related thrombosis	OASIS 6
Bivalirudin	Direct antithrombin	Half-life of 25 min	More reliable thrombin-inhibitory effect than heparin Does not activate platelets Short half-life No associated thrombocytopenia	Expensive Not reversible Short half-life Acute stent thrombosis risk	HORIZONS EUROMAX HEAT-PCI

Modified from Dauerman HL. Anticoagulation strategies for primary percutaneous coronary intervention: current controversies and recommendations. *Circ Cardiovasc Interv.* 2015;8.

ADMIRAL, Abciximab Before Direct Angioplasty and Stenting in Myocardial Infarction Regarding Acute and Long-Term Follow-up; *ATOLL,* Acute STEMI Treated with Primary PCI and IV Enoxaparin or UFH to Lower Ischemic and Bleeding Events at Short- and Long-Term Follow-up; *CADILLAC,* Controlled Abciximab and Device Investigation to Lower Late Angioplasty Complications; *EUROMAX,* European Ambulance Acute Coronary Syndrome Angiography; *HEAT-PCI,* How Effective Are Antithrombotic Therapies in Primary Percutaneous Coronary Intervention; *HORIZONS,* Harmonizing Outcomes with RevascularIZatiON and Stents; *OASIS-6,* Sixth Organization to Assess Strategies in Acute Ischemic Syndromes; *PAMI,* Primary Angioplasty in Myocardial Infarction *PCI,* percutaneous coronary intervention.

> **BOX 2.1 ■ European and US Recommendations for Anticoagulation in Primary PCI**
>
> UFH: Class I recommended, level of evidence C
> - With GP IIb/IIIa receptor antagonist planned: 50–70 U/kg IV bolus to achieve therapeutic ACT
> - With no GP IIb/IIIa receptor antagonist planned: 70–100 U/kg bolus to achieve therapeutic ACT
>
> Bivalirudin: Class I recommended, level of evidence B
> - 0.75 mg/kg IV bolus, then 1.75 mg/kg/h infusion with or without prior treatment with UFH. An additional bolus of 0.3 mg/kg can be given if needed
> - Reduce infusion to 1 mg/kg/h with estimated CrCl <30 mL/min
> - Preferred over UFH with GP IIb/IIIa receptor antagonist in patients at high risk of bleeding class IIA, level of evidence B
>
> Fondaparinux: not recommended as sole anticoagulant for primary PCI class III: not recommended, B
> Enoxaparin: not mentioned; no recommendation level given
> Bivalirudin: Class I recommended, level of evidence B
> - With use of GP IIb/IIIa blocker, restricted to bailout
> - Recommended over UFH and a GP IIb/IIIa blocker
> - Bivalirudin 0.75 mg/kg IV bolus followed by IV infusion of 1.75 mg/kg/h for up to 4 hours after the procedure as clinically warranted. After cessation of the 1.75 mg/kg/h infusion, a reduced infusion dose of 0.25 mg/kg/h may be continued for 4–12 hours as clinically necessary
>
> Enoxaparin: Class IIB, level of evidence B
> - With or without routine GP IIb/IIIa blocker
> - May be preferred over UFH
> - Enoxaparin 0.5 mg/kg IV bolus
>
> UFH: Class I recommended, level of evidence C
> - With or without routine GP IIb/IIIa blocker
> - Must be used in patients not receiving bivalirudin or enoxaparin
> - UFH 70–100 U/kg IV bolus when no GP IIb/IIIa inhibitor is planned
> - 50–60 U/kg IV bolus with GP IIb/IIIa inhibitors
>
> Fondaparinux is not recommended for primary PCI; class III, level of evidence B.
>
> ---
>
> *ACT,* Activated clotting time; *CrCl,* creatinine clearance; *GP,* glycoprotein; *IV,* intravenous; *PCI,* percutaneous coronary intervention; *UFH,* unfractionated

- Clopidogrel was the most commonly used $P2Y_{12}$ antagonist in primary PCI: clopidogrel is a prodrug that undergoes processing in the liver, yielding an active metabolite.
- Its effect on platelet inhibition may not occur for as long as 12 hours with a load of 300 mg.
- A 600-mg load has been shown to be more effective in rapidly inhibiting platelet aggregation.
- Thus, patients who are to undergo primary PCI should probably be given a loading dose of 600 mg immediately (i.e., in the emergency department) and 75 mg daily thereafter.
- Similar to clopidogrel, prasugrel is a thienopyridine prodrug requiring conversion to an active metabolite by the hepatic cytochrome P-450 system, but prasugrel inhibits platelet activation more rapidly, more consistently, and to a greater extent.
- Prasugrel is administered 60 mg orally once as loading dose, then 10 mg/day orally in combination with aspirin 81 to 325 mg/day.
- Patients who are elderly, have a prior history of cerebrovascular events, or are of low body weight do not derive a benefit from more aggressive platelet inhibition with prasugrel resulting in a US Food and Drug Administration (FDA) warning urging caution regarding

prasugrel treatment for elderly and low-body-weight patients and a strict contraindication for patients with prior stroke.

■ Unlike the other two inhibitors of the $P2Y_{12}$ platelet receptor, ticagrelor is a nonthienopyridine that does not require conversion into an active metabolite. Ticagrelor (180 mg loading dose followed by 90 mg twice per day) was compared with clopidogrel (300 mg or 600 mg loading dose followed by 75 mg per day) in the Platelet Inhibition and Patient Outcomes (PLATO) trial of patients with acute coronary syndrome.

■ The prespecified subgroup of patients ($n = 7544$) presenting for primary PCI for STEMI or new LBBB had lower risks of major adverse cardiovascular events at 1 year of follow-up, with significant reductions in the risk of cardiovascular death and stent thrombosis.

■ However, patients randomized to ticagrelor had higher risks of stroke and intracranial hemorrhage.

■ Additionally, the benefit of ticagrelor appeared to be related to the dose of aspirin, resulting in a warning from the FDA recommending that patients taking ticagrelor receive less than 100 mg of aspirin daily.

■ Although the American College of Cardiology/American Heart Association guidelines give all three oral $P2Y_{12}$ inhibitors equal (class 1B) recommendations for the treatment of patients with STEMI, the European Society of Cardiology guidelines favor ticagrelor over clopidogrel owing to the favorable outcomes in trials in direct comparison with clopidogrel.

VASCULAR APPROACH FOR PRIMARY PCI

■ The approach to primary PCI was routinely via femoral access for the first 20 years of this reperfusion modality.

■ Trials over the past 5 years have emphasized the potential benefits of a radial artery access approach to limit bleeding and, potentially, mortality among patients undergoing primary PCI.

CHAPTER 3

Acute Myocardial Infarction: Adjunctive Pharmacologic Therapies

Common Misconceptions

- β-blockers are contraindicated in patients with acute myocardial infarction with chronic obstructive pulmonary disease.
- Proton pump inhibitors (PPI) should not be given concomitantly with clopidogrel.
- Prasugrel improved outcomes compared with clopidogrel, with no increase in fatal bleeding.
- This chapter focuses on evidence-based adjunctive medical therapies indicated for patients with acute myocardial infarction (MI), both ST elevation MI (STEMI) and non-ST elevation acute coronary syndromes (NSTE ACS).

Antiplatelet Therapy

- Because platelets play a critical role in thrombus formation at sites of coronary atherosclerotic plaque rupture or erosion, inhibiting platelets plays a central role in the treatment of STEMI and NSTE ACS.
- The involvement of platelets in the initiation of thrombus is a multistep process of adhesion, activation, and aggregation (Fig. 3.1).
- The current standard of care for treatment of patients with ACS endorses multireceptor inhibition by routine use of aspirin in combination with a $P2Y_{12}$ antagonist, a combination commonly termed *dual antiplatelet therapy (DAPT)*.

ASPIRIN

- One pathway that participates in the regulation of platelet activity involves the conversion of arachidonic acid to thromboxane A_2 (TXA_2) and other prostaglandins by the platelet cyclooxygenase (COX) enzymes, COX-1 and COX-2.
- Constitutive COX-1 promotes platelet aggregation, thrombosis, and vasoconstriction, and protects gastrointestinal mucosa.
- In contrast, inducible COX-2 is proinflammatory via prostaglandin E_2 (PGE_2) and antithrombotic and vasodilatory via prostaglandin I_2 (PGI_2 [prostacyclin]).
- Aspirin (acetylsalicylic acid) exerts antiplatelet actions through acetylation of a serine residue on COX-1 to irreversibly block the production of TXA_2 which, in turn, inhibits platelet activation and aggregation.
- The effect of aspirin can be detected within 30 to 40 minutes of ingestion and lasts for the life of the platelet (7 to 10 days).
- Low-dose aspirin appears to selectively inhibit COX-1, whereas higher doses inhibit both COX-1 and COX-2.
- Low-dose aspirin may therefore block TXA_2 production while sparing PGI_2 synthesis.

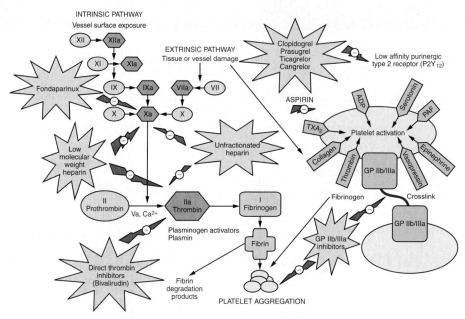

Fig. 3.1   Sites of action of antiplatelet and antithrombin agents. Low-molecular-weight heparin produces more potent inhibition of factor Xa than thrombin, whereas unfractionated heparin produces equal inhibition of factor Xa and thrombin. Direct thrombin inhibitors inhibit thrombin, but have little effect on its generation. Thrombin amplifies generation of factors VIIIa and Va, enhancing thrombus formation. Thrombin also promotes platelet activation by binding to platelet thrombin receptor. Crosslinks, via ligands such as fibrinogen (factor I) to platelet glycoprotein (GP) IIb/IIIa receptors, lead to platelet aggregation. GP IIb/IIIa inhibitors act at these sites. *ADP*, Adenosine triphosphate; *PAF*, platelet-activating factor; *TXA₂*, thromboxane A₂.

- The efficacy of aspirin in acute STEMI was established in the randomized ISIS-2 trial, which assessed the effects of a 1-hour intravenous infusion of streptokinase (1.5 million U) or oral aspirin (160 mg) or both in patients within 24 hours of symptoms.
  - At 5 weeks, aspirin reduced total cardiovascular mortality by 23% (absolute risk reduction of 2.4%).
- Aspirin is generally well tolerated, but has an increased risk of bleeding, more frequent at higher doses (e.g. aspirin dose above 100 mg per day).
- When aspirin is combined with other antiplatelet therapy, such as $P2Y_{12}$ antagonists, the risk of bleeding is increased.
- Results from the Clopidogrel in Unstable Angina to Prevent Recurrent Events (CURE) trial suggest there is an interaction between the dose of aspirin and the risk of bleeding with combined aspirin plus clopidogrel such that the risk was mitigated by use of low-dose aspirin (<100 mg).
- For secondary prevention, the absolute benefits of aspirin are considered to far outweigh the risk of major bleeding; collective evidence supports low-dose aspirin (drug dose is a range e.g. 75-81 mg per day) for long-term use.
- Some patients are unable to tolerate aspirin owing to hypersensitivity from one of three types of reactions: respiratory, cutaneous, or systemic.
  - Patients with aspirin allergy presenting with ACS should undergo desensitization, if at all feasible.

- Aspirin desensitization is not feasible for individuals known to have an anaphylactoid response.
- For patients with irremediable intolerance to aspirin, use of another antiplatelet agent, such as a $P2Y_{12}$ antagonist, is recommended.
- Aspirin is also contraindicated in patients with active bleeding or with high-risk bleeding conditions (e.g., retinal hemorrhage, active peptic ulcer, other serious gastrointestinal or urogenital bleeding, hemophilia, and untreated severe hypertension).
- In patients with prior gastrointestinal bleeding attributed to peptic ulcer disease, addition of a proton pump inhibitor to low-dose aspirin has been shown to reduce the risk of recurrent bleeding.
- Based on these results and evidence of the large benefit of aspirin after MI, aspirin combined with a PPI should be continued if possible, unless bleeding is life threatening or uncontrollable.

RECOMMENDATIONS

- Aspirin should be administered as soon as possible to all patients with ACS without a known intolerance.
- On presentation, patients with STEMI should be treated with 162 to 325 mg of aspirin followed by 81 mg daily indefinitely.
- Non–enteric-coated aspirin should be used initially and chewed to ensure rapid absorption.
- Currently, recommendations endorse low-dose aspirin daily indefinitely for all patients following an MI.

$P2Y_{12}$ Platelet Antagonists

- The oral $P2Y_{12}$ antagonists include the thienopyridines, ticlopidine, clopidogrel, and prasugrel, which are prodrugs whose active metabolites irreversibly bind to and inhibit the $P2Y_{12}$ receptor and the direct acting, nonthienopyridine, reversible antagonist, ticagrelor (Table 3.1).
- Ticlopidine, the oldest member of this class, was replaced by clopidogrel for the reduction of atherothrombotic events following stent implantation, due to a risk of serious neutropenia, thrombotic thrombocytopenic purpura (TTP) and aplastic anemia.
- A parenteral short-acting reversible $P2Y_{12}$ antagonist, cangrelor, is also available for early infusion to support PCI among patients who have not been pretreated with an oral $P2Y_{12}$ antagonist (see Table 3.1) prior to intervention.

CLOPIDOGREL

- Clopidogrel is an oral agent that blocks activation of platelets by irreversibly inhibiting the binding of adenosine diphosphate (ADP) to the $P2Y_{12}$ receptor.
- Clopidogrel is a prodrug that is metabolized in the liver in a multistep process, predominantly through the cytochrome P450 isoform CYP2C19, to a short-lived active metabolite that binds to the ligand-binding site of the $P2Y_{12}$ receptor (see Table 3.1).
- Clopidogrel produces significant platelet inhibition after 2 to 3 days, but may take 4 to 7 days to achieve its full effect, reinforcing the need for a loading dose.
- The onset of clopidogrel antiplatelet action is reported at 2 to 6 hours after a loading dose and persists for 7 to 10 days after therapy is stopped.
- Clopidogrel monotherapy has been shown to have benefits in reducing the risk of adverse ischemic events among patients with a history of or at high risk for atherosclerotic heart disease.

TABLE 3.1 ■ **Properties of Platelet P2Y$_{12}$ ADP Receptor Antagonists**

	Clopidogrel	Prasugrel	Ticagrelor	Cangrelor
P2Y$_{12}$ receptor blockade	Irreversible	Irreversible	Reversible	Reversible
Route of administration	Oral	Oral	Oral	Intravenous
Frequency of administration	Once daily	Once daily	Twice daily	Bolus plus infusion
Prodrug	Yes	Yes	No	No
Onset of action	2–8 h	30 min–4 h	30 min–4 h	2 min
Offset of action	7–10 d	7–10 d	3–5 d	30–60 min
Interactions with CYP-metabolized drugs	CYP2C19	No	CYP3A4/5	No
Indications for use	ACS and stable CAD undergoing PCI	ACS undergoing PCI	ACS (full spectrum)	PCI not pretreated with oral P2Y$_{12}$ antagonist
Loading dose	300–600 mg	60 mg	180 mg	30 μg/kg bolus
Maintenance dose	75 mg daily	10 mg daily	90 mg twice daily	4 μg/kg/min infusion

ACS, Acute coronary syndrome; *CAD*, coronary artery disease; *PCI*, percutaneous coronary intervention.

- In the Clopidogrel versus Aspirin in patients at Risk of Ischaemic Events (CAPRIE) trial, clopidogrel was modestly more effective in reducing the combined risk of ischemic stroke, MI, or vascular death than aspirin.
- Clopidogrel may be substituted in patients with aspirin allergy or intolerance.
- The effect of adding clopidogrel to aspirin in the early phase of ACS was studied in the landmark Clopidogrel in Unstable Angina to Prevent Recurrent Events (CURE) trial.
  - Cardiovascular death, MI, and stroke was reduced by 20% among patients randomized to clopidogrel (300 mg is a loading dose given initially on admission then the patient will get 75 mg per day thereafter) plus aspirin, within 24 hours.
- The Clopidogrel as Adjunctive Reperfusion Therapy—Thrombolysis in Myocardial Infarction (CLARITY-TIMI) 28 study tested the effect of clopidogrel on angiographic and clinical outcome among patients younger than 75 years with STEMI who were treated with fibrinolytic therapy.
  - The results demonstrated that the addition of clopidogrel for patients with STEMI who were receiving fibrinolytic therapy improved the patency rate of the infarct-related artery and significantly reduced adverse ischemic events with no significant increase in bleeding complications.
- The effect of the addition of clopidogrel to aspirin for patients with STEMI was further studied in the Clopidogrel and Metoprolol in Myocardial Infarction Trial/Second Chinese Cardiac Study (COMMIT/CCS-2).
  - This study showed that adding clopidogrel (75 mg/day) to aspirin (162 mg/day) significantly reduced death, reinfarction, or stroke by 9% and mortality by 7% with no significant excess risk of fatal or cerebral bleeding.
- Although these studies employed clopidogrel with a loading dose of 300 mg or no loading dose, subsequent studies suggested a faster onset of action and an added benefit with a

higher loading dose of 600 mg, particularly among higher-risk patients undergoing percutaneous coronary intervention (PCI).

- In the Clopidogrel and Aspirin Optimal Dose Usage to Reduce Recurrent Events—Seventh Organization to Assess Strategies in Ischemic Syndromes (CURRENT-OASIS-7) trial, double-dose clopidogrel reduced the rate of cardiovascular death, MI, or stroke, and stent thrombosis in patients undergoing PCI, but major bleeding was more common.
- The cumulative data suggest that, for clopidogrel, the recommended loading dose is 600 mg with a maintenance dose of 75 mg.
- Wide interindividual variability in the degree of inhibition of ADP-induced platelet function has been observed with clopidogrel; so-called "high on-treatment platelet reactivity" is reported in up to 35% of patients.
    - The mechanisms for this variability are likely multifactorial, including drug, environmental, and genetic interactions.
- Proton pump inhibitors, such as omeprazole and esomeprazole, which are strong inhibitors of CYP2C19, are associated with decreased inhibition of platelet aggregation by clopidogrel, however, most clinical studies, have not confirmed an adverse effect on clinical outcomes.
- Clopidogrel combined with aspirin increases bleeding risk, has been associated with gastrointestinal upset, and a rare incidence of thrombotic thrombocytopenic purpura.
- Clopidogrel plus aspirin has been associated with significant increases in major bleeding with coronary artery bypass graft (CABG) surgery and so should be withheld for 5 to 7 days before surgery.

PRASUGREL

- Prasugrel is another thienopyridine antagonist of the platelet $P2Y_{12}$ receptor and is a prodrug that is metabolized into an active metabolite that irreversibly binds to and blocks the ligand binding site of the $P2Y_{12}$ receptor (see Table 3.1).
- Prasugrel inhibits greater than 80% of *in vitro* ADP-induced platelet aggregation and has less interpatient variability than clopidogrel.
- The efficacy of prasugrel as compared with clopidogrel on outcomes among patients with ACS undergoing PCI was examined in the Trial to Assess Improvement in Therapeutic Outcomes by Optimizing Platelet Inhibition with Prasugrel–Thrombolysis in Myocardial Infarction (TRITON-TIMI) 38 trial.
    - Patients with STEMI or high-risk NSTE ACS due to undergo planned PCI were randomly assigned to prasugrel or clopidogrel.
    - Treatment with prasugrel resulted in a significant reduction in cardiovascular death, MI, and stroke, and stent thrombosis, but a 32% increased risk of bleeding, including fatal bleeding.
- Prasugrel is administered as a 60-mg loading dose followed by a maintenance dose of 10 mg/day.
- A lower maintenance dose of 5 mg/day has been recommended in patients who weigh less than 60 kg or who are older than 75 years.
- It is recommended that prasugrel be discontinued 7 days prior to CABG surgery.

TICAGRELOR

- Ticagrelor is an oral cyclopentyltriazolopyrimidine that reversibly inhibits the platelet $P2Y_{12}$ receptor (see Table 3.1).
- Ticagrelor is not a prodrug and does not bind to the ADP-binding site; instead, it binds to a separate site of the $P2Y_{12}$ receptor, thereby inhibiting G-protein activation and signaling.

- The onset of action of ticagrelor is faster than clopidogrel, with 40% platelet inhibition in 30 minutes after dosing, with a peak effect in approximately 2 hours.
- Ticagrelor has a plasma half-life of 8 to 12 hours.
- The offset of ticagrelor action is faster than with thienopyridines.
- The effect of ticagrelor compared with clopidogrel for treatment of patients with ACS was examined among 18,624 patients treated with aspirin in the Platelet Inhibition and Patient Outcomes (PLATO) study.
  - At 1 year, patients randomly assigned to receive ticagrelor had a significant reduction in overall mortality and also death from vascular causes, MI, or stroke.
  - No significant difference in rate of major bleeding was observed between ticagrelor and clopidogrel.
  - Ticagrelor was generally well tolerated, but adverse effects included increased non–CABG-related bleeding, dyspnea, ventricular pauses (mostly asymptomatic), and increased serum creatinine.
- Ticagrelor also has non-$P2Y_{12}$ receptor–mediated effects that include blocking the equilibrative nucleoside transporter-1, which can result in increased plasma concentrations of adenosine.
- The clinical significance of this observation is unknown, but adenosine stimulates of pulmonary vagal C fibers that can cause dyspnea and an increased incidence of dyspnea was observed in the PLATO trial among patients receiving ticagrelor (14.5%), but severe in only 0.4% of patients.
- Ticagrelor is administered as a loading dose of 180 mg followed by a maintenance dose of 90 mg twice per day.
- When ticagrelor is prescribed for DAPT, the aspirin dose should be 81 mg/day.
- It is recommended that ticagrelor be withheld 5 days prior to CABG surgery.

CANGRELOR

- After oral administration of a loading dose of a $P2Y_{12}$ antagonist, clinically effective platelet inhibition may be delayed by hours, particularly among patients with STEMI.
- Administered intravenously, it is a potent, direct-acting, rapidly reversible $P2Y_{12}$ antagonist with predictable plasma levels and linear dose-dependent receptor inhibition (see Table 3.1).
- An effective level (> 80%) of platelet inhibition with cangrelor is achieved within minutes after start of intravenous infusion and recovers within 60 to 90 minutes after discontinuation.
- Cangrelor has been studied in a number of trials, the most important of which was the Cangrelor versus Standard Therapy to Achieve Optimal Management of Platelet Inhibition (CHAMPION) PHOENIX trial, in which 10,942 patients who were clopidogrel-naive with coronary artery disease requiring PCI for stable angina, NSTE ACS, or STEMI received a bolus and subsequent infusion of cangrelor or placebo.
  - The composite rate of death, MI, ischemia-driven revascularization, or stent thrombosis at 48 hours was significantly lower in the cangrelor group than in the clopidogrel group and was not accompanied by a significant increase in severe bleeding or in the need for transfusions compared with patients on clopidogrel.
- In light of these favorable results, cangrelor may be considered for use in patients with STEMI or high-risk ACS undergoing urgent PCI who have not been adequately preloaded with an oral $P2Y_{12}$ antagonist.
- Cangrelor is administered as a 30-μg/kg intravenous bolus infused over 1 minute before PCI, followed by a 4 μg/kg/min infusion for the duration of the procedure or at least 2 hours.

RECOMMENDATIONS

- Collective evidence indicates that all patients with ACS and all patients undergoing PCI with stent implantation should receive DAPT, with aspirin and a $P2Y_{12}$ antagonist, in the absence of contraindications.
- Aspirin should be administered immediately and the $P2Y_{12}$ antagonist should be administered as early as feasible after presentation.
- The selection of the $P2Y_{12}$ antagonist should be individualized with attention to clinical syndrome, comorbidities, timing, and a careful assessment of ischemic risk and bleeding risk.

Glycoprotein IIb/IIIa Antagonists

- The final common pathway of platelet aggregation involves crosslinking of activated platelets via binding of the platelet glycoprotein IIb/IIIa (GP IIb/IIIa) receptor to the divalent ligand, fibrinogen (see Fig. 3.1).
- The GP IIb/IIIa receptor emerged as a therapeutic target to treat cardiovascular events with the isolation of monoclonal antibodies that block the binding of the receptor to fibrinogen and improved patency rates after fibrinolysis and reduced rethrombosis.
- These early studies eventually led to the clinical development of the three currently available GP IIb/IIIa antagonists, abciximab, eptifibatide, and tirofiban.

ABCIXIMAB

- The humanized chimeric monoclonal antibody, abciximab binds to the GP IIb/IIIa receptor with high avidity after intravenous administration.
- Several trials showed that administration of abciximab as a bolus followed by a 12-hour infusion significantly reduced the incidence of adverse ischemic events among patients undergoing PCI.
- A meta-analysis of trials of abciximab use during primary PCI reported that abciximab was associated with significant reductions in mortality and recurrent MI.
- Nevertheless, abciximab has been associated with significantly increased rates of bleeding, raising questions regarding the utility of abciximab in the era when patients are commonly pretreated with a $P2Y_{12}$ antagonist.
- However, abciximab may be useful as adjunctive therapy to reduce acute ischemic events among select patients at high risk undergoing PCI for STEMI with stenting or as a provisional "bail-out" agent for thrombotic complications during PCI.

TIROFIBAN

- Tirofiban is a small molecule inhibitor of the GP IIb/IIIa receptor on platelets. In the Platelet Receptor Inhibition in Ischemic Syndrome Management in Patients Limited by Unstable Signs and Symptoms (PRISM-PLUS) trial, intravenous tirofiban reduced adverse ischemic events in patients with NSTE ACS requiring revascularization procedures.
- In early PCI trials, concern was that tirofiban dosing was inadequate to achieve optimal platelet inhibition and so a higher-dose regimen was developed and tested, with potentially improved outcomes and is recommended in guidelines to support primary PCI.

EPTIFIBATIDE

- Eptifibatide is a cyclic heptapeptide inhibitor of the GP IIb/IIIa receptor.
- In the Platelet Glycoprotein IIb/IIIa in Unstable Angina: Receptor Suppression Using Integrilin Therapy (PURSUIT) trial, patients with NSTE ACS were randomized to receive eptifibatide (a bolus dose of 180 μg/kg, followed by an infusion of 2.0 μg/kg/min) versus placebo with a mean duration of infusion of 72 hours.
  - Treatment with eptifibatide resulted in reduced rates of death or MI, but with an increased risk of bleeding.
- In the Early Glycoprotein IIb/IIIa Inhibition in Non–ST-Segment Elevation Acute Coronary Syndrome (EARLY ACS) trial, a strategy of early administration of eptifibatide was compared with administration after angiography, which showed that ischemic outcomes were not significantly improved and bleeding rates were increased.

RECOMMENDATIONS

- Recent guidelines suggest a limited role for GP IIb/IIIa antagonists, such as in the setting of large thrombus burden, inadequate loading with a P2Y$_{12}$ antagonist, or for provisional bail-out use for thrombotic complications.
- Eptifibatide or tirofiban may be considered for patients with NSTE ACS awaiting angiography in addition to a P2Y$_{12}$ antagonist for those at very high risk or potentially instead of a P2Y$_{12}$ antagonist in select patients when there is reluctance to load with a P2Y$_{12}$ antagonist owing to concern about the need for urgent CABG surgery.

β-Blockers

- β-adrenergic receptor blockers (β-blockers) compete with catecholamines for binding to β-adrenergic receptors:
  - β$_1$ receptors are primarily located in the myocardium and affect sinus node rate, atrioventricular (AV) node conduction velocity and contractility.
  - β$_2$ receptors are primarily located in bronchial and vascular smooth muscle.
- β-Blockers slow the heart rate, reduce blood pressure, and reduce cardiac contractility, resulting in decreased cardiac workload and reduced myocardial oxygen consumption.
- The prolongation of diastolic filling time increases coronary perfusion.
- Given acutely, β-blockers decrease infarct size in patients who do not receive reperfusion therapy, reduce the rate of reinfarction in patients who receive reperfusion therapy, and decrease the frequency of arrhythmias.
- The effects of β-blockers on outcome following an acute MI have been extensively tested in randomized clinical trials.
  - In the pre-fibrinolytic era, the Norwegian multicenter study randomized 1884 patients to receive timolol versus placebo started at 7 to 28 days after infarction.
    - At 33 months, the timolol-treated group showed lower rates of mortality (39%) and reinfarction (28%).
  - In the Beta-Blocker Heart Attack Trial (BHAT), the nonselective β-blocker propranolol was initiated orally 5 to 21 days following an MI.
    - At an average 25-month follow up, there was a highly significant (26%) reduction in total mortality.
- The benefit of early administration of β-blockers for acute MI was also tested in three major trials.

- The International Studies of Infarct Survival-1 (ISIS-1) study compared intravenous followed by oral administration of atenolol with placebo in patients within 12 hours of presentation with STEMI, with a significant (15%) relative reduction in mortality at 7 days.

- In the Metoprolol in Acute Myocardial Infarction (MIAMI) trial, intravenous initiation of metoprolol followed by oral dosing within 24 hours of onset of symptoms was compared with placebo among patients hospitalized with acute MI. After 15 days, there was a nonsignificant (13%) lower rate of death ($P = .29$).

- In the later Thrombolysis In Myocardial Infarction Phase II (TIMI-II) trial, patients with STEMI who were treated with alteplase were randomly assigned to receive immediate intravenous followed by oral metoprolol or deferred metoprolol (orally after day 6). At 6 weeks, no overall difference was seen in mortality between the immediate intravenous and deferred groups, but the immediate intravenous group showed a lower incidence of reinfarction and recurrent chest pain at 6 days.

- Many of the early trials of β-blocker use after acute MI did not enroll patients with heart failure (HF) or left ventricular systolic dysfunction (LVSD), an important high-risk group.
  - The Carvedilol Post-Infarct Survival Control in Left-Ventricular Dysfunction (CAPRICORN) trial compared carvedilol, initiated 3 to 21 days after MI with placebo in patients after an acute MI with an LV ejection fraction (LVEF) of 40% or less.
    - At a mean follow up of 15 months, all-cause mortality was 23% lower in the carvedilol group than in the placebo group ($P = .03$) and a later study showed a 59% reduction in atrial tachyarrhythmias and a 76% reduction in ventricular tachyarrhythmias.
  - More recently, the COMMIT/CCS-2 study randomized 45, 852 patients within 24 hours of onset of suspected MI to receive metoprolol (intravenous followed by oral) or placebo.
    - At a mean of 15 days follow up, no difference was observed for death, reinfarction, and cardiac arrest.

- A retrospective analysis of 201, 752 patients in the Cooperative Cardiovascular Project concluded that after acute MI, even patients with conditions that are traditionally considered contraindications to β-blockers—such as congestive heart failure (CHF), pulmonary disease, and older age—benefited significantly from β-blocker therapy.

- A meta-analysis of the effect of intravenous followed by oral β-blocker therapy on death, reinfarction, and cardiac arrest during the scheduled treatment periods tested in over 50,000 patients in randomized trials, demonstrated highly significant (13% to 22%) relative risk reduction for adverse events from β-blocker therapy.

- Only β-blockers without intrinsic sympathomimetic activity have been shown to reduce mortality after MI; β-blockers with intrinsic sympathomimetic activity are not indicated for secondary prevention.

- The American College of Cardiology/American Heart Association (ACC/AHA) guidelines recommend caution with the use of intravenous β-blockade, especially in patients who are at risk for cardiogenic shock, but the long-term use of oral β-blockers is recommended for secondary prevention in patients at high risk, after they have been stabilized, with gradual dose titration.

- No adequate trials have been conducted of head-to-head comparisons of different β-blockers in the setting of STEMI or ACS.

- One therapeutic target is a heart rate of 50 to 60 beats/min and/or a blunting of the rise in heart rate with light activity, unless there are side effects.

- The dose of β-blocker can be titrated up to specified targets (Table 3.2).

- The major side effects of β-blocker therapy include hypotension, bradycardia, AV block, worsening of CHF, and exacerbation of reactive airways disease.

TABLE 3.2 ■ Target Doses for β-Blockers

β-Blocker	β Selectivity	Partial Agonist Activity	Target Dose
Acebutolol	β_1	Yes	200–600 mg twice daily
Atenolol	β_1	No	50–200 mg daily
Betaxolol	β_1	No	10–20 mg daily
Bisoprolol	β_1	No	10 mg daily
Carvedilol[a]	None	No	6.25 mg twice daily up to 25 mg twice daily
Esmolol (intravenous)	β_1	No	50–300 µg/kg/min
Labetalol[a]	None	Yes	200–600 mg daily
Metoprolol	β_1	No	50–200 mg twice daily
Nadolol	None	No	40–80 mg daily
Pindolol	None	Yes	2.5–7.5 mg three times daily
Propranolol	None	No	20–80 mg twice daily
Timolol	None	No	10 mg twice daily

[a]Labetalol and carvedilol are combined α- and β-blockers. Drugs are listed alphabetically and not in order of preference.
Modified from Gibbons RJ, Chatterjee K, Daley J, et al. ACC/AHA/ACP-ASIM guidelines for the management of patients with chronic stable angina. *J Am Coll Cardiol*. 1999;33:2092–2197.

- Relative contraindications include chronic obstructive pulmonary disease (COPD) or asthma.
  - Patients with mild pulmonary disease not taking β-agonists benefit from β-blockers after acute MI, but patients with severe COPD or asthma taking β-agonists do not benefit.
  - After 2 years, patients with COPD receiving β-blocker therapy had a higher survival rate than patients who did not receive therapy.
  - Cardioselective β-blockers do not worsen pulmonary function tests in patients with mild to moderate COPD or reactive airways disease.
  - Because the benefit of β-blockers is significant, lower initial doses of cardioselective β-blockers and careful uptitration are recommended.
- β-blockers improve survival and produce benefits in patients after MI patients with preserved or decreased EF.
- In patients with peripheral artery disease, there is no evidence of worsening of claudication with β-blockers.
- Long-term β-blocker therapy in STEMI survivors shows mortality benefit despite revascularization with CABG or PCI.

RECOMMENDATIONS

- β-Blocker therapy is recommended for all patients who have had an acute MI without a history of intolerance or contraindications.
- If tolerated, oral β-blocker therapy should be continued indefinitely.
- Relative contraindications to β-blocker therapy include heart rate less than 60 beats/min, systolic blood pressure less than 100 mm Hg, moderate to severe LVSD with CHF, shock, AV block, active asthma, reactive airways disease, and MI induced by cocaine use.

Nitrates

- Administration of nitrates results in an endothelium-independent release of nitric oxide, direct relaxation of vascular smooth muscle, and dose-related vasodilation.
- Nitrates may also produce vasodilation indirectly through the endothelial release of PGI_2 and may exert antiplatelet and antithrombotic effects.
- Nitroglycerin directly dilates coronary arteries, which may relieve vasoconstriction at or adjacent to sites of thrombotic obstruction or at sites occluded owing to primary coronary vasospasm and promotes collateral flow to ischemic regions, resulting in improved myocardial perfusion.
- Nitrates promote venodilation, resulting in a reduction in LV preload, chamber size, and wall stress.
- Reducing preload and afterload decreases myocardial oxygen demand, which reduces myocardial ischemia and, therefore, potentially limiting myocardial infarct size.
- However, nitrates may also cause hypotension, resulting in decreased coronary perfusion that could be detrimental in the acute phase of acute MI.
- Prolonged nitroglycerin infusions at high doses may produce tolerance.
- Low-dose intravenous nitroglycerin can be administered safely to patients with evolving anterior STEMI; however, patients with inferior STEMI are more sensitive to preload reduction, especially if right ventricular infarction is present.
- Guidelines support the use of nitroglycerin for suppressing ongoing myocardial ischemic pain and for managing acute MI complicated by CHF or pulmonary edema.
- The ACC/AHA guidelines recognized the usefulness of low-dose intravenous nitroglycerin infusion in titrating therapy to the blood pressure response and suggested that the infusion should begin at 5 to 10 µg/min with increases of 5 to 20 µg/min until symptoms are relieved or mean blood pressure is reduced by 10% in patients who are normotensive and by up to 30% in those who are hypertensive, but not below a systolic pressure of 90 mm Hg.
- Nitrates should be avoided in patients with STEMI with hypotension, bradycardia, tachycardia, or right ventricular MI.
- Nitrates are contraindicated in patients taking phosphodiesterase inhibitors.
- Tolerance to nitrate therapy typically develops after 24 hours and so the dosage may need to be increased, but lower doses or nitrate-free intervals prevent tolerance.

RECOMMENDATIONS

- Routine nitrate therapy is not recommended for patients with STEMI.
- Selective use should be considered to ameliorate symptoms and signs of myocardial ischemia and may be useful to treat patients with STEMI and hypertension or CHF.
- Rarely, methemoglobinemia can develop.

Angiotensin-Converting Enzyme (ACE) Inhibitors and Other Renin-Angiotensin-Aldosterone System Inhibitors

- Inhibition of the conversion of angiotensin I to angiotensin II by ACE inhibition, and of the binding of angiotensin to its receptor, result in vasodilation and a reduction in LV afterload.
- These hemodynamic effects, as well as putative local effects within the myocardium and vasculature, may result in beneficial effects on LV wall stress and remodeling, translating into clinical benefit.

- ACE inhibitors and angiotensin receptor blocker (ARBs) have emerged as effective adjunctive agents for preventing LV remodeling and improving survival after MI, and are recommended for the early management of acute STEMI.

ANGIOTENSIN-CONVERTING ENZYME INHIBITORS

- The beneficial physiologic effects of ACE inhibitors are related mainly to inhibition of ACE and kininase.
  - ACE inhibition results in decreased activity of the renin-angiotensin-aldosterone system (RAAS); decreased formation of angiotensin II; decreased catecholamine secretion, inotropic stimulation, heart rate, and vasoconstrictor tone; and improved collateral flow.
  - Kininase inhibition contributes to vasodilation.
  - The net results include increased venous capacitance and decreased preload, decreased afterload, improved perfusion, decreased infarct size, decreased chamber size and wall stress, and decreased ventricular dilation.
  - ACE inhibitors do not block the formation of angiotensin II that occurs via alternate pathways, and they do not prevent all aldosterone formation.
  - ARBs selectively block the effects of angiotensin II via AT_1 receptors, and aldosterone antagonists block the mineralocorticoid receptor, aldosterone.
  - Angiotensin II degradation by ACE_2 leads to formation of angiotensin-(1–7), a vasodilator that is increased during ACE inhibitor and ARB therapy and may contribute to their cardioprotective effects.
- Several clinical studies have examined the effect of very early and prolonged ACE inhibition after MI.
  - In the Survival and Ventricular Enlargement (SAVE) trial, 2231 patients with an EF of 40% or less but without overt heart failure or symptoms of myocardial ischemia were randomly assigned to receive captopril or placebo, at 42 months there was a significant (19%) reduction in all-cause mortality, a 37% reduction in severe CHF, and a 25% reduction in recurrent MI.
  - Early administration of an ACE inhibitor in the acute phase of MI was tested in the second Cooperative New Scandinavian Enalapril Survival Study (CONSENSUS II), in which 6090 patients presenting with acute MI were randomized to receive enalapril or placebo.
    - At 6 months, there was no difference in all-cause mortality but the incidence of death owing to progressive heart failure was increased by 26% in the enalapril group ($P = .06$), which raised significant concerns for ACE inhibitor administration early post acute myocardial infarction (AMI).
  - Two subsequent large-scale studies (GISSI-3 and ISIS-4), compared an oral ACE inhibitor initiated within 24 hours of symptom onset with placebo, demonstrated benefit for early initiation of oral ACE inhibitor therapy among patients with AMI with or without evidence of CHF or LVSD.
  - Beneficial effects of oral ACE inhibitors that were started early after onset of MI were also demonstrated for ramipril in the Acute Infarction Ramipril Efficacy (AIRE) trial and zofenopril in the Survival of Myocardial Infarction Long-Term Evaluation (SMILE) trial.
  - In total, 11 studies have shown improved survival (Table 3.3), and randomized clinical trials involving more than 100, 000 patients have demonstrated that early use among patients with MI results in 4.6 fewer deaths for every 1000 patients.
- Based on data showing early benefit of oral ACE inhibitor therapy in STEMI, therapy should be given early, within 24 hours, provided that there is no contraindications.
- The dose of ACE inhibitor should be rapidly titrated upward to achieve the full dose by 24 to 48 hours.

TABLE 3.3 ■ Major Trials of Angiotensin-Converting Enzyme Inhibitors in Heart Failure and Myocardial Infarction

Trial	N	Disease	Drug	Onset	Duration	Outcome
CONSENSUS, 1987	253	HF	Enalapril	—	20 mo	27% ↓ mortality; ↓ morbidity
SOLVD (symptomatic), 1991	2569	HF	Enalapril	≥4 wk	41.4 mo	16% ↓ mortality; ↓ morbidity
SOLVD (asymptomatic), 1992	4228	HF	Enalapril	≥4 wk	37.4 mo	8% ↓ mortality (NS); ↓ morbidity
CONSENSUS II, 1992	6090	MI	Enalapril	<24 h	6 mo	No decrease in mortality; hypotension
SAVE, 1992	512	MI	Captopril	3–16 d	42 mo	19% ↓ mortality; ↓ morbidity
AIRE, 1993	2006	MI	Ramipril	3–10 d	15 mo	27% ↓ mortality; ↓ morbidity
GISSI-3, 1994	19, 394	MI	Lisinopril	≤24 h	6 wk	11% ↓ mortality; ↓ morbidity
ISIS-4, 1995	58, 050	MI	Captopril	≤24 h	35 d	7% ↓ mortality; ↓ morbidity
TRACE, 1995	6676	MI	Trandolapril	3–7 d	24 mo	34.7% ↓ mortality; ↓ morbidity
CCS-1, 1995	13, 634	MI	Captopril	≤36 h	1 mo	6% ↓ mortality; ↓ morbidity
SMILE, 1995	1556	MI	Zofenopril	≤24 h	6 wk	29% ↓ mortality; ↓ morbidity
GISSI-3 (6-mo effects), 1996	19, 394	MI	Lisinopril	≤24 h	6 wk	6.2% ↓ mortality and LV dysfunction combined
HEART, 1997	352	MI	Ramipril	≤24 h	1–14 d	↓ LV remodeling

HF, Heart failure; *LV*, left ventricular; *MI*, myocardial infarction; *NS*, nonsignificant.

- Besides reperfusion and aspirin, ACE inhibitor therapy is the only other therapy shown to reduce 30-day mortality when CHF complicates STEMI, which is a class effect.
- Although the optimal duration of ACE inhibitor therapy has not been determined, for patients with STEMI, the general consensus is that it should be continued indefinitely.

ANGIOTENSIN RECEPTOR BLOCKERS

- Despite proven clinical efficacy of ACE inhibitors for patients with CHF and MI, not all patients tolerate them, often owing to an intractable cough because of the effect on kininases in the lungs.
- It also has been recognized that ACE inhibitors are capable of blocking only part of the total production of angiotensin II.
- And so, several trials investigated the benefits of ARBs in patients with MI and CHF, using an ACE inhibitor as comparator and on top of background therapy (Table 3.4).
  - In the Optimal Trial in Myocardial Infarction with Angiotensin II Antagonist Losartan (OPTIMAAL), 5477 patients with CHF after acute MI were randomly assigned to losartan or captopril.

TABLE 3.4 ■ Major Trials of Angiotensin Receptor Blockers in Heart Failure and Myocardial Infarction

Trial	N	Disease	Angiotensin Receptor Blocker	Comparator	Outcome
ELITE, 1997	722	HF	Losartan	Captopril	Unexpected 46% ↓ in mortality (secondary endpoint)
RESOLVD, 1999	768	HF	Candesartan	Enalapril	Early trend in ↑ mortality and HF (secondary endpoint)
ELITE II, 2000	3152	HF	Losartan	Captopril	Not superior
Val-HeFT, 2001	5010	HF	Valsartan	ACE inhibitor	Not superior; ↓ composite endpoint
OPTIMAAL, 2002	5477	MI	Losartan	Captopril	Not superior (noninferiority criteria not met)
CHARM—Overall, 2003	7601	HF	Candesartan	ACE inhibitor	Improved primary outcome (mortality and morbidity)
CHARM—Added, 2003	2548	HF	Candesartan	ACE inhibitor	Improved primary outcome (clinical, morbidity)
CHARM—Alternative, 2003	2028	HF	Candesartan	ACE inhibitor	Improved primary outcome (mortality and morbidity)
CHARM—Preserved, 2003	3023	HF	Candesartan	ACE inhibitor	Similar primary outcome (improved secondary outcome)
VALIANT, 2003	14,703	MI	Valsartan	Captopril	Not superior, noninferior

ACE, Angiotensin-converting enzyme; *HF*, heart failure; *MI*, myocardial infarction.

- Unexpectedly, at an average of 2.7 years, a nonsignificant ($P = 0.07$) relative (13%) increase was seen in the rate of all-cause death in the losartan group.
- In the subsequent Valsartan in Acute Myocardial Infarction Trial (VALIANT), valsartan was compared with captopril and the combination of valsartan and captopril by random assignment of 14,808 patients with acute MI complicated by LVSD, CHF, or both.
- At 25 months, no difference was observed between valsartan and captopril with respect to mortality or cardiovascular events, but combining valsartan with captopril increased the rate of adverse events without improving survival.
- Therefore, ARBs represent an alternative approach to the inhibition of the RAAS for patients after MI who do not tolerate ACE inhibitors.

ALDOSTERONE ANTAGONISTS

- Aldosterone appears to affect multiple processes that may be deleterious to cardiovascular physiology, including plasma volume homeostasis, electrolyte balance, inflammation, collagen formation, myocardial fibrosis, and remodeling.
- The aldosterone blocker, spironolactone, was shown to reduce adverse events, including death in patients with severe HF owing to chronic LVSD.

- With this as background, the Eplerenone Post–Acute Myocardial Infarction Heart Failure Efficacy and Survival Study (EPHESUS) tested the use of the aldosterone antagonist eplerenone in patients with acute MI complicated by LVSD.
  - EPHESUS recruited 6632 patients following an acute MI with an LVEF of 40% or less and CHF, or at high risk by the presence of diabetes.
  - Patients with serum creatinine greater than 2.5 mg/dL, with serum potassium greater than 5.0 mmoL/L or receiving a potassium-sparing diuretic were excluded.
  - At a mean follow-up of 16 months, eplerenone was associated with a highly significant (15%) lower rate of all-cause mortality and 21% reduction in sudden cardiac death compared with placebo.
  - The rate of serious hyperkalemia was increased by 1.6% in the eplerenone group.
  - The benefit of eplerenone was observed among patients who were already treated optimally with ACE inhibitors, ARBs, diuretics, and β-blockers at the time of randomization.
- Given the relatively high risk of sudden death within the first 30 days following an acute MI complicated by LVSD recently highlighted by data from VALIANT and the lack of proven benefit of implantable cardioverter defibrillators to reduce that risk, it is notable that additional analyses of the EPHESUS data suggested that within 30 days after randomization, eplerenone reduced the risk of sudden cardiac death by 37% ($P = .051$) and, among those at very high risk (EF$\leq$30%), by 58% ($P = .008$).

ADVERSE EFFECTS OF ACE INHIBITORS, ARBS, AND ALDOSTERONE BLOCKERS

- ACE inhibitors and ARBs can cause hypotension that may be symptomatic or hazardous in the setting of acute MI, acute renal failure, hyperkalemia, and, rarely, angioedema.
- The risk of first-dose hypotension can be minimized by starting with a low dose or not beginning therapy if the patient is volume depleted and by holding or discontinuing diuretic therapy.
- An elevation in serum creatinine and a reduction in glomerular filtration rate may be observed in some patients treated with ACE inhibitors or ARBs and is more common among patients who have bilateral renal artery stenosis, hypertensive nephrosclerosis, CHF, polycystic kidney disease, or chronic kidney disease.
- The rate of acute renal failure is 1% to 2%.
- With a glomerular filtration rate (GFR) decline of more than 30%, ACE inhibitor or ARB therapy should be stopped and the GFR allowed to return to normal.
- ACE inhibitors and ARBs reduce aldosterone secretion, thereby impairing the efficiency of urinary potassium excretion, which can result in hyperkalemia in 3% to 4% of patients.
- Hyperkalemia is more common in patients who are diabetic taking nonsteroidal anti-inflammatory drugs, patients taking potassium-sparing diuretics, and elderly patients.
- The risk of acute renal failure and hyperkalemia mandate serial monitoring of serum potassium and creatinine after the initiation of these agents.
- Angioedema is a rare but potentially fatal complication that occurs in 0.1% to 0.7% of patients treated with ACE inhibitors.
  - Angioedema usually develops within the first week of therapy, but delayed reactions several years later have been reported.
  - There is a high risk of recurrence if ACE inhibitor therapy is resumed after stopping owing to angioedema.
  - Angioedema has also been associated with ARB therapy and so careful risk–benefit assessment should be done before starting a patient who had angioedema from an ACE inhibitor on ARB therapy.

- A dry, hacking cough has been described in 5% to 10% of patients treated with an ACE, which appears to be related to increased local concentrations of kinins, substance P, prostaglandins, and thromboxane from ACE inhibitor actions on converting enzyme and kininases in the lungs.
    - Cough is much less common with ARBs, which can be substituted.
- The side effects of aldosterone receptor blockers include hyperkalemia and hypotension.
- Spironolactone can result in painful gynecomastia in men or menstrual irregularities in women, but eplerenone does not have those side effects.

RECOMMENDATIONS

- ACE inhibitors remain the preferred RAAS inhibitor; ARBs are used in patients who are ACE inhibitor–intolerant.
- Among patients with STEMI, early initiation (within 24 hours) of oral ACE inhibitors and continued long-term treatment are recommended but, if intolerant, ARBs also have demonstrated efficacy.
- The aldosterone blocker eplerenone is recommended for patients with STEMI with LVSD and an LVEF of 40% or less and either symptomatic CHF or diabetes without significant renal dysfunction or hyperkalemia who are already receiving an ACE inhibitor or ARB.
- Recommendations for initial and target doses of ACE inhibitors, ARBs, and aldosterone blockers are shown in Table 3.5.

Calcium Channel Blockers

- Calcium channel blockers (CCBs) block the entry of calcium into cells or transmembrane calcium flux through voltage-dependent L-type and T-type calcium channels.

TABLE 3.5 ▓ Initial and Target Doses for Renin-Angiotensin-Aldosterone System Inhibitors

Drug	Initial Dose	Target Dose
ACE Inhibitors		
Captopril	6.25 mg three times daily	50 mg three times daily
Enalapril	2.5 mg twice daily	10–20 mg twice daily
Fosinopril	5–10 mg daily	40 mg daily
Lisinopril	2.5–5 mg daily	20–40 mg daily
Perindopril	2 mg daily	8–16 mg daily
Quinapril	5 mg twice daily	20 mg twice daily
Ramipril	1.25–2.5 mg daily	10 mg daily
Trandolapril	1 mg daily	4 mg daily
Angiotensin Receptor Blockers		
Candesartan	4–8 mg daily	32 mg daily
Losartan	25–50 mg daily	50–100 mg daily
Valsartan	20–40 mg daily	160 mg daily
Aldosterone Antagonists		
Eplerenone	25 mg daily	50 mg daily
Spironolactone	12.5–25 mg daily	25 mg daily or twice daily

Drugs are listed alphabetically and not in order of preference.

- The major sites of action are the vascular smooth muscle cells, cardiomyocytes, and sino-atrial and atrioventricular (AV) node cells.
- CCBs inhibit the slow inward calcium current, exert a negative inotropic effect on myocardium, and dilate vascular smooth muscle.
- As vasodilators, CCBs reduce myocardial oxygen demand and increase supply and are effective antiischemic and spasmolytic agents.
- They also reduce myocardial oxygen demand by decreasing heart rate and contractility.
- However, clinical trials and systematic reviews have raised concern about increased mortality with routine use of CCBs in acute MI.
- The effect of early administration of the short-acting dihydropyridine CCB nifedipine on outcome after acute MI was compared with placebo in two randomized trials involving 1177 patients; short-term mortality was significantly increased (60%), and so short-acting nifedipine should not be administered to patients in the early phase of STEMI.
- The effects of administration of the non-dihydropyridine CCBs, verapamil and diltiazem, initiated later after acute MIs, were studied in the Danish Verapamil Infarction Trial (DAVIT II) and the Multicenter Diltiazem Post-Infarction Trial (MDPIT), respectively.
  - In DAVIT II, 1775 patients were randomly assigned to verapamil or placebo, and at a mean follow-up of 16 months, a nonsignificant (20%) lower rate of death was seen in the verapamil group.
  - In MDPIT, 2466 patients were randomly assigned to receive diltiazem or placebo after acute MI and followed for a mean of 25 months.
    - Overall mortality and adverse cardiac events were similar, but a significant interaction was observed between diltiazem and pulmonary congestion or LVSD.
- A meta-analysis of the trials indicated that CCBs did not reduce mortality or morbidity in acute MI.
- The main side effects of CCBs are hypotension, bradycardia, AV block, and worsening HF.

RECOMMENDATIONS

- The non-dihydropyridine CCBs verapamil and diltiazem may be beneficial after acute MI for patients without CHF or LVSD, but the weight of evidence favors long-term use of β-blockers for all patients without contraindications.
- Routine use of CCBs in patients with STEMI is not recommended.

Morphine and Other Analgesic Agents

- Pain relief is an important aspect of the early management of acute MI; morphine sulfate is the analgesic of choice for managing pain in these patients.
  - In acute MI, morphine relieves pain that contributes to the hyperadrenergic state, decreases blood pressure via arterial dilation and venodilation, decreases heart rate via increased vagal tone and withdrawal of sympathetic tone, decreases myocardial oxygen demand, and relieves pulmonary edema.
  - A dose of 1 to 4 mg intravenously, repeated at 5- to 15-minute intervals, is commonly used.
  - The most common side effects of morphine are nausea and vomiting, seen in 20% of patients.
  - Adverse effects include hypotension, especially prominent in patients who are volume depleted, have been given vasodilator therapy, or have right ventricle (RV) MI.

- Treatment of morphine-induced hypotension includes placing the patient in a supine or Trendelenburg position and administering intravenous saline boluses, with the addition of atropine (0.5 to 1.5 mg intravenously) for concomitant bradycardia.
- Rarely, the narcotic antidote naloxone (0.4 to 2 mg intravenously) or an inotropic agent may be needed.

RECOMMENDATIONS

- Morphine remains recommended for the relief of continuing pain in patients with STEMI.

Anticoagulants

- Current parenteral anticoagulants potentially useful during the acute phase of STEMI include unfractionated heparin (UFH), low-molecular-weight heparin (LMWH), fondaparinux, and bivalirudin (Table 3.6).
- Thrombin is a key protease of the coagulation system.
    - Thrombin inhibitors (UFH and LMWH) prevent the formation of thrombin and inhibit the activity of already formed thrombin.

TABLE 3.6 ▦ **Duration of Antiplatelet and Anticoagulant Therapy Following ST Elevation Myocardial Infarction**

	Duration of Therapy
Oral Antiplatelet Therapy	
Aspirin	Lifelong
Clopidogrel/prasugrel/ticagrelor	If patient had bare metal stent, minimum 1 month, or 1 year post-ACS
	If patient had drug-eluting stent, minimum 1 year, longer for select cases
	If patient has not been revascularized, can continue clopidogrel or ticagrelor for up to 1 year
Anticoagulant Therapy	
Unfractionated heparin (intravenous)	Up to 48 h, provided no other contraindications to discontinuation
	Can discontinue when patient has been revascularized by stenting
Low-molecular-weight heparin	Up to 8 d or duration of hospitalization, provided no other contra-indications to discontinuation
	Can discontinue when patient has been revascularized by stenting
Fondaparinux	Up to 8 d or duration of hospitalization, provided no other contra-indications to discontinuation
	Can discontinue when patient has been revascularized by stenting
Bivalirudin	Up to 3 days, provided no other contraindications to discontinuation
	Can discontinue when patient has been revascularized by stenting
Warfarin	If patient has left ventricular thrombus or aneurysm, 3 months to lifelong therapy

- ▪ UFH is a mixture of glycosaminoglycan chains that produces its anticoagulant effect by binding to antithrombin III, which inactivates factor IIa (thrombin), factor IXa, factor Ia, and factor Xa (see Fig. 3.1).
- ▪ UFH prevents growth of existing thrombus, but does not lyse clot.
- ▪ LMWH produces more potent inactivation of factor Xa than thrombin.
- ▪ UFH produces equal inhibition of factor Xa and thrombin.
- ▪ Fondaparinux is a synthetic heparin polysaccharide that binds to antithrombin with higher affinity than either UFH or LMWH and causes a conformational change that results in a preferential increase in the ability of the antithrombin–fondaparinux complex to inactivate factor Xa.
- ▪ Direct thrombin inhibitors, such as hirudin and bivalirudin, bind and inactivate thrombin without need for a cofactor, but have little effect on generation of thrombin.
- ▪ In GUSTO-1, in which intravenous and subcutaneous heparin and systemic alteplase and streptokinase were studied, an optimal activated partial thromboplastin time of between 60 and 70 seconds was associated with the lowest mortality, fewest bleeding complications, lowest reinfarction rate, and lowest frequency of hemorrhagic shock.
- ▪ Intravenous heparin should be given cautiously or not at all when streptokinase is used, unless it is specifically indicated.
- ▪ Prolonged heparin is effective in preventing LV thrombus after an acute MI.
- ▪ Side effects with both types of heparin include bleeding, thrombocytopenia, and osteoporosis.
- ▪ Patients at high risk for bleeding include women, patients over 65 years of age, and patients with comorbid states such as peptic ulcer, liver disease, and malignancy.
- ▪ Intravenous protamine can be used to reverse UFH but only partially reverses LMWH.
- ▪ Heparin-induced thrombocytopenia (HIT) is a well-known complication of UFH and LMWH therapy.
  - ▪ Two types of HIT are recognized.
    - ▪ HIT type I occurs in the first 4 days with a platelet nadir of 100, 000/mL, resolves even with continued therapy, and is not thought to be immune related.
    - ▪ HIT type II occurs within 5 to 10 days in 1% to 3% of patients and is immune mediated. It should be suspected when the platelet count decreases more than 50%, if venous or arterial thrombosis develops, or if there is necrosis noted at heparin injection sites.
  - ▪ Monitoring of platelet counts is recommended for patients on heparin or LMWH.
  - ▪ Patients exposed to heparin during the previous 3 months can develop early HIT type II mediated by circulating antibodies.
  - ▪ Management of HIT type II includes immediate discontinuation of LMWH or UFH.
  - ▪ Patients who have a history of HIT type II should not be reexposed to either type of heparin because a recurrence can be expected.
  - ▪ Patients with STEMI with HIT or a history of HIT who require anticoagulation should be treated with a nonheparin anticoagulant, such as bivalirudin or argatroban.
- ▪ For patients receiving fibrinolytic therapy, clinical trials support the use of unfractionated heparin, enoxaparin, and fondaparinux.
- ▪ For patients receiving primary PCI, evidence supports the adjunctive use of UFH and bivalirudin.
- ▪ Fondaparinux is not recommended in patients undergoing primary PCI owing to an increased risk of thrombotic procedural complications.
- ▪ It is recommended that patients with STEMI who require anticoagulation be given UFH as an intravenous infusion, with a bolus of 60 U/kg (maximum 4000 U) followed by an infusion of 12 U/kg/hr (maximum 1000 U/hr).

- Weight-based initial dosing for intravenous heparin is preferred because of evidence that the effects of heparin are primarily mediated by weight.
- Low-molecular-weight heparin for the management of STEMI has also been studied.
  - The Clinical Trial of Reviparin and Metabolic Modulation in Acute Myocardial Infarction Treatment Evaluation (CREATE) randomly assigned 15, 570 patients in India and China presenting with STEMI or new left bundle branch block, who had reperfusion therapy with either primary PCI or thrombolytic therapy, to LMWH (reviparin) or placebo.
  - LMWH improved 30-day survival and reduced reinfarction regardless of therapy.
- The effect of the factor Xa inhibitor fondaparinux (2.5 mg/day) was studied in the Organization for the Assessment of Strategies for Ischemic Syndromes (OASIS-6) trial of 12, 092 patients with STEMI.
  - Fondaparinux reduced 30-day mortality or reinfarction from 11.2% to 9.7% compared with controls with benefits apparent at 9 days without increasing bleeding and strokes.

RECOMMENDATIONS

- Patients with STEMI who undergo primary PCI should receive anticoagulation with UFH or bivalirudin.
- Anticoagulation should generally be discontinued following revascularization.
- Patients with STEMI receiving fibrinolytic therapy should receive anticoagulation using UFH, enoxaparin, or fondaparinux for at least 48 hours or until revascularization.

CHAPTER 4

Right Ventricular Myocardial Infarction

Common Misconceptions

- Right-sided electrocardiogram (ECG) in inferior myocardial infarction (MI) has no value.
- Cardiogenic shock is not possible with preserved left ventricular (LV) function.
- Intravenous nitroglycerin or morphine should be given to all patients with acute MI and ongoing chest pain.
- Infarction of the right ventricle (RV) is a common clinical event, occurring in one-third of patients with inferior MI.
- Right ventricular MI confers a worse prognosis in patients with inferior wall MI.
- Because of the requirement for different treatment strategies in RVMI, prompt recognition and appropriate treatment require a thorough understanding of the unique anatomy and pathophysiology of the RV.

Coronary Circulation and the Right Ventricle

- In the 85% of patients with right dominant coronary circulation, the RV receives its blood supply almost exclusively from the right coronary artery (RCA), with the septum and part of the posterior wall supplied by the posterior descending artery and the anterior and lateral RV walls supplied by acute marginal branches of the RCA.
- The left anterior descending artery supplies a small portion of the anterior wall of the right ventricle.
- In left dominant circulation, the left circumflex coronary artery supplies the posterior descending artery, and a nondominant RCA supplies the acute marginal branches.
- Isolated RV infarct without any LV involvement can occur with occlusion of a nondominant RCA.
- The angiographic hallmark of RVMI is thrombotic occlusion of the RCA proximal to the origin of the acute marginal branches.
- Not every case of proximal RCA occlusion results in RVMI.
- This relative protection of the right ventricle from infarction is thought to be a consequence of its lower oxygen demand, its continued perfusion during systole, and the potential presence of collaterals from the left anterior descending coronary artery, which, because of the lower systolic pressure on the right side, are more capable of supplying blood in the direction of the right ventricle than in the reverse direction.

Ventricular Interdependence

- The concept of ventricular interdependence in RVMI is central to understanding the pathogenesis of the resultant low cardiac output state.
- Ventricular interdependence is mediated through the common pericardium and shared septum.
- In RVMI, acute RV dilation occurs, and because the RV shares a relatively fixed space with the LV, the pericardial pressure abruptly increases, leading to impaired LV filling.

- Except in rare cases of isolated RVMI, some degree of LVMI accompanies RVMI.
- The pericardial constraint and alterations in septal geometry lead to reduced LV filling; cardiac output is diminished further by the decrease in LV systolic function.
- Development of shock syndrome with isolated RVMI proves that LV systolic dysfunction is not necessary for the development of shock.

The Hemodynamic Hallmarks of right ventricular myocardial inraction (Table 4.1) (Fig. 4.1)

Clinical Presentation

- RVMI is a syndrome of RV diastolic and systolic failure that, in its extreme form, is characterized by a triad of signs: hypotension that can progress to cardiogenic shock, elevated neck veins, and clear lung fields.
- Associated findings include a high frequency of bradycardia, atrioventricular (AV) block, and atrial arrhythmias, including supraventricular tachycardias and atrial fibrillation or flutter.
- The differential diagnosis (Table 4.2).

Diagnosis

- The ECG remains the most useful tool for the diagnosis of RVMI.
- The hallmark of acute RV ischemia is ST segment elevation in the right precordial leads.

TABLE 4.1 ▦ Hemodynamic Findings in Cases of Right Ventricular Myocardial Infarction

Elevated right atrial pressure (>10 mm Hg)
Right atrial pressure/pulmonary wedge pressure ratio >0.8
Noncompliant jugular venous pattern (prominent *y* descent)
Dip and plateau right ventricular diastolic pressure pattern
Depressed and delayed (often bifid) right ventricular systolic pressure
Decreased cardiac output
Hypotension

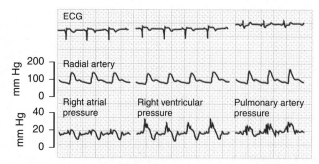

Fig. 4.1 Hemodynamic tracings in right ventricular myocardial infarction (RVMI). Noncompliant pattern of RVMI, with elevated right atrial pressure, a deep *y* descent in the atrial tracing, dip and plateau diastolic pattern in the right ventricle, and relatively low pulmonary artery pressure. (From Lorrell B, Leinbach RC, Pohost GM, et al. Right ventricular infarction: clinical diagnosis and differentiation from cardiac tamponade and pericardial constriction. Am J Cardiol. 1979;43:465–471.)

TABLE 4.2 ■ Differential Diagnosis of Right Ventricular Myocardial Infarction

Cardiac tamponade (rule out with echocardiography)

Tension pneumothorax
Acute pulmonary embolism (PE; suggested by echo findings of 60/60 sign, McConnell sign—confirm
   with computed tomography PE protocol)
Acute tricuspid regurgitation (rule out with echocardiography, assess for endocarditis and vegetations)
Pulmonary hypertension with right ventricular failure
Mass obstruction on the right side of the heart (rule out with echocardiography, other imaging techniques)
Constriction/restriction (rule out with clinical presentation and history—most often not an acute process)
Right ventricular variant Takotsubo cardiomyopathy (consider if coronary arteries are normal on
   angiography)

- The importance of obtaining right-sided chest leads on presentation in patients with suspected acute MI, particularly with evidence of inferior wall involvement, cannot be overemphasized (Fig. 4.2).
- It is important to obtain a right-sided ECG soon after the patient's presentation because ST segment elevations in lead V4R resolve within 10 hours after the onset of chest pain in half of patients.
- ST segment elevation in lead V4R is a strong predictor of in-hospital morbidity and mortality.
- Major complications (ventricular fibrillation, sustained ventricular tachycardia, cardiogenic shock, cardiac rupture, high-grade AV block, reinfarction) are markedly more common in patients with ECG evidence of RV involvement.

ATRIOVENTRICULAR BLOCK

- High-degree AV block is more common in inferior wall MI with RV involvement.
- Because cardiac output depends on preload and right atrial function, RV pacing alone may be inadequate to improve hemodynamics in complete heart block. In that case, AV sequential pacing should be implemented.

ARRHYTHMIA

- Atrial arrhythmias, including atrial fibrillation, are common complications of RVMI.
- Because of the propensity for low cardiac output and preload dependence, these arrhythmias are poorly tolerated and should be treated aggressively with early cardioversion and antiarrhythmic therapy.

Echocardiography (Table 4.3).

Treatment

The goals of treatment for RV infarction are volume resuscitation to maintain arterial pressure, electrical stabilization, revascularization, and, if needed, mechanical or pharmacologic support.

Pharmacologic therapies that reduce preload should be avoided, including nitrates, morphine sulphate, and diuretics (Table 4.4).

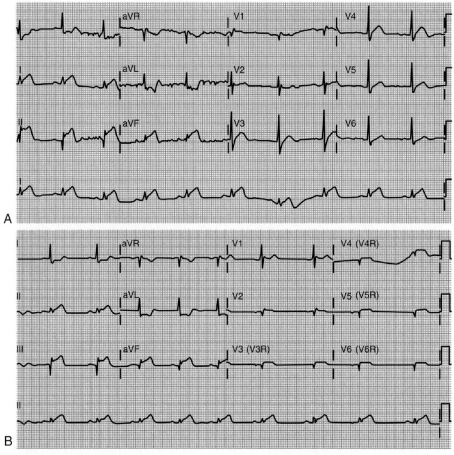

Fig. 4.2 (A) 12-Lead electrocardiogram from a 63-year-old man with chest discomfort after running on a treadmill, demonstrating ST elevation in lead III greater than in lead II; ST depression in leads I and aVL; and ST elevation in lead aVF greater than ST depression in lead V_2. Findings are suggestive of a right ventricular myocardial infarction. (B) 12-Lead electrocardiogram from the patient in (A) using right-sided precordial leads, demonstrating ST segment elevation in leads V3R to V6R, consistent with a right ventricular myocardial infarction. Adapted from Nagam MR, Vinson DR, Levis JT. ECG diagnosis: right ventricular myocardial infarction. Perm J. 2017;21:16–105, with permission from The Permanente Federation. www.thepermanentejournal.org.

TABLE 4.3 ▓ Echocardiographic Findings in Right Ventricular (RV) Myocardial Infarction

RV free wall dilatation and wall motion abnormalities (hypokinesis, akinesis)
Flattened interventricular septum (D-shaped septum) and paradoxic movement
Reduced septal wall thickening
Reduced tissue Doppler peak systolic velocity (S'), and early peak diastolic velocity (E')
Reduced RV ejection fraction

TABLE 4.4 ■ **Treatment Strategies for Right Ventricular Myocardial Infarction**

Consider invasive hemodynamic monitoring
Volume resuscitation (goal: right atrial pressure 14 mm Hg)
Electrical stabilization and synchrony (may need atrioventricular sequential pacing)
Reperfusion therapy (early, primary percutaneous coronary intervention preferred)
Inotropic support for persistent hypotension with low output (dobutamine, dopamine, norepinephrine)
Right ventricular assist devices (Impella RP, Tandem Heart, extracorporeal membrane oxygenation [ECMO])

TABLE 4.5 ■ Complications of Right Ventricular Myocardial Infarction

Atrioventricular block
Atrial tachyarrhythmias
Tricuspid regurgitation
Right-to-left shunting
Right ventricular thrombus
Pulmonary embolism
Paradoxical embolism
Septal rupture
Free wall rupture

Complications

Patients with inferior wall MI and accompanying RVMI have a much higher rate of complications than patients with inferior wall MI without RV involvement, accounting for part of the adverse prognostic implications of RVMI (Table 4.5).

Prognosis

■ After RVMI, RV function generally improves.
■ Long-term prognosis is determined, however, by residual LV rather than RV function.

CHAPTER 5

Mechanical Complications of Acute Myocardial Infarction

Common Misconceptions

- The mechanical complications of acute myocardial infarction are more common in large infarctions.
- The mechanical complications of acute myocardial infarction can be treated medically.
- Patients with ventricular septal rupture should be stabilized for several weeks before surgical repair.
- Early and effective reperfusion of acute myocardial infarction (MI) has resulted in a substantial decline in the incidence of mechanical complications, including free wall rupture, ventricular septal rupture, and papillary muscle rupture resulting in acute mitral regurgitation.
- However, mechanical complications remain important causes of morbidity and mortality in the peri-infarct setting.
- Mechanical complications are frequently associated with cardiogenic shock; approximately 12% of patients with cardiogenic shock have these complications.
- Because in many patients the MI may not be large, if patients can be diagnosed early and treated effectively, they can often be discharged with reasonably preserved left ventricular (LV) function and have an acceptable quality of life.
- The mechanical complications of acute MI are described in this chapter and summarized in Table 5.1.

Free Wall Rupture

- Acute rupture of a cardiac free wall is a sudden, usually catastrophic complication of acute MI.
- It is the second most common cause of post-MI death after cardiogenic shock without mechanical defects.
- Free wall rupture accounts for up to 20% of all deaths resulting from an acute MI.
- The overall incidence of free wall rupture is about 1% to 2%.
- Risk factors for free wall rupture include female sex, advanced age, single-vessel disease, hypertension, transmural MI, and late reperfusion therapy.

The incidence of rupture for patients with successful reperfusion (0.9%) is less than that without reperfusion treatments (2.7%).

Pathophysiology

- The most frequent site of post-MI cardiac rupture is the LV free wall (80% to 90% of cases) (Fig. 5.1).
- Less commonly, the LV posterior wall, right ventricle (RV), or atria may rupture.
- Rupture may rarely occur at more than one site and occur in combination with papillary muscle or septal rupture.

TABLE 5.1 ▦ **Mechanical Complications of Acute Myocardial Infarction**

Left ventricular free wall rupture
  ▪ Acute
  ▪ Subacute
  ▪ Pseudoaneurysm secondary to contained rupture
Right ventricular free wall rupture (very rare)
Interventricular septal rupture
Papillary muscle rupture
  ▪ Posteromedial
  ▪ Anterolateral (rare)
  ▪ Tricuspid (very rare)

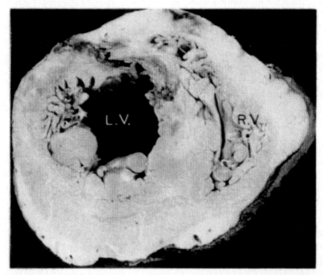

Fig. 5.1 Acute anteroseptal myocardial infarction with a rupture of the anterior wall of the left ventricle (L.V.) in a 72-year-old woman. Death from hemopericardium. *R.V.*, Right ventricle. (From Van Tasssel RA, Edwards J. Rupture of heart complicating myocardial infarction: analysis of 40 cases including nine examples of left ventricular false aneurysm. Chest 1972;61:104–116.)

■ The path of the rupture through the wall may be direct (through the center of the necrotic area), but is often serpiginous and frequently seen at an eccentric position, near the "hinge point" of mobility between the normally contracting and dyskinetic myocardium.

CLINICAL FEATURES

■ Free wall rupture occurs within 24 hours in 25% to 35% of cases and within the first week in 87% of patients following the onset of the acute coronary syndrome.
■ There are no specific symptoms or signs of acute or subacute free wall rupture.
■ Patients may present with syncope or signs and symptoms of cardiogenic shock.
■ Sudden onset of severe chest pain during or after some types of physical stress, such as coughing or straining at stool, may suggest the onset of free wall rupture.

- Some patients have premonitory symptoms, such as unexplained chest pains that are not typical of ischemia or pericarditis-related chest pains, repeated emesis, restlessness, and agitation.
- Rapid onset of tamponade owing to hemopericardium, resulting in severe hypotension and electromechanical dissociation, characterizes acute rupture; antemortem diagnosis is almost impossible in these patients.
- In patients with subacute rupture, relatively slower development of tamponade may allow antemortem diagnosis and corrective surgical therapy with salvage of these patients.
- In some patients, a pseudoaneurysm may develop.
- Elevated jugular venous pressure, pulsus paradoxus, muffled heart sounds, and a pericardial friction rub may indicate subacute rupture.
- A new systolic, diastolic, or "to-and-fro" murmur may be present in these patients with or without pseudoaneurysm.

DIAGNOSIS

- In acute free wall rupture, the electrocardiogram (ECG) reveals electromechanical dissociation and terminal bradycardia.
- In subacute rupture, several ECG findings have been described, including the presence of Q waves; recurrent ST-segment elevation or depression; pseudonormalization of inverted T waves, particularly in the precordial leads; persistent ST segment elevation; and new Q waves in two or more leads.
- None of the ECG findings are sufficiently specific or sensitive to be of value for early diagnosis of impending rupture.
- Transthoracic echocardiography should be performed as soon as the subacute rupture is suspected.
- Color Doppler may be useful for the diagnosis of the rupture site.
- The most frequent echocardiographic finding is pericardial effusion.
- Contrast echocardiography may show extravasation of the contrast material into the pericardial space, confirming the diagnosis of free wall rupture.

MANAGEMENT

- Surgical repair is the definitive treatment for subacute rupture or pseudoaneurysm and, salvage rates may be considerable.
- The operative mortality has been reported to be 24% to 35%, with a total in-hospital mortality rate of 50% to 60%.

Currently, conservative surgical techniques using simple sutures supported with felt or application of a patch to the epicardial surface with biologic glue are used.

Mitral Regurgitation

- Although mild mitral regurgitation is common in patients with acute MI, severe mitral regurgitation owing to papillary muscle and LV wall dysfunction with or without rupture of the papillary muscle is much less frequent.
- The incidence of severe mitral regurgitation complicating MI is approximately 10%, and the incidence of mitral regurgitation resulting from papillary muscle rupture is 1%.
- In patients without papillary muscle rupture, prior MI, large infarct size, multivessel coronary artery disease, recurrent myocardial ischemia, and heart failure on admission are more prevalent.
- In contrast, in patients with papillary muscle rupture, absence of previous angina, inferoposterior MI, absence of diabetes, and single-vessel disease are more common.

PATHOPHYSIOLOGY

- Acute transient papillary muscle ischemia is associated with impaired shortening of the muscle, which usually causes only mild mitral regurgitation.
- Ischemic dysfunction of anterior and posterior papillary muscles may be associated with more severe mitral regurgitation.
- Ischemia of only papillary muscles without involvement of the adjacent LV walls seldom results in severe mitral regurgitation.
- The subendocardial position of the papillary muscles and their characteristic vascular anatomy (supplied by coronary end-arteries) predispose them to ischemia.
- The posteromedial papillary muscle receives its blood supply from only the posterior descending coronary artery, whereas the anterolateral papillary muscle receives its blood supply from the left anterior descending and left circumflex coronary arteries.
- As a result, ischemia of the posteromedial papillary muscle is more common than ischemia of the anterolateral papillary muscle.
- A large posterior MI that involves the anchoring area of the posteromedial papillary muscle may be associated with severe mitral regurgitation.
- A small inferior or inferoposterior MI with involvement of the posteromedial papillary muscle can also produce severe mitral regurgitation as a result of severe leaflet prolapse.
- Rupture of the posteromedial papillary muscle is 6 to 12 times more frequent than rupture of the anterolateral papillary muscle, which explains the higher incidence of severe mitral regurgitation in patients with inferior MI.
- Severe mitral regurgitation imposes a sudden additional hemodynamic burden on LV dynamics and function.
- Sudden large-volume overload resulting from regurgitation to a left atrium (LA) with normal compliance and size causes a marked increase in LA and pulmonary capillary wedge pressure (PCWP), causing severe pulmonary edema.
- Because of postcapillary pulmonary hypertension, which increases RV afterload, the RV also fails.
- LV forward stroke volume decreases, resulting in a reduction in cardiac output and systemic hypotension.
- The hemodynamic features of cardiogenic shock develop rapidly and, usually, abruptly.
- The ejection fraction is usually reduced owing to dysfunctional ischemic or infarcted myocardium.

CLINICAL FEATURES

- Severe mitral regurgitation secondary to papillary muscle rupture occurs at a median of 1 day (range, 1 to 14 days) after the onset of the index infarction; approximately 20% of papillary muscle ruptures occur within 24 hours of the onset of infarction.
- In patients with mild mitral regurgitation secondary to papillary muscle dysfunction, the only clinical indication may be the presence of a pansystolic (holosystolic) or, more often, a late systolic murmur.
- In patients with rupture of a papillary muscle, the clinical presentation is characterized by the abrupt onset of severe respiratory distress resulting from "flash" pulmonary edema.
- Hypotension and reflex tachycardia rapidly develop along with other clinical features of preshock or shock.
- Although the sudden appearance of a pansystolic or early systolic murmur radiating to the left axilla, to the base, or both is a characteristic physical finding, a palpable thrill is uncommon.

- In some patients, the murmur may be abbreviated or absent owing to a rapid decrease in the pressure gradient between the LA and the LV.
- "Bubbling" rales of pulmonary edema are present bilaterally and make cardiac auscultation difficult.

DIAGNOSIS

- The ECG most frequently reveals recent inferior or inferoposterior MI (55%); however, the location of the index infarction is anterior (34%) or posterior (32%) in patients with severe mitral regurgitation and cardiogenic shock.
- Radiographic evidence of acute severe pulmonary edema is invariably present.
- Transthoracic echocardiography is less sensitive than transesophageal echocardiography for visualization of the disrupted mitral valve (45% to 50% vs. 100%), but it is 100% sensitive for the detection by color Doppler of the resultant severe mitral regurgitation.
- Echocardiography shows the underlying regional LV wall motion at the site of ischemia/infarction and excludes ventricular septal or free wall rupture.
- A partial papillary muscle rupture may be detectable by echocardiography.
- A complete rupture is diagnosed when the head of the papillary muscle is seen as a freely moving mobile mass attached to the mitral valve chordae.
- Although pulmonary artery (PA) catheterization is unnecessary for the diagnosis of severe mitral regurgitation, if it is undertaken, it reveals giant "v" waves in the PCWP tracing (Fig. 5.2).

Management

- Severe mitral regurgitation complicating acute MI with cardiogenic shock requires surgical intervention for mitral valve replacement or repair.
- In the Should We Emergently Revascularize Occluded Coronaries for Cardiogenic Shock (SHOCK) trial registry, in-hospital mortality without valve surgery was 71% versus 40% with surgery, indicating a significant improvement in the short-term prognosis.

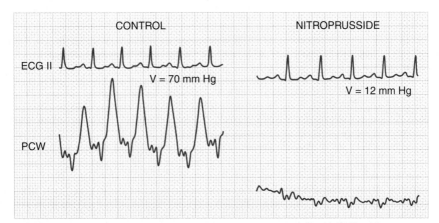

Fig. 5.2   Acute mitral regurgitation. *Left tracings:* Large "v" waves in the pulmonary capillary wedge *(PCW)* tracing. *Right tracings:* Reduction in magnitude of the v wave during sodium nitroprusside infusion. *ECG,* Electrocardiogram.

- Supportive and stabilizing treatments consist of mechanical ventilation, diuretics, vasodilators, inotropic agents, and, if possible, an intraaortic balloon pump.
- Vasodilator drugs, such as sodium nitroprusside, reduce regurgitant volume, decrease PCWP and PA pressures, and increase forward stroke volume and cardiac output.
- The therapeutic approach for mitral regurgitation complicating an MI is outlined in Table 5.2.

Ventricular Septal Rupture

- The incidence of ventricular septal rupture complicating acute MI is approximately 0.2% in the reperfusion era.
- Before the introduction of reperfusion therapy for MI, the incidence was 0.5% to 2%.
- Patients with ventricular septal rupture tend to be older, more often female, and less often have previous MI, diabetes mellitus, or a smoking history.

PATHOPHYSIOLOGY

- Most commonly, ventricular septal rupture occurs after a first MI.
- The rupture usually occurs in thin akinetic areas; it may be direct or "complex."
- The complex rupture forms a dissection plane in a serpiginous path in the septum.
- Ventricular septal rupture seems to occur with almost equal frequency in anterior and inferior MI.
- Ventricular septal rupture usually produces a large, left-to-right shunt (pulmonary-to-systemic flow > 3:1) that places a volume load on the RV, pulmonary circulation, LA, and LV.
- The LV performance, which is depressed by ischemia, is compromised further by the volume overload.
- In the SHOCK trial registry, the range of ejection fraction in patients with post-MI ventricular septal rupture was 25% to 40%.
- LV forward stroke volume declines, but RV stroke volume and pulmonary flow increase.
- There is a reflex increase in heart rate and systemic vascular resistance, which increases LV ejection impedance, further increasing the magnitude of left-to-right shunt.
- RV performance also declines because of the volume load and postcapillary pulmonary hypertension.

TABLE 5.2 ■ Suggested Management of Mitral Regurgitation Complicating Acute Myocardial Infarction

Mild Mitral Regurgitation
  Reperfusion treatments
  Adjunctive treatments
  Angiotensin-converting enzyme inhibitors or angiotensin receptor blockers, β-blockers, aldosterone antagonists, lipid-lowering agents, antiplatelet agents
Severe Mitral Regurgitation
  Corrective valve surgery
  Stabilizing and supportive treatments
  Mechanical ventilation, diuretics, intraaortic balloon pump, vasodilators, vasopressors, inotropic agents
  Adjunctive treatments in survivors
  Angiotensin-converting enzyme inhibitors or angiotensin receptor blockers, β-blockers, aldosterone antagonists, lipid-lowering agents, antiplatelet agents

CLINICAL FEATURES

- In more than 70% of patients, the clinical presentation is characterized by circulatory collapse with hypotension, tachycardia, and low cardiac output along with other clinical features of shock that may develop abruptly or within a few hours after the occurrence of a new systolic murmur.
- The murmur is best heard over the left lower sternal border and may be associated with a palpable thrill in approximately half of cases.
- Right-sided and left-sided S_3 gallops with an accentuated pulmonic component of S_2 are often present along with findings of tricuspid regurgitation.
- Pulmonary edema is less abrupt and fulminant than is seen with papillary muscle rupture.
- The chest radiograph shows a combination of pulmonary edema and increased pulmonary flow.
- The ECG shows evidence of MI with or without evidence of ischemia.

DIAGNOSIS

- Echocardiography with Doppler reveals the septal defect in most cases.
- Regional wall motion abnormalities and changes in RV and LV function are also visualized.
- Doppler echocardiography increases diagnostic yield by demonstrating transseptal flow.
- Color flow imaging during echocardiography is very sensitive for diagnosing and characterizing ventricular septal rupture.
- Agitated saline can be used to identify the defect and may show negative contrast in the RV. PA catheterization, although not required for the diagnosis of ventricular septal rupture, if undertaken, shows a step-up in oxygen saturation in the RV and PA compared with RA saturation (Fig. 5.3).

Management

- Urgent surgical repair of the ventricular septal rupture is a class I indication of the American College of Cardiology Foundation/American Heart Association guideline committee.

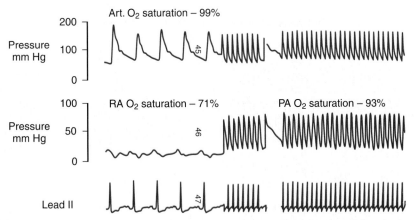

Fig. 5.3 Ventricular septal defect. Oxygen saturation step-up between the right atrium *(RA)* and pulmonary artery *(PA)*. *Art.*, arterial.

- In the SHOCK trial registry, surgical repair of ventricular septal rupture was undertaken in 31 of 55 patients with cardiogenic shock; 21 of these 31 patients also had concomitant coronary artery bypass graft surgery.
- Overall mortality in the surgical group was 81%; only 1 of 24 patients not undergoing surgery survived.
- Surgical repair should be considered if not absolutely contraindicated.
- The mythology that waiting weeks to allow patients to stabilize will improve survival actually just selects out for patients who would survive without surgery.
- Catheter-based percutaneous closure of the ventricular septal rupture may be considered for patients who cannot undergo surgery, but the technique is challenging given the necrotic ventricular septum at the site of rupture.
- Survivors of surgery usually have improved functional class and a 10-year survival rate of 50% has been reported.
- Medical therapy is required to stabilize patients before surgery.
- The goal of medical therapy is to reduce the magnitude of the left-to-right shunt, improve cardiac output and systemic perfusion, and decrease pulmonary congestion.
- The magnitude of the left-to-right shunt in ventricular septal defect is determined by the resistance at the defect and the relative resistances in the pulmonary and systemic vascular beds.
- When the size of the defect is large, as in patients with post-MI ventricular septal rupture, the magnitude of the left-to-right shunt is principally determined by the ratio of pulmonary to systemic resistance.
- Vasodilators, such as sodium nitroprusside, may increase the magnitude of left-to-right shunt owing to vasodilation of the pulmonary artery.
- Vasodilators with less vasodilatory effects on the pulmonary vascular bed but significant systemic vasodilatory effect, such as hydralazine or phentolamine, may be more effective in reducing the magnitude of left-to-right shunt.
- The most effective nonsurgical treatment to decrease the magnitude of left-to-right shunt is intraaortic balloon counterpulsation, which selectively reduces LV ejection impedance.
- The therapeutic approach for the management of ventricular septal rupture is outlined in Table 5.3.

TABLE 5.3 ▧ Suggested Therapeutic Approach for Patients With Postinfarction Ventricular Septal Rupture

Corrective surgery as soon as feasible if not contraindicated
Intraaortic balloon pump to decrease magnitude of left-to-right shunt
Vasopressors and inotropic agents
Arteriolar dilators
Diuretics
Survivors: Angiotensin-converting enzyme inhibitors or angiotensin receptor blockers, β-blockers, aldosterone antagonists, lipid-lowering agents, antiplatelet agents

CHAPTER 6

Cardiogenic Shock

Common Misconceptions

- Cardiogenic shock only occurs in patients with left ventricular systolic function.
- An intraaortic balloon pump (IABP) reduces mortality in cardiogenic shock.
- Cardiac function is a key predictor of survival of patients with cardiogenic shock.

Clinical Presentation

- Circulatory shock is characterized by the inability of blood flow and oxygen delivery to meet metabolic demands.
- Cardiogenic shock is a type of circulatory shock resulting from severe impairment of ventricular function, the diagnosis of which should include:
  - Systolic blood pressure (BP) less than 80 mm Hg without inotropic or vasopressor support, or less than 90 mm Hg with inotropic or vasopressor support, for at least 30 minutes
  - Low cardiac output (< 2.0 L/min/m^2) not related to hypovolemia (pulmonary artery capillary wedge pressure < 12 mm Hg), arrhythmia, hypoxemia, acidosis, or atrioventricular block
  - Tissue hypoperfusion manifested by oliguria (< 30 mL/h), peripheral vasoconstriction, or altered mental status
- The most common cause of cardiogenic shock is acute myocardial infarction (MI).
  - Often, anterior MI due to acute thrombotic occlusion of the left anterior descending artery results in extensive infarction.
  - Alternatively, a smaller MI in a patient with borderline left ventricle (LV) function may be responsible for insufficient cardiac output (CO).
  - Large areas of ischemic, nonfunctioning but viable myocardium or right ventricular (RV) MI from occlusion of a proximal large right coronary artery (CAD) can occasionally lead to shock (see Chapter 4).
  - Mechanical complications account for approximately 12% of cases (see Chapter 5), which include:
    - Infarction or rupture of the mitral valve papillary muscle causing acute, severe mitral regurgitation (see Chapter 14)
    - Rupture of the interventricular septum causing ventricular septal defect (VSD)
    - Rupture of the LV free wall producing pericardial tamponade
- Other cardiac causes include end-stage cardiomyopathy, myocardial contusion, myocarditis, hypertrophic cardiomyopathy, valvular heart disease, pericardial disease, RV myocardial infarction, and post-cardiopulmonary bypass.
- LV dysfunction is not a requirement for cardiogenic shock as evidenced in RV MI, cardiac tamponade, massive pulmonary embolism, acute mitral regurgitation, and acute aortic regurgitation.
- Noncardiac causes include aortic dissection, tension pneumothorax, massive pulmonary embolism, ruptured viscus, hemorrhage, and sepsis.

- Approximately 50% of patients with acute MI develop cardiogenic shock within 6 hours and 72% within 24 hours of symptoms.
- Others first develop a preshock state manifested by systemic hypoperfusion without hypotension and may benefit from aggressive supportive therapy aborting the onset of cardiogenic shock.
- Risk factors for cardiogenic shock complicating acute MI, include older age, anterior MI, hypertension, diabetes mellitus, multivessel CAD, prior MI, prior LV failure, ST segment elevation myocardial infarction, or left bundle branch block.
- Patients usually appear ashen or cyanotic, with cold and clammy skin.
- They may be agitated, disoriented, or lethargic from cerebral hypoperfusion.
- The pulses are rapid and faint, the pulse pressure narrow, and arrhythmias are common.
- Jugular venous distention and pulmonary rales are usually present in LV shock.
- Jugular venous distention, Kussmaul sign (a paradoxic increase in jugular venous pressure during inspiration), and absent rales are found in RV shock.
- A systolic thrill along the left sternal border is consistent with mitral regurgitation (MR) or VSD.
- The heart sounds are distant.
- Third and fourth heart sounds or a summation gallop may be present.
- The systolic murmur of MR is often present; VSD also produces a systolic murmur.
- The Society for Cardiovascular Angiography and Interventions (SCAI) shock stages, akin to the AHA/ACC stages A-D of heart failure, help visualise the progression and improvement of patients from those patients merely at risk (A) of cardiogenic shock to those in extremis (E), see Figs. 6.1 and 6.2.

Pathophysiology of Cardiogenic Shock in Acute MI

- The early development of cardiogenic shock is usually caused by acute thrombosis of a coronary artery supplying a large myocardial distribution, with no collateral flow recruitment; frequently, this is the left anterior descending artery, but multivessel disease is present in two thirds of patients.

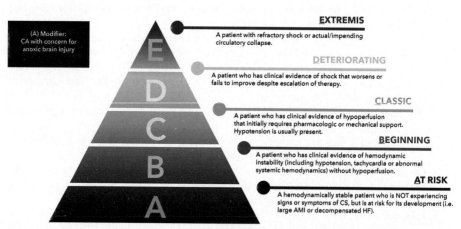

Fig. 6.1 The SCAI SHOCK classification pyramid. AMI, acute myocardial infarction; CS, cardiogenic shock; HF, heart failure; SCAI, Society for Cardiovascular Angiography and Interventions. Antman EM, Braunwald E. Acute myocardial infarction. In: Braunwald E, Fauci A, Kasper D, et al, eds. Harrison's Principles of Internal Medicine. 15th ed. New York, NY: McGraw-Hill; 2001:1395.

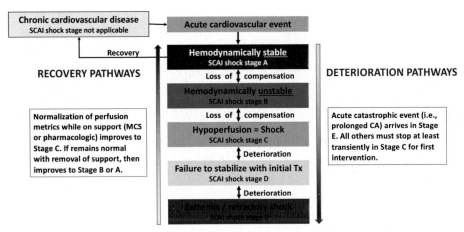

Fig. 6.2 Cardiogenic shock is a dynamic process. CA, cardiac arrest; MCS, mechanical circulatory support; SCAI, Society for Cardiovascular Angiography and Interventions. Tehrani B, Truesdell A, et al. A Standardized and Comprehensive Approach to the Management of Cardiogenic Shock. JACC: Heart Failure. 2020;8(11):879-891.

- Autopsy studies have consistently shown that at least 40% of the myocardium is infarcted in patients who die of cardiogenic shock.
  - The infarct border zone in patients without hypotension is clearly demarcated. In patients succumbing to shock, however, it is irregular, with marginal extension.
  - Focal areas of necrosis remote from the infarct zone are also present.
  - These findings result from progressive cell death owing to poor coronary perfusion, are reflected by prolonged release of cardiac enzymes, and contribute to hemodynamic deterioration.
- Progressive hemodynamic deterioration resulting in cardiogenic shock results from a sequence of events (Fig. 6.3).
  - A critical amount of diseased myocardium decreases contractile mass and CO.
  - When CO is low enough that arterial BP falls, coronary perfusion pressure decreases in the setting of an elevated LV end-diastolic pressure.
  - The resulting reduction in coronary perfusion pressure gradient from epicardium to endocardium exacerbates myocardial ischemia, further decreasing LV function and CO, perpetuating a vicious cycle.
  - The speed with which this process develops is modified by the infarct zone, remaining myocardial function, neurohumoral responses, and metabolic abnormalities.
- The infarct zone can be enlarged by reocclusion of a previously patent infarct artery, side branch occlusion from coronary thrombus propagation or embolization, or by thrombosis of a second stenosis stimulated by low coronary blood flow and hypercoagulability.
- This promotes LV dilation, increasing wall stress and oxygen demand in the setting of low CO.
- Preclinical and clinical studies have demonstrated the importance of hypercontractility of remaining myocardial segments in maintaining CO in the setting of a large MI.
- This compensatory mechanism is lost when multivessel disease is present and severe enough to produce demand ischemia in noninfarcted segments.
- A series of neurohumoral responses is activated in an attempt to restore CO and vital organ perfusion (see Chapter 7).

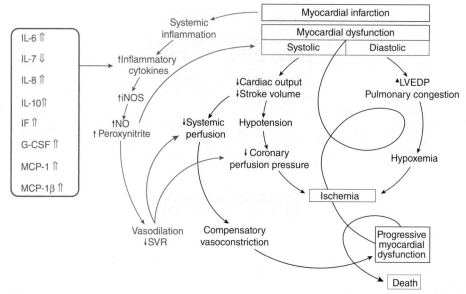

Fig. 6.3 Prognostically relevant components of cardiogenic shock complicating myocardial infarction. In addition to severe systolic and diastolic cardiac dysfunction compromising macrocirculation and micro-circulation, systemic inflammatory response syndrome and even sepsis may develop, finally resulting in multiorgan dysfunction syndrome. The proinflammatory and antiinflammatory cytokines mentioned have prognostic significance, with either higher (↑) or lower (↓) serum levels in nonsurvivors compared with survivors. *G-CSF,* Granulocyte colony-stimulating factor; *IF,* interferon; *IL,* interleukin; *LVEDP,* left ventricular end-diastolic pressure; *MCP,* monocyte chemotactic protein; *MIP,* macrophage inflammatory protein; NO, nitric oxide; iNOS, inducible macrophage-type nitric oxide synthase; *SVR,* systemic vascular resistance. From Hochman. Cardiogenic Shock Complicating Acute Myocardial Infarction Expanding the Paradigm, Circulation 2003;107:2998–3002 (502).

- Decreased baroreceptor activity owing to hypotension increases sympathetic outflow and reduces vagal tone.
- This increases heart rate, myocardial contractility, venous tone, and arterial vasoconstriction.
- Vasoconstriction is most pronounced in the skeletal, splanchnic, and cutaneous vascular beds to redistribute CO to the coronary, renal, and cerebral circulations.
- An increase in the ratio of precapillary to postcapillary resistance decreases capillary hydrostatic pressure, facilitating movement of interstitial fluid into the vascular compartment.
- Increased catecholamine levels and decreased renal perfusion lead to renin release and angiotensin production.
- Elevated angiotensin levels stimulate peripheral vasoconstriction and aldosterone synthesis.
- Aldosterone increases sodium and water retention by the kidney, raising blood volume.
- Release of antidiuretic hormone from the posterior pituitary by baroreceptor stimulation also increases water retention.
- Enhanced anaerobic metabolism, lactic acidosis, and depleted adenosine triphosphate stores result when compensatory neurohumoral responses are overwhelmed, further depressing ventricular function.
- Loss of vascular endothelial integrity because of ischemia culminates in multiorgan failure.
- Pulmonary edema impairs gas exchange.

- Renal and hepatic dysfunction results in fluid, electrolyte, and metabolic disturbances.
- Gastrointestinal ischemia can lead to hemorrhage or entry of bacteria into the bloodstream, causing sepsis.
  - Microvascular thrombosis owing to capillary endothelial damage with fibrin deposition and catecholamine-induced platelet aggregation further impairs organ function.
- A systemic inflammatory state with high plasma levels of cytokines and inappropriate nitric oxide production may also depress myocardial function or impair catecholamine-induced vasoconstriction, respectively.
- All of these factors, in turn, lead to diminished coronary artery perfusion and thus trigger a vicious cycle of myocardial ischemia and necrosis resulting in even lower BP, lactic acidosis, multiorgan failure, and ultimately death.
- The SCAI SHOCK stage is an indication of cardiogenic shock severity and
- comprises one component of mortality risk prediction in such patients (see Table 6.1). A helpful SCAI 3-axis model of risk stratification in cardiogenic shock helps one to consider the risk factors, etiology and phenotype and severity of shock (see Fig. 6.4).

INVESTIGATIONS

Electrocardiography and Laboratory Testing
- A large anterior or anterolateral MI pattern is often present.
- Old anterior Q waves or new ST segment elevation in the right precordial leads consistent with RV MI may be noted with acute inferior MI.
- Multiple lead ST segment depression, often with ST elevation in lead aVR, is another pattern that can occur with multivessel or left main CAD.
- New left or right bundle branch block and third-degree atrioventricular conduction block are ominous findings.
- A relatively normal electrocardiogram should alert one to other causes of shock.
- Troponin and creatine kinase levels are high, may peak late because of prolonged washout or ongoing necrosis, and can rise secondarily with infarct extension.
- Lactic acidosis, hypoxemia, and mixed venous oxygen desaturation are usually present.

ECHOCARDIOGRAPHY

- Bedside echocardiography, which can be performed rapidly, offers valuable information on the extent of LV dysfunction.
- A dilated, hypokinetic LV suggests LV shock, whereas a dilated RV suggests RV involvement.
- Normal ventricular function, low CO, and MR are consistent with acute severe MR.
- Pericardial tamponade from hemorrhagic effusion or free wall rupture can be detected quickly.
- Doppler evaluation can easily confirm the presence of significant MR or VSD.

Management
GENERAL MEASURES

- A number of supportive measures need to be instituted quickly (Fig. 6.5).
  - Patients with a history of inadequate fluid intake, diaphoresis, diarrhea, vomiting, or diuretic use may not have pump failure and will improve dramatically with fluid administration.
  - Because preload is critical in patients with RV shock, fluid support and avoidance of nitrates and morphine are indicated (Table 6.2).

TABLE 6.1 ■ Descriptors of shock stages: Physical examination, biochemical markers, and hemodynamics.

Stage	Description	Physical examination/bedside findings		Biochemical markers		Hemodynamics	
		Typically includes	**May include**	**Typically includes**	**May include**	**Typically includes**	**May include**
A At risk	A patient who is **not currently experiencing signs or symptoms of CS, but is at risk for its development.** These patients may include those with large acute myocardial infarction or prior infarction and/or acute or acute-on-chronic heart failure symptoms.	Normal JVP **Warm and well-perfused** • Strong distal pulses • Normal mentation	Clear lung sounds	**Normal lactate**	Normal labs • Normal (or at baseline) renal function	**Normotensive** (SBP ≥ 100 mmHg or at baseline)	If invasive hemodynamics are assessed: • Cardiac Index ≥ 2.5 L/min/m² (if acute) • CVP ≤ 10 mmHg • PCWP ≤ 15 mmHg • PA saturation ≥ 65%
B Beginning CS	A patient who has **clinical evidence of hemodynamic instability** (including relative hypotension or tachycardia) **without hypoperfusion.**	Elevated JVP **Warm and well-perfused** • Strong distal pulses • Normal mentation	Rales in lung fields	**Normal lactate**	Minimal acute renal function impairment Elevated BNP	**Hypotension** • SBP < 90 mmHg • MAP < 60 mmHg • > 30 mmHg drop from baseline	
C Classic CS	A patient who manifests with **hypoperfusion and who requires one intervention (pharmacological or mechanical) beyond volume resuscitation.** These patients typically present with relative hypotension (but hypotension is not required).	**Volume overload**	Looks unwell Acute alteration in mental status Feeling of impending doom Cold and clammy Extensive rales Ashen mottled, dusky, or cool extremities Delayed capillary refill Urine Output <30 mL/h	**Lactate ≥ 2 mmol/L**	Creatinine increase to 1.5 x baseline (or 0.3 mg/dL) or > 50% drop in GFR Increased LFTs Elevated BNP	**Tachycardia** • Heart rate ≥ 100 bpm • If invasive hemodynamics assessed **(strongly recommended)** • Cardiac index <2.2 L/min.m² • PCWP >15 mmHg	

Stage	Description	Physical Exam	Biochemical Markers	Hemodynamics
D Deteriorating	A patient who is similar to category C but is getting worse. **Failure of initial support strategy to restore perfusion** as evidenced by worsening hemodynamics or rising lactate.	**Any of stage C and worsening (or not improving) signs/symptoms of hypoperfusion despite the initial therapy.**	**Any of stage C and lactate rising and persistently >2 mmol>L** / Deteriorating renal function Worsening LFTs Rising BNP	**Any of stage C and requiring escalating doses or increasing numbers of pressors or addition of a mechanical circulatory support device to maintain perfusion**
E Extremis	**Actual or impending circulatory collapse**	**Typically unconscious** / Near pulselessness Cardiac collapse Multiple defibrillations	**Lactate ≥ 8 mmol/L**[a] / CPR (A-modifier) Severe acidosis • pH <7.2 • Base deficit >10 mEg/L	**Profound hypotension despite maximal hemodynamic support** / Need for bolus doses of vasopressors

BNP, B-type natriuretic peptide; CPR, cardiopulmonary resuscitation; CVP, central venous pressure; GFR, glomerular filtration rate; JVP, jugular venous pressure; LFT, liver function tests; MAP, mean arterial pressure; PA, pulmonary artery; PCWP, pulmonary capillary wedge pressure; SVP, systolic ventricular pressure.

[a]Stage E prospectively is a patient with cardiovascular collapse or ongoing CPR.
From SCAI SHOCK Stage Classification Expert Consensus Update: A Review and Incorporation of Validation Studies Naidu, Srihari S. et al. JCAI; Volume 1, Issue 1, 100008

Proposed 3-axis model of cardiogenic shock evaluation and prognostication

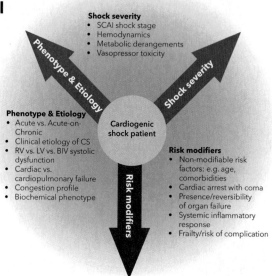

Shock severity
- SCAI shock stage
- Hemodynamics
- Metabolic derangements
- Vasopressor toxicity

Phenotype & Etiology
- Acute vs. Acute-on-Chronic
- Clinical etiology of CS
- RV vs. LV vs. BIV systolic dysfunction
- Cardiac vs. cardiopulmonary failure
- Congestion profile
- Biochemical phenotype

Cardiogenic shock patient

Risk modifiers
- Non-modifiable risk factors: e.g. age, comorbidities
- Cardiac arrest with coma
- Presence/reversibility of organ failure
- Systemic inflammatory response
- Frailty/risk of complication

Fig. 6.4 The SCAI 3-axis model of cardiogenic shock evaluation and prognostication. (From SCAI SHOCK Stage Classification Expert Consensus Update: A Review and Incorporation of Validation Studies Naidu, Srihari S. et al. JCAI; Volume 1, Issue 1, 100008)

- Oxygenation and airway protection are critical.
- Intubation and mechanical ventilation may be required, followed by sedation, and often muscular paralysis.
- Positive end-expiratory pressure decreases preload and afterload.
- These interventions also improve the safety of electrical cardioversion or cardiac catheterization, if needed, and decrease oxygen demand.
- Hypokalemia and hypomagnesemia predispose patients to ventricular arrhythmias and should be corrected.
- Because metabolic acidosis decreases contractile function, hyperventilation should be considered, but sodium bicarbonate should be avoided given its short half-life and the large sodium load.
- Arrhythmias and atrioventricular heart block have a major influence on CO.
  - Sustained tachyarrhythmias should be electrically cardioverted promptly rather than treated with pharmacologic agents.
  - Severe bradycardia owing to excess vagotonia can be corrected with atropine.
  - Temporary pacing should be initiated for high-degree heart block, preferably with a dual-chamber system.
  - This is especially important in patients with RV infarction who depend on the preload contribution of synchronous right atrial contraction.
- Morphine sulfate decreases pain and anxiety, excessive sympathetic activity, preload, and afterload, but should only be administered in small increments.
- Diuretics decrease filling pressures and should be used to control volume.
- Beta-blockers and calcium channel blockers should be avoided because they are negative inotropic agents.
- An insulin infusion may be required to control hyperglycemia.

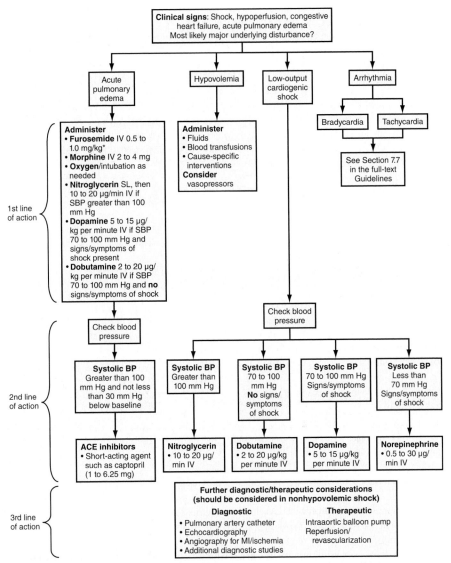

Fig. 6.5 Emergency management of complicated ST-elevation myocardial infarction. ACE, Angiotensin-converting enzyme; BP, blood pressure; IV, intravenous; MI, myocardial infarction; SBP, systolic blood pressure; SL, sublingual. (From Antman EM, Anbe DT, Armstrong PW, et al. ACC/AHA guidelines for the management of patients with ST-elevation myocardial infarction: a report of the American College of Cardiology/American Heart Association Task Force on Practice Guidelines. Circulation. 2004;110;e82.)

HEMODYNAMIC MONITORING

- Central hemodynamic monitoring is critical for confirming the diagnosis and guiding pharmacologic therapy (Table 6.3; see Chapter 23).
- Urine output needs to be monitored hourly through an indwelling urinary catheter.
- An arterial catheter allows constant monitoring of the BP.

TABLE 6.2 ■ **Conventional Therapy for Cardiogenic Shock**

1.	Maximize volume	e.g. RAP 10–14 mm Hg, PAWP 18–20 mm Hg
2.	Maximize oxygenation	e.g. ventilator
3.	Correct electrolyte and acid-base imbalances	
4.	Control rhythm	e.g. pacemaker, cardioversion
5.	Sympathomimetic amines	e.g. dobutamine, dopamine, norepinephrine
6.	Phosphodiesterase inhibitors	e.g. milrinone
7.	Vasodilators	e.g. nitroglycerin, nitroprusside
8.	Intraaortic balloon counterpulsation	

PAWP, Pulmonary artery wedge pressure; *RAP*, right atrial pressure.

TABLE 6.3 ■ **Hemodynamic Profiles**

Left ventricular shock	High PCWP, low CO, high SVR
Right ventricular shock	High RA RA/PCWP > 0.8 Exaggerated RA "y" descent RV square root sign
Mitral regurgitation	Large PCWP "v" wave
Ventricular septal defect	Large PCWP "v" wave, oxygen saturation step-up (> 5%) from RA to RV
Pericardial tamponade	Equalization of diastolic pressures ~20 mm Hg

CO, Cardiac output; *PCWP*, pulmonary capillary wedge pressure; *RA*, right atrial; *RV*, right ventricular; *SVR*, systemic vascular resistance.

- A pulmonary artery catheter should be considered to measure intracardiac pressures, CO, systemic vascular resistance, and mixed venous oxygen saturation.
- The hemodynamic profile of LV shock, as defined by Forrester and coworkers, includes pulmonary artery wedge pressure greater than 18 mm Hg and a cardiac index less than 2.2 L/min/m^2.
- Others have used a pulmonary wedge pressure of 15 or 12 mm Hg and a cardiac index of 2.0 or 1.8 L/min/m^2.
- The hemodynamic profile of RV shock includes RA pressure of 85% or more of the pulmonary artery wedge pressure, steep Y descent in the RA pressure tracing, and the dip and plateau (i.e., square root sign) in the RV wave form.
- Large V waves in the pulmonary artery wedge tracing suggest the presence of severe MR.
- An oxygen saturation step-up (> 5%) from the RA to the RV confirms the diagnosis of VSD.
- Equalization of RA, RV end-diastolic, pulmonary artery diastolic, and pulmonary capillary wedge pressures occurs with severe RV infarction or pericardial tamponade owing to free wall rupture or hemorrhagic effusion.
- Cardiac power (mean arterial pressure × cardiac output/451) is the strongest hemodynamic predictor of hospital mortality.

PHARMACOLOGIC SUPPORT

- Vasopressor and inotropic drugs are the major initial interventions for reversing hypotension and improving vital organ perfusion (Table 6.4).
    - Failure to improve BP with these agents is an ominous prognostic sign.
    - Continued hypotension results in progressive myocardial ischemia and deterioration of ventricular function.
- Dobutamine, a synthetic catecholamine with predominantly β_1-adrenergic effects, is the initial inotropic agent of choice for patients with systolic pressures greater than 70 mm Hg.
    - CO is increased and filling pressures are decreased.
    - Dobutamine is particularly effective in RV shock.
- Norepinephrine is a natural catecholamine with predominantly peripheral α-adrenergic effects.
    - It is used when the systolic pressure is less than 70 mm Hg, because it is a potent venous and arterial vasoconstrictor.
    - Many now prefer norepinephrine over dopamine as initial therapy.
- Dopamine, a natural catecholamine, is the initial vasopressor of choice when the systolic pressure is greater than 70 mm Hg. Low doses (2–5 µg/kg/min) increase stroke volume (SV) and renal perfusion by stimulating dopamine receptors.
    - Intermediate doses have a dose-dependent β_1-adrenergic receptor effect, increasing inotropy and chronotropy.
    - High doses (15–20 µg/kg/min) activate α-adrenergic receptors, increasing vascular resistance.
- Catecholamine infusions should be carefully titrated.
    - A delicate balance must be obtained between increasing coronary perfusion pressure and increasing oxygen demand so that myocardial ischemia is not exacerbated.
    - Moreover, excessive peripheral vasoconstriction decreases tissue perfusion, increased afterload increases filling pressures, and excessive tachycardia or arrhythmias can be stimulated.
- Cardiac glycosides have no significant inotropic effect in patients with severe pump failure and increased oxygen consumption and should be avoided.

TABLE 6.4 ■ **Pharmacologic Treatment for Cardiogenic Shock**

Drug	Dose	Side Effects
Dobutamine	5–15 µg/kg/min IV	Tolerance
Dopamine	2–20 µg/kg/min IV	Increased oxygen demand
Norepinephrine	0.5–30 µg/min IV	Peripheral and visceral vasoconstriction
Nitroglycerin	10 µg/min, increased by 10 µg every 10 min, maximum 200 µg/min IV	Headache, hypotension, tolerance
Nitroprusside	0.3–10 µg/min IV	Hypotension, cyanide toxicity
Milrinone	50 µg/kg over 10 min IV, then 0.375–0.75 µg/kg/min	Ventricular arrhythmia
Furosemide	20–160 mg/IV	Hypokalemia, hypomagnesemia
Bumetanide	1–3 mg IV	Nausea, cramps

IV, intravenous.

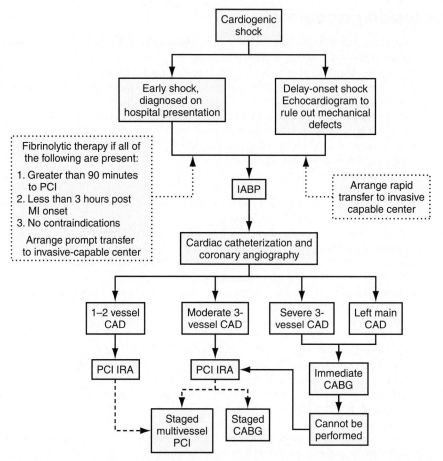

Fig. 6.6 Recommendations for initial reperfusion therapy. *CABG*, coronary artery bypass graft surgery; *CAD*, coronary artery disease; *IABP*, intraaortic balloon counterpulsation; *IRA*, infarct-related artery; *LBBB*, left bundle branch block; *MI*, myocardial infarction; *PCI*, percutaneous coronary intervention. (From Antman EM, Anbe DT, Armstrong PW, et al. ACC/AHA guidelines for the management of patients with ST-elevation myocardial infarction: a report of the American College of Cardiology/American Heart Association Task Force on Practice Guidelines. Circulation. 2004;110;e82.)

- Ischemic myocardium is susceptible to the arrhythmogenic effects of digoxin, and intravenous administration causes coronary and peripheral vasoconstriction.
- Vasodilators are useful if adequate BP and coronary artery perfusion pressure can be restored.
  - Nitroprusside is an arterial dilator and a venodilator, whereas nitroglycerin is predominantly a venodilator.
  - Afterload reduction increases SV and is especially important when MR or VSD is present.
  - Preload reduction decreases filling pressures and oxygen demand by reducing wall tension.
  - The major hazard is that a reduction in preload and afterload could decrease diastolic arterial pressure, compromising coronary artery perfusion pressure and resulting in extension of ischemic myocardial injury.

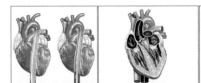

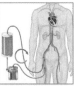

	IABP	IMPELLA	TANDEMHEART	VA-ECMO
Cardiac Flow	0.3-0.5 L/ min	1-5L/ min (Impella 2.5, Impella CP, Impella 5)	2.5-5 L/min	3-7 L/min
Mechanism	Aorta	LV → AO	LA → AO	RA → AO
Maximum Implant Days	Weeks	7 days	14 days	Weeks
Sheath Size	7-8 Fr	13-14 Fr Impella 5.0 - 21 Fr	15-17 Fr Arterial 21 Fr Venous	14-16 Fr Arterial 18-21 Fr Venous
Femoral Artery Size	>4 mm	Impella 2.5 & CP - 5-5.5 mm Impella 5 - 8 mm	8 mm	8 mm
Cardiac Synchrony or Stable Rhythm	Yes	No	No	No
Afterload	↓	↓	↑	↑↑↑
MAP	↑	↑↑	↑↑	↑↑
Cardiac Flow	↑	↑↑	↑↑	↑↑
Cardiac Power	↑	↑↑	↑↑	↑↑
LVEDP	↓	↓↓	↓↓	↔
PCWP	↓	↓↓	↓↓	↔
LV Preload	---	↓↓	↓↓	↓
Coronary Perfusion	↑	↑	---	---
Myocardial Oxygen Demand	↓	↓↓	↔↓	↔

Fig. 6.7 Comparison of mechanical support devices. *AO,* Aorta; *IABP,* intraaortic balloon pump; *LA,* left atrium; *LV,* left ventricle; *LVEDP,* left ventricular end-diastolic pressure; *MAP,* mean arterial pressure; *PCWP,* pulmonary capillary wedge pressure; *RA,* right atrium; *VA-ECMO,* venoarterial extracorporeal membrane oxygenation. (From Atkinson TM, Ohman EM, O'Neill WW, et al. A practical approach to mechanical circulatory support in patients undergoing percutaneous coronary intervention: an interventional perspective. JACC Cardiovasc Interv. 2016;9:871–883.)

- Reflex tachycardia increases oxygen demand.
- Nitroglycerin and nitroprusside can be started at low-dose infusions and titrated against BP and pulmonary capillary wedge pressure.
- Phosphodiesterase inhibitors (e.g., milrinone) are not indicated for acute cardiogenic shock, but can be useful in low-output states when the patient is relatively stable by augmenting myocardial contractility and producing peripheral vasodilation.

MECHANICAL SUPPORT

- When pharmacologic therapy provides insufficient hemodynamic support, mechanical circulatory assistance can be instituted (see Chapters 24 and 25), especially when revascularization or surgical repair of mechanical complications is planned (Figs. 6.6 and 6.7).

CHAPTER 7

Acute Heart Failure and Pulmonary Edema

Common Misconceptions

- Acute decompensated heart failure (ADHF) typically presents with hypotension or shock.
- The diagnosis of ADHF is made on the basis of imaging studies and natriuretic peptide levels.
- ADHF is a single disease entity.
- All patients with ADHF require a pulmonary artery catheter.
- The predominant effect of low-dose nitroglycerin infusion in ADHF is mediated through afterload reduction.

Clinical Presentation

- Acute decompensated heart failure (ADHF) is a clinical syndrome of new or worsening signs and symptoms of HF, leading to hospitalization or a visit to the emergency department.
- Patients with ADHF represent a heterogeneous population with high readmission rates.
- The average patient has had symptoms for about 5 to 7 days before seeking medical attention.
- ADHF is the most common cause of hospital admission in patients older than 65 years, accounting for 1 million admissions annually and with a 20% to 30% mortality rate within 6 months after admission.
- The onset and severity of symptoms vary and depend on the nature of the underlying etiology and the rate of development.
- The largest proportion of patients (70%) with ADHF are admitted because of worsening HF; up to 15% to 20% of patients present with HF for the first time and approximately 5% are admitted for advanced or end-stage HF.
- Few patients with ADHF present with low BP (<8%) or shock (<3%).
- Most patients are elderly, with an average age of 70 to 75 years and almost half will have preserved left ventricular ejection fraction (LVEF).
- A history of coronary artery disease is present in 60% of patients, 45% of whom have had a prior myocardial infarction (MI), hypertension in 70%, atrial fibrillation (AF) in 30%, diabetes mellitus in 40%, and chronic obstructive pulmonary disease in 30%.
- The European Society of Cardiology guidelines for the diagnosis and treatment of ADHF classifies patients into one of six groups on the basis of the clinical and hemodynamic profiles (Table 7.1).

GROUP 1: ACUTE-ON-CHRONIC DECOMPENSATED HEART FAILURE

- This syndrome is seen in patients with an established diagnosis of HF who develop increasing signs or symptoms of decompensation after a period of relative stability.

TABLE 7.1 ■ **Acute Heart Failure Syndromes**

Phenotype	Rate of Onset	Signs and Symptoms	Hemodynamic Profile	Diagnostics
1a. Acute-on-chronic HF	Gradual	Dyspnea and fluid overload	Normal or low normal BP	CR: normal or mild interstitial edema
		Adequate tissue perfusion	Possible pleural effusion	
1b. New-onset ADHF	Gradual or rapid	Dyspnea, variable fluid overload	Normal or low BP	CR: normal or mild interstitial edema
		Variable tissue perfusion	Possible pleural effusion	
2. Hypertensive ADHF	Rapid	Acute dyspnea	SBP >180 mm Hg	CR: interstitial lung edema
	Minimal fluid overload	Adequate tissue perfusion		
3. ADHF and pulmonary edema	Rapid or gradual	Severe dyspnea, tachypnea	Low normal BP	Hypoxic on room air
	Tachycardia	Variable tissue perfusion		
4a. Cardiogenic shock (low output syndrome)	Usually gradual	Weakness/fatigue Altered mental status Poor tissue perfusion	Low normal BP	Echo shows severe LV dysfunction
4b. Severe cardiogenic shock	Rapid	Weakness/fatigue Oliguria/anuria	Low BP (<90 mm Hg)	
5. High-output HF	Rapid or gradual	Dyspnea; tachycardia and warm periphery	Normal BP	
6. Acute right HF	Rapid or gradual; marked fluid overload	Variable tissue perfusion	Severe dyspnea	Low normal BP

Modified from Nieminen MS, Bohm M, Cowie MR, et al. for the ESC Committee for Practice Guideline: Executive summary of the guidelines on the diagnosis and treatment of acute heart failure: The Task Force on Acute Heart Failure of the European Society of Cardiology. *Eur Heart J* 2005;26:384–416; and Joseph SM, Cedars AM, Ewald GA, et al. Acute decompensated heart failure: contemporary medical management. *Tex Heart Inst J.* 2009;36(6):510–20.
BP, Blood pressure; *CR*, chest radiograph; *HF*, heart failure; *SBP*, systolic blood pressure.

- Progressive dyspnea is the most common complaint of patients, along with lower extremity edema, epigastric tenderness, or abdominal fullness.
- An elevated jugular venous pressure, positive hepatojugular reflux test, and a tender, enlarged liver are frequent findings.
- Rales and wheezing may be heard with significant pulmonary congestion, but the absence of rales does not imply that the pulmonary venous pressures are not elevated.
- Diminished air entry at the lung bases is usually caused by a pleural effusion, which is often more frequent on the right.

- Leg edema is frequently evident in both legs, particularly in the pretibial region and ankles in ambulatory patients.
- The cardiac examination may be entirely normal in patients with heart failure with preserved LVEF, whereas many patients with advanced LV systolic dysfunction (LVSD) exhibit a third heart sound and a laterally displaced point of maximal impulse.
- A murmur of mitral regurgitation is often audible when the LV is markedly enlarged, whereas a tricuspid regurgitation murmur is present when the right ventricle (RV) is volume or pressure overloaded.

GROUP 2: HYPERTENSIVE ACUTE HEART FAILURE

- The syndrome of ADHF is characterized by the rapid onset of symptoms or signs of HF.
- This phenotype is more common in females and the systolic BP on admission usually exceeds 180 mm Hg.
- There is usually predominant pulmonary congestion and minimal weight gain prior to admission.
- Virtually all patients have a preserved LVEF.

GROUP 3: ACUTE HEART FAILURE WITH SEVERE PULMONARY EDEMA

- Severe pulmonary edema is seen in less than 3% of all patients admitted with ADHF.
- Patients typically experience a sudden and overwhelming sensation of suffocation and air hunger accompanied by extreme anxiety, cough, expectoration of a pink frothy liquid, and a sensation of drowning.
- The patient sits bolt upright, is unable to speak in full sentences owing to a marked respiratory rate, and may also thrash about.
- An ominous sign is obtundation, which may be a sign of severe hypoxemia.
- Sweating is profuse, and the skin tends to be cool, ashen, and cyanotic.
- The oxygen saturation is usually less than 90% on room air before treatment.
- Auscultation of the lung usually reveals coarse airway sounds bilaterally with rhonchi, wheezes, and moist fine crepitant rales that are detected first at the lung bases, but then extend upward to the apices as the lung edema worsens.
- Cardiac auscultation may be difficult in the acute situation, but third and fourth heart sounds may be present.

GROUP 4: CARDIOGENIC SHOCK AND LOW-OUTPUT SYNDROME

- Systolic BP is less than 90 mm Hg in approximately 8% of patients with acute decompensated HF.
- Low-output HF is characterized by symptoms and signs that are related to decreased end-organ perfusion.
- A typical patient with this clinical syndrome has severe LVSD and usually presents with symptoms of fatigue, altered mental status, or signs of organ hypoperfusion.
- The patient may present with tachypnea at rest, tachycardia, and a cold and cyanotic periphery.
- The degree of peripheral hypoperfusion may be so advanced that the skin over the lower extremities is mottled and cool.
- Occasionally, the clinician may detect *pulsus alternans*—when a strong or normal pulse alternates with a weak pulse during normal sinus rhythm, a sign of severe LVSD.

GROUP 5: HIGH-OUTPUT HEART FAILURE

- The phenotype is uncommon and generally presents with warm extremities, pulmonary congestion, tachycardia, and a wide pulse pressure.
- Underlying conditions include anemia, thyrotoxicosis, advanced liver failure, and Paget disease.

GROUP 6: RIGHT-SIDED HEART FAILURE

- This syndrome occurs commonly in patients with severe isolated tricuspid regurgitation, RV dysfunction, chronic lung disease, or long-standing pulmonary hypertension.
- These patients present with signs and symptoms of right-sided volume overload.

Pathophysiologic Considerations

- Integral to the understanding of the pathogenesis and treatment of ADHF is an understanding of the forces involved in fluid retention, capillary–interstitial fluid exchange (Starling relationship), and myocardial pump performance.

CHRONIC PROGRESSIVE FLUID AND WATER RETENTION

- Arterial underfilling is sensed by mechanoreceptors in the LV, carotid sinus, aortic arch, and renal afferent arterioles, caused by a decrease in systemic arterial pressure, stroke volume, renal perfusion, or peripheral vascular resistance.
- This leads to an increase in sympathetic outflow from the central nervous system, activation of the renin-angiotensin-aldosterone system, and the nonosmotic release of arginine vasopressin, as well as the stimulation of thirst.
- These factors—together with increased release of vasoconstrictors, such as endothelin and vasopressin, and resistance to endogenous natriuretic peptides—contribute to sodium and water retention leading to decompensation of HF.

PULMONARY EDEMA

- The flux of fluid out of any vascular bed results from the sum of forces promoting extravasation of fluid from the capillary lumen versus forces acting to retain intravascular fluid.
- Under normal conditions, the sum of the forces is slightly positive, producing a small vascular fluid flux into the precapillary interstitium of the lung that is drained as lymph into the systemic veins.
- Because the intravascular pressure in the pulmonary capillaries is always higher than plasma osmotic pressure, transcapillary fluid flux out of the pulmonary capillary is continuous.
- When the interstitial fluid exceeds the interstitial space capacity, fluid floods into the alveoli.
- The interstitial space is drained by a rich bed of lymphatics and pulmonary lymph flow may increase threefold before fluid extravasates into the alveolar airspaces.
- Table 7.2 lists the causes of pulmonary edema based on the initiating mechanism.
- Pulmonary edema occurs if the pulmonary capillary pressure exceeds the plasma colloid osmotic (oncotic) pressure, which is approximately 28 mm Hg in humans.
- The normal pulmonary capillary wedge pressure is approximately 8 mm Hg, which allows a margin of safety of about 20 mm Hg.

TABLE 7.2 ■ Classification of Acute Pulmonary Edema

Cardiogenic Pulmonary Edema

A. Acute increase in pulmonary capillary pressure
  1. Increased LA pressure with normal LV diastolic pressure
    a. Thrombosed prosthetic mitral valve
    b. Obstructive left atrial myxoma
  2. Increased LA pressure owing to elevated LV diastolic pressure
    a. Increased myocardial stiffness or impaired relaxation
      i. Myocardial ischemia
      ii. Acute myocardial infarction
      iii. Hypertrophic heart disease complicated by tachycardia or ischemia
      iv. Stress-induced cardiomyopathy
    b. Acute volume load
      i. Acute mitral or aortic regurgitation
      ii. Ischemic myocardial septal rupture
    c. Acute increases in LV afterload
      i. Hypertensive crisis
      ii. Thrombosed prosthetic aortic valve
B. Exacerbation of chronically elevated pulmonary capillary pressures
  1. Increase in elevated LA pressure with normal LV diastolic pressure
    a. Mitral stenosis and atrial fibrillation with rapid heart rate
    b. Left atrial myxoma
  2. Increase in elevated LA pressure caused by a further increase in LV diastolic pressure
    a. Further increases in myocardial stiffness or impaired relaxation
      i. Cardiomyopathy complicated by myocardial ischemia or infarction
      ii. Hypertrophic heart disease complicated by tachycardia or ischemia
    b. Volume load imposed on preexisting LV diastolic dysfunction
      i. Worsening mitral regurgitation
      ii. Vigorous postoperative fluid administration
      iii. Dietary indiscretion
    c. Pressure load imposed on preexisting LV systolic dysfunction
      i. Accelerated hypertension

Noncardiogenic Pulmonary Edema

A. Altered alveolar capillary membrane permeability (adult respiratory distress syndrome)
  1. Infectious or aspiration pneumonia
  2. Septicemia
  3. Acute radiation or hypersensitivity pneumonitis
  4. Disseminated intravascular coagulopathy
  5. Shock lung
  6. Hemorrhagic pancreatitis
  7. Inhaled or circulating toxins
  8. Massive trauma
B. Acute decrease in interstitial pressure of the lung
  1. Rapid removal of unilateral pleural effusion
C. Unknown mechanisms
  1. High-altitude pulmonary edema
  2. Neurogenic pulmonary edema
  3. Narcotic overdose
  4. Pulmonary embolism
  5. After cardioversion
  6. After anesthesia or cardiopulmonary bypass

LA, Left atrial; *LV*, left ventricular.

- Although pulmonary capillary pressure must be abnormally high to increase the flow of the interstitial fluid, these pressures may not correlate with the severity of pulmonary edema when edema is clearly present.
- Pressures may return to normal when there is still considerable pulmonary edema because of the time required for removal of interstitial and pulmonary edema.
- Chronic elevations in left atrial pressure are associated with hypertrophy in the lymphatics, which then clear greater quantities of capillary filtrate during acute increases in pulmonary capillary pressure.
- The removal of edema fluid from the alveolar and interstitial compartments of the lung depends on active transport of sodium and chloride across the alveolar epithelial barrier.
- Reabsorption of these electrolytes is mediated by the epithelial ion channels located on the apical membrane of alveolar epithelial type I and type II cells and distal airway epithelia.
- Water follows passively, probably through aquaporins that are found predominantly on alveolar epithelial type I cells.

LEFT VENTRICULAR PUMP PERFORMANCE IN ADHF

- The relationship between pressure and volume throughout the cardiac cycle can be presented as a pressure-volume (PV) loop (Fig. 7.1).
- The PV loop can provide a simple, but comprehensive, description of LV pump function as it encapsulates the systolic and diastolic functions of the heart.
- Because these loops also circumscribe end-systolic volume (ESV) and end-diastolic volumes (EDV), the stroke volume (SV) and EF can be derived.
- The bottom limb of the loop, also termed" diastolic pressure-volume curve," describes LV diastolic compliance.
- Progressive increases in systolic pressure produce a nearly linear increase in ESV.
- By matching the end-systolic pressure (ESP) and volume coordinates from multiple, variably loaded beats, a near-linear relationship is established.
- The slope of this relationship (E_{max}), determined by altering load, reflects LV contractility (see Fig. 7.1).
- A positive inotropic intervention is associated with an increased ESP and SV and a decreased EDV.
- This results in an increased E_{max} and a shift of the PV relationship to the left (Fig. 7.2A).
- Conversely, a negative inotropic intervention decreases ESP and SV and increases EDV.
- This results in a decrease in E_{max} and a shift of the PV relationship to the right (see Fig. 7.2B).
- In the intact human heart, an increase in systolic pressure is associated with an increase in ESV and, if the LV fails to dilate, stroke volume decreases (Fig. 7.3A).
- An increase in preload is accompanied by an increase in SV and a modest increase in ESP (see Fig. 7.3B).
- Acute and chronic changes in the PV relationship in the failing heart depend on the underlying myocardial structure and function, the type and extent of injury, and the severity and nature of the hemodynamic load.

CHAMBER STIFFNESS

- Chamber stiffness is determined by analyzing the curvilinear diastolic PV relationships (Fig. 7.4).
- The slope of the tangent (dP/dV) to this curvilinear relationship defines the chamber stiffness at a given filling pressure.

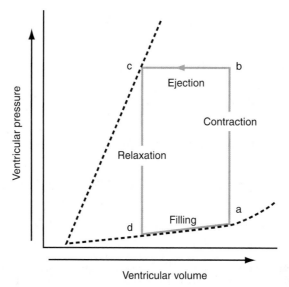

Fig. 7.1 Schematic representation of the left ventricular (LV) pressure-volume loop. The aortic valve opens at *b* and closes at *c*. The mitral valve opens at *d* and closes at *a*. The slope of the *broken line* through *c* represents the end-systolic pressure-volume relationship (E_{max}), and the *broken line* through *d* and *a* represents the end-diastolic pressure-volume relationship. As contractile force develops in the LV in systole, the pressure rapidly increases in the ventricular chamber (*a* → *b*) without changing its volume (i.e., isovolumic phase of systole). When the pressure exceeds the diastolic aortic pressure, the aortic valve opens and the ventricle ejects its contents into the arterial circulation (*b* → *c*, the ejection phase of systole). At the end of ejection (point *c*), LV pressure decreases and the aortic valve closes. Pressure rapidly declines at a constant volume (*c* → *d*, isovolumic relaxation) to levels below that of the left atrium. At this point, the mitral valve opens (point *d*), and the relaxing LV fills along the segment *d* → *a*. The trajectory *a* → *b* → *c* represents the contractile or inotropic function of the LV at any given end-diastolic volume, whereas the trajectory *c* → *d* → *a* represents the lusitropic function (relaxation and filling) of the heart at any given end-systolic pressure. The area within the loop graphically depicts the external work (i.e., stroke work) of the ventricle.

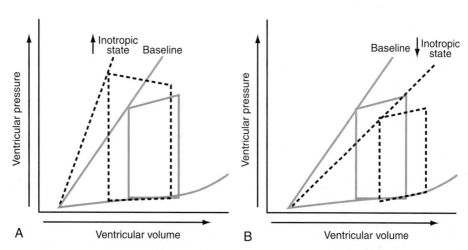

Fig. 7.2 Schematic diagrams illustrating the effects of inotropic interventions on the pressure-volume loop. (A) With a positive inotropic intervention, the pressure-volume loop *(broken line)* is shifted to the left and the slope of the end-systolic pressure-volume line is increased. (B) With a negative inotropic intervention, the pressure-volume loop is shifted to the right and the slope of the end-systolic pressure-volume line is decreased.

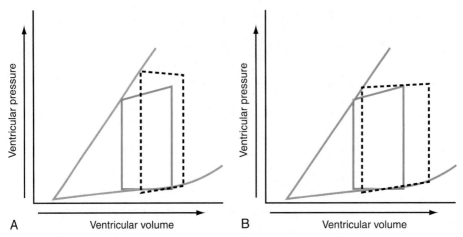

A   Ventricular volume   B   Ventricular volume

Fig. 7.3 Schematic diagrams illustrating the effects of changing loading conditions on the pressure-volume loop in the intact heart. (**A**) An increase in afterload shifts the pressure-volume loop *(broken line)* to the right, increasing the end-systolic and end-diastolic volumes and the end-systolic and end-diastolic pressures while decreasing the stroke volume. The slope of the end-systolic pressure-volume line is usually not affected by a pure change in afterload. (**B**) An increase in preload also shifts the pressure-volume loop *(broken line)* to the right, increasing the end-diastolic volume and end-diastolic pressure. The increase in preload may be associated further with a small increase in end-systolic volume and a modest increase in end-systolic pressure; in contrast to the case with an increase in afterload; however, the stroke volume increases. Similar to an increase in afterload, the slope of the end-systolic pressure-volume line is not affected by a change in preload.

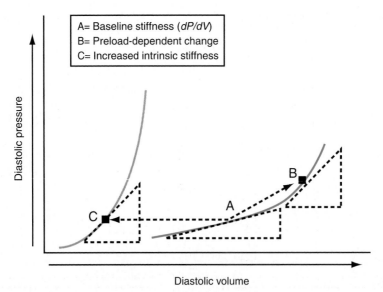

Fig. 7.4 Schematic diagram of the diastolic left ventricular pressure-volume curve. The slope of the tangent (dP/dV) to this curvilinear relationship defines chamber stiffness at a given filling pressure. An increase in dP/dV owing to an increase in volume, shown diagrammatically as $A \rightarrow B$, has been termed a preload-dependent change in stiffness. When the pressure-volume relationship shifts to the left, $A \rightarrow C$, the tangent is steeper (increased chamber stiffness) at the same diastolic pressure.

- An increase in dP/dV owing to an increase in volume, shown in Fig. 7.4 (A → B), has been called a "preload-dependent change in stiffness."
- When the pressure-volume relationship shifts to the left (A → C), the tangent is steeper at the same diastolic pressure.
- The latter may be caused by an increase in myocardial mass or intrinsic myocardial stiffness or by changes in several extramyocardial factors.
- Chamber stiffness of the LV is determined by static factors (e.g., chamber volume, wall mass, stiffness of the wall) and dynamic factors (e.g., pericardium, RV, myocardial relaxation, erectile effects of the coronary vasculature).
- Most acute alterations in LV chamber stiffness result from a preload-dependent increase in chamber stiffness, a shift to a different PV curve, or a combination of the two.
- All can result in elevated left atrial pressure, pulmonary venous hypertension, and the signs and symptoms of ADHF.

MECHANISTIC CONSIDERATIONS IN ADHF SYNDROMES

- During the early phase of myocardial infarction or with acute ischemia, reduced ventricular ejection increases ESV (residual volume) and, together with reduced LV compliance, leads to rapid increases in LV filling pressures.
- It is thought that lusitropic dysfunction associated with ischemia is the result of an increase in stiffness in the ischemic myocardial segment (possibly caused by slowing and incompleteness of the relaxation process) and dilation of the nonischemic segment, causing a preload-dependent increase in chamber stiffness.
- The increase in LV filling pressure that occurs with acute infarction or ischemia is caused by the combination of a preload-dependent increase in chamber stiffness and a leftward shift of the diastolic PV curve.
- Increased diastolic pressures after an acute ischemic insult may also result from the redistribution of blood from the periphery to the central blood pool.
- The effects of these changes on the PV relationship are shown in Figure 7.5A.
- In acute volume overload, as seen in patients with sudden and severe valvular regurgitation or after ischemic ventricular septal rupture, the LV dilates, causing the ventricle to operate on the steeper portion of the pressure-volume curve.
- Consequently, small increments in volume result in a marked increase in filling pressures.
- The effects of these changes on the PV relationship are shown in Figure 7.5B.
- The lusitropic abnormalities of LV hypertrophy secondary to aortic stenosis, severe hypertension, or hypertrophic cardiomyopathy are caused by abnormalities of the static and dynamic determinants of chamber stiffness.
- Increased passive stiffness of the hypertrophied heart results in part from the increased myocardial mass and the low volume-to-mass ratio; abnormal intrinsic myocardial stiffness also may contribute to increased chamber stiffness.
- Abnormalities of myocardial relaxation further impair filling in the hypertrophied heart.
- The effects of these changes on the pressure-volume relationship are shown in Figure 7.5C.
- Chronic HF is characterized by a compressed PV.
- This compressed loop, characterized by a decrease in ESP and an increase in end diastolic pressure (EDP), means that the work of the failing heart is reduced while maintaining a near-normal SV.
- Comparable to the changes with ischemia, the elevated filling pressures in HF are caused by a combination of a preload-dependent increase in chamber stiffness (i.e., the LV operates at higher end-diastolic volumes to optimize the Starling relationship) and a preload-independent increase in chamber stiffness (see Fig. 7.5D).

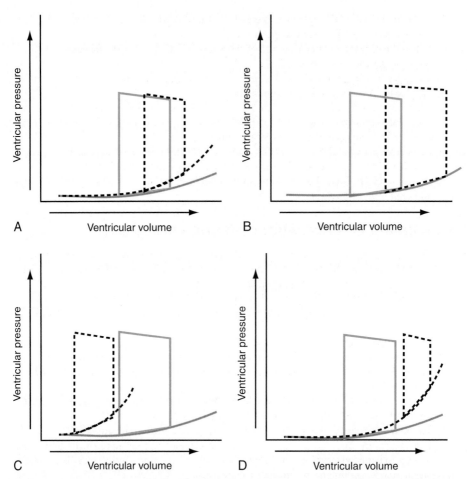

Fig. 7.5 Schematic diagrams of four different pathophysiologic states. In each diagram, the control pressure-volume loop and the diastolic pressure-volume relationship *(curve)* are shown in *solid lines*. The effects of different pathologic states on the pressure-volume relationship are depicted by the *broken lines* (**A**). With acute ischemia or infarction, the pressure-volume curve is shifted upward and to the right. (**B**) In a volume-overloaded heart (i.e., valvular regurgitation), the pressure-volume relationship is shifted to the right along the same diastolic pressure-volume curve. The increase in diastolic pressure is the result of the left ventricle operating on the steeper portion of the diastolic pressure-volume relationship. (**C**) With excessive hypertrophy, the pressure-volume relationship is shifted to the left, so that the heart operates at smaller end-diastolic and end-systolic volumes. The increase in chamber stiffness is reflected by the steep diastolic pressure-volume curve. (**D**) In chronic advanced heart failure, the pressure-volume loop is often compressed and shifted to the right. This compressed loop, characterized by a lower end-systolic and an increased end-diastolic pressure, implies that the work of the heart is reduced, while maintaining a near-normal stroke volume. Comparable to the situation in (**A**), the elevated diastolic pressure is caused by preload-dependent and preload-independent increases in chamber stiffness.

Investigations

- The diagnosis of ADHF is generally straightforward, especially when a patient presents with the triad of fluid retention, exertional dyspnea, and a history of HF.
- However, worsening exertional dyspnea could also be owing to a range of other conditions, including pulmonary embolism, pneumonia, chronic obstructive pulmonary disease, asthma, pleural effusion, anemia or hyperthyroidism.

- The diagnosis of ADHF should be based primarily on signs and symptoms and supported by appropriate investigations, such as electrocardiogram, chest radiograph, cardiac biomarkers, and echocardiography according to the American Heart Association/American College of Cardiology and European Society of Cardiology Guidelines.
- The electrocardiogram is rarely normal in ADHF.
- The chest radiograph can be helpful for the diagnosis of acute HF (Fig. 7.6), but up to 20% of patients with ADHF may have normal chest radiographs.
- When the diagnosis, of ADHF, is uncertain, determination of plasma B-type natriuretic peptide (BNP) or N-terminal pro-B-type natriuretic peptide (NT-proBNP) concentration should be considered, but interpreted in the context of all available clinical data.
  - Because many conditions increase natriuretic peptide levels, low values of BNP (<100 pg/mL) or NT-proBNP (<300 pg/mL) are most useful because the diagnosis of ADHF is very unlikely.

EVALUATION AND TRIAGE OF PATIENTS WITH ADHF

- Several steps are necessary for a comprehensive evaluation of a patient with ADHF.

Step 1: Define Clinical Severity of ADHF

- Several grading classifications of the severity of ADHF have been in place for many years; the Killip classification, based on clinical signs and chest radiography findings, and the Forrester classification, based on clinical signs and hemodynamic characteristics, are discussed elsewhere.
- Other authors have proposed a classification based on an assessment of adequacy of perfusion (warm or cold) and of fluid volume status (wet or dry).
  - Patients can be classified as warm and dry, warm and wet, cold and dry, and cold and wet (Fig. 7.7).
- A pragmatic approach is simply to define the severity of ADHF based on oxygen requirements and BP.
- The most critical patient is the patient with the lowest BP and highest oxygen requirement.

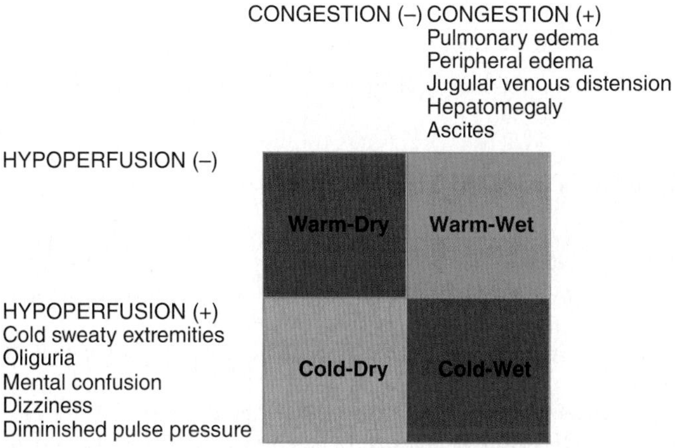

Fig. 7.6 Clinical phenotype based on the presence of congestion and/or hypoperfusion in acute heart failure.

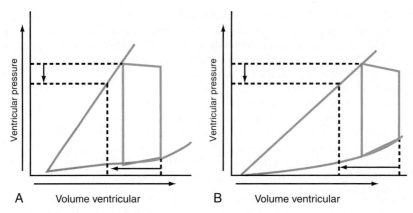

Fig. 7.7 Schematic diagram of the left ventricular wall stress-volume relationship. The loop has the same configuration as the pressure-volume relationship. (**A**) With mild heart failure, a decrease in wall stress *(arrows)* results in an increase in stroke volume. (**B**) With more advanced heart failure, a similar decrease in wall stress is accompanied by a marked increase in stroke volume. Vasodilator therapy (i.e., afterload reduction) produces a larger increase in stroke volume in advanced heart failure than in mild heart failure.

- A subset of patients with decompensated end-stage HF present to the emergency department in occult shock and may be clinically indistinguishable from patients with mildly decompensated HF and stable HF.
- The only parameter differentiating patients with occult shock from those who are non-shock is a significantly elevated lactic acid level.

Step 2: Establish Etiology of ADHF

- The most common causes of ADHF are listed in Table 7.2.

Step 3: Identify Precipitating Causes of ADHF

- Patients with HF are susceptible to infections, which often manifest atypically in patients with ADHF.
- Identifying the precipitating causes of acute hemodynamic decompensation has obvious therapeutic implications.
- Table 7.3 lists common precipitating causes.

Step 4: Decide on Disposition of Patient

- Patients with severe respiratory failure and patients in shock should be admitted to the cardiac intensive care unit.

ONGOING EVALUATION OF THE PATIENT

- Generally, the following parameters should be measured in all critically ill patients with ADHF: mental status, BP, temperature, respiratory rate, heart rate, and urine output.
- Some laboratory tests should be done repeatedly (i.e., electrolytes, creatinine, and glucose, or markers for infection or other metabolic disorders).
- Liver function tests and lactate levels should be measured when there is evidence of hypoperfusion.
- Routine arterial blood gas analysis is generally not needed.
- Patients with ADHF should be carefully monitored to ensure that the treatment goals (summarized in Table 7.4) are met, and continued progress is made toward a stable state.

TABLE 7.3 ▓ **Precipitants of Heart Failure**

Dietary indiscretion
Vigorous fluid administration
Noncompliance to medical regimen
Worsening renal failure
Uncontrolled hypertension
Anemia
Systemic infection
Pulmonary embolism
Myocardial ischemia
Tachyarrhythmias and bradyarrhythmias
Electrolyte disturbances
Severe emotional or physical stress
Hyperthyroidism and hypothyroidism
Cardiodepressant and other drugs
Antiarrhythmic drugs
Calcium channel blockers
β-Adrenergic blocking agents

Pulmonary Artery Catheter (see chapter 23)

- The routine use of pulmonary artery catheters in patients with ADHF is unnecessary and unlikely to lead to a better outcome.
- However, they may be of utility in select patients, such as those with cardiogenic shock, rapidly decompensating HF, heart transplantation candidates, obese patients who are difficult to assess and monitor, and patients with severe LV and RV dysfunction.

Management

- The management of patients with ADHF is primarily aimed at restoring perfusion of vital organs and relieving congestion.

GENERAL MEASURES

- Bed rest should be enforced, usually in the semiupright position, with legs dependent.

Oxygenation

- When there is hypoxia (PaO_2 <60 mm Hg or SpO_2 <90%) without hypercapnia, oxygen-enriched inspired gas may suffice via nasal prongs, Venturi masks, or reservoir bag masks, depending on the severity of gas exchange abnormality.
- Noninvasive ventilation by either continuous positive airway pressure breathing or bilevel positive airway pressure may become necessary when oxygenation cannot be maintained or there is evidence of progressive hypercapnia.
- Failing these interventions, intubation and mechanical ventilation may be needed to improve oxygenation and reverse hypercapnia.

TABLE 7.4 ▦ **Treatment Goals for Acute Heart Failure Syndromes**

Acute Heart Failure Syndrome	Systolic Blood Pressure	First-Line Treatment	Second-Line Treatment	Third-Line Treatment
Hypertensive	>140 mm Hg	Oxygen CPAP if needed IV loop diuretic IV nitroglycerin	Increase doses of nitroglycerin or diuretic or both	Intravenous nitroprusside
Normotensive	100–140 mm Hg	Oxygen CPAP if needed Loop diuretic Vasodilators	Increase doses of nitroglycerin or diuretic or both Add thiazide diuretic	Milrinone when there is evidence of prerenal azotemia
Preshock	85–100 mm Hg	Oxygen CPAP Vasodilator and diuretics	Dobutamine or milrinone	Add norepinephrine
Cardiogenic shock	<85 mm Hg	Oxygen CPAP Volume-loading Norepinephrine	Norepinephrine Vasopressin	Mechanical support IABP Consider LVAD

CPAP, Continuous positive airway pressure; *IABP*, intraaortic balloon pump; *IV*, intravenous; *LVAD*, left ventricular assist device.

Deep Venous Thrombosis Prophylaxis

- Patients with ADHF who are bedridden or with limited physical mobility are at high risk for developing deep venous thrombosis.
- Routine prophylactic treatment should be given unless there are contraindications to such therapy.

Diabetes

- Hyperglycemia occurs commonly in patients with ADHF owing to impaired metabolic control.
- Routine hypoglycemic drugs should be discontinued, glycemic control using short-acting insulin titrated to response, and intensive insulin therapy should be avoided.

MEDICATIONS

- The use of opiates in ADHF should largely be avoided.
- If morphine is used, the patient should be monitored for respiratory depression, which can be reversed by naloxone.

TREATMENT OF TRIGGERS OF DECOMPENSATION

Acute Coronary Syndrome

- The coexistence of an acute coronary syndrome and ADHF identifies a very high-risk group in which early revascularization is recommended.

Rapid Arrhythmias and Severe Bradycardia

- Unstable rhythm disturbances should be treated promptly with either cardioversion or temporary pacing.

Acute Mechanical Instability

- Patients usually require circulatory support with surgical or percutaneous interventions following acute and sudden valvular regurgitation, free wall or septal wall rupture, or fulminant myocarditis.

HEMODYNAMIC GOALS OF TREATMENT

- Reduction of LV preload is intended to shift central blood volume to the periphery, reducing LV diastolic volume and pressure.
- When ADHF is associated with an expanded circulating volume, substantial preload reduction can be achieved without a significant decline in arterial pressure.
- In the setting of hypertension and normovolemia, aggressive reduction in preload may lead to hypotension.
- It is important to decide in advance whether a patient who presents with ADHF is likely to be at increased risk of developing hypotension with reductions in LV preload.
- Ventricular afterload is increased in most patients with HF; the detrimental effects of afterload excess are proportional to the degree of LVSD.
- Afterload reduction with vasodilator therapy is directed at reducing excessive LV wall stress, with a resultant increase in SV and a decrease in EDP.
- A reduction in afterload provides the greatest hemodynamic benefit for patients with the most advanced HF; a far greater increase in SV and decrease in EDP are achieved with similar reductions in wall stress in patients with severe LVSD compared with patients with milder forms of HF (Fig. 7.8).
- A simple treatment algorithm for the management of ADHF according to the different hemodynamic phenotypes is outlined in Fig. 7.9.

SPECIFIC INTERVENTIONS

Vasodilators

- Reasonable hemodynamic endpoints include a reduction in LV filling pressure to 15 mm Hg or less and an increase in CO that would ensure adequate tissue oxygen delivery (usually a cardiac index >2.5 L/min/m^2) while maintaining a systemic BP of 90 mm Hg or greater.

Nitroglycerin

Actions

- Nitroglycerin causes vasodilation by stimulating guanylate cyclase within the vascular smooth muscle of arterial resistance and venous capacitance vessels.
- At lower doses, nitroglycerin acts principally on the peripheral veins and reduces RV and LV filling pressures.
- At higher doses, nitroglycerin causes modest arterial vasodilation; consequently, it may improve CO.

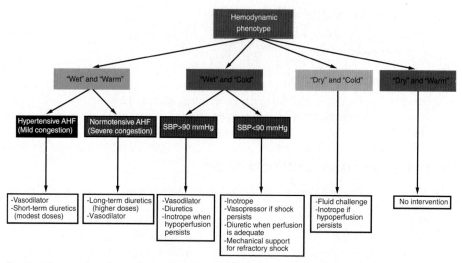

Fig. 7.8 Management of acute heart failure based on the clinical phenotype. (Modified from Ponikowski P, Voors AA, Anker SD, et al. 2016. ESC Guidelines for the diagnosis and treatment of acute and chronic heart failure: The Task Force for the diagnosis and treatment of acute and chronic heart failure of the European Society of Cardiology (ESC). Developed with the special contribution of the Heart Failure Association (HFA) of the ESC. Eur J Heart Fail. 2016;18:891–975.)

Use in ADHF

- Randomized trials in ADHF have shown that titration to the highest hemodynamically tolerable dose of nitrates with low-dose furosemide is superior to high-dose diuretic treatment alone.
- Nitroglycerin is effective in relieving the symptoms of acute pulmonary edema and is often the vasodilatory agent of choice in patients with underlying coronary artery disease.
- The intravenous route generally is preferred, the initial infusion rate is 5 μg/min, and may be increased to 200 μg/min to achieve the desired effects.
- The dose of nitroglycerin should not be increased when the systolic arterial pressure is less than 90 mm Hg. From a practical perspective, a reduction of 10 mm Hg in mean arterial pressure should be achieved.

Nitroprusside

Actions

- Nitroprusside infusion improves ventricular performance by decreasing all the major components of LV afterload.
- Proper dose selection achieves a reduction in afterload and preload with little change in systemic BP.
- Vasodilators that are associated with a decrease in LV filling pressures invariably unload the right heart.

Use in ADHF

- Nitroprusside is the vasodilator of choice when a substantial reduction in LV afterload is required.

- Because of the magnitude of arterial vasodilation achieved with nitroprusside, it has the greatest potential to produce hypotension which may lead to more neurohormonal activation and rebound hemodynamic effects after abrupt withdrawal.
- Nitroprusside is most beneficial for patients who are hypertensive or patients with an elevated LV filling pressure ($\geq$20 mm Hg) and a systemic arterial pressure of 100 mm Hg or greater.
- This clinical picture is commonly encountered in patients with a large MI, with ADHF, with acute valvular regurgitation, or after cardiopulmonary bypass.
- The use of nitroprusside in those with low-output, advanced HF (cold and wet) has been demonstrated to be safe when titrated for a mean arterial pressure of 65 to 70 mm Hg benefiting both hemodynamic measurements and possibly also mortality.
- The initial dose of 5 to 10 μg/min is gradually increased as needed (up to 300 μg/min) to attain the desired clinical and hemodynamic effects.

DECONGESTIVE THERAPY

- Persistent congestion remains at discharge in more than a quarter of patients and recognition and avoidance is important because residual congestion at discharge is associated with increased rehospitalization and mortality.

Diuretics

Actions

- Loop diuretics block the Na^+/$2Cl^-$/K^+ transporter, resulting in increased urine volume by enhancing the excretion of water, sodium chloride, and other ions.
- This, in turn, leads to a decrease in plasma and extracellular fluid volume, total body water, and sodium, resulting in a reduction in ventricular filling pressures and also congestion.
- In patients with ADHF, the diuretic dose-response curve shifts downward and to the right to the extent that higher doses are required to achieve a therapeutic effect.
- Intravenous administration of loop diuretics also exerts a vasodilating effect, manifested by an early (5 to 30 minutes) decrease in right atrial and pulmonary wedge pressure and pulmonary resistances.
- It is thought that vasodilation rather than diuresis is the principal early mechanism by which diuretics alleviate symptoms of pulmonary edema.
- High bolus doses (>1 mg/kg of furosemide) of diuretics may lead to reflex vasoconstriction.
- In severe ADHF, the use of diuretics improves loading conditions and may reduce neurohormonal activation in the short term.

Use in ADHF

- Intravenous loop diuretics are initiated without delay and titrated according to the diuretic response and relief of congestive symptoms.
- The diuretic doses for patients with mild congestion and new-onset ADHF are generally much lower than doses for patients with advanced fluid overload or patients with renal dysfunction.
- The doses of diuretics in ADHF are summarized in Table 7.5.

Diuretic resistance

- This is defined as the clinical state in which diuretic response is diminished or lost before the goal of treatment has been achieved and is associated with a poor prognosis.
- Mechanisms underlying include the "braking phenomenon," "rebound" effect, and hyperaldosteronism.

- The braking phenomenon occurs when long-term diuretic use results in a reduced natriuretic response caused, in part, by nephron adaptations that lead to avid sodium reabsorption at more distal sites.
- The rebound effect involves postdiuretic sodium retention, typically in the setting of inadequate dosing frequency and insufficient sodium restriction.
- To overcome inadequate response to diuretics, it is important to adhere to the following principles (see Table 7.5).

Worsening renal failure (WRF)

- Decongestive therapy with diuretics is complicated by WRF (defined as an increase in serum creatinine of ≥ 0.3 mg/dL during hospitalization) in one-third of HF admissions and is associated with an increased length of stay, readmission rate, and mortality.
- However, recent data have suggested that transient WRF during ADHF therapy may not negatively effect outcomes after discharge.
- The differential diagnosis of WRF should include the possibility of inadequate decongestion and progressive cardiorenal syndrome.
- These two ends of the volume spectrum are distinguishable by history and physical examination.

Vasopressin Antagonists

- Elevations of arginine vasopressin (AVP) in ADHF promote water retention, with resultant congestive symptoms and hyponatremia.
- AVP antagonists have been developed to block the action of AVP at the V2 receptor in renal tubules to promote aquaresis.

TABLE 7.5   Diuretic Dosing

Clinical Scenario	Diuretic	Dose
Moderate fluid overload	Furosemide	20–40 mg IV q12h[a]
	Bumetanide	0.5–1 mg IV q12h[a]
Severe fluid overload	Furosemide	40–80 mg IV q12h[b,c] or
		Bolus of 60 mg IV + continuous infusion at 10–20 mg/h
	Bumetanide	1–2 mg IV q12h[b] or bolus of 2 mg IV + continuous infusion at 0.25–0.5 mg/h
Severe fluid overload *and* renal dysfunction (GFR <30 mL/min)	Furosemide	80–200 mg IV q12h or bolus + continuous infusion at 20–40 mg/h
Diuretic resistance	Add hydrochlorothiazide or metolazone	25 mg or 50 mg 5 mg or 10 mg 30 min prior to loop diuretic

Adapted from Ponikowski P, et al. 2016 ESC guidelines for the diagnosis and treatment of acute and chronic heart failure: the Task Force for the Diagnosis and Treatment of Acute and Chronic Heart Failure of the European Society of Cardiology (ESC) developed with the special contribution of the Heart Failure Association (HFA) of the ESC. *Eur Heart J.* 2016;37(27):2129–2200.
The IV loop diuretic dose should be equal to or double the outpatient oral dose for patients with decompensated chronic HF.
[a]Double dose if goal not attained.
[b]If goal not attained, add a thiazide (see diuretic resistance).
[c]Lower dose if systolic blood pressure <100 mm Hg.
GFR, Glomerular filtration rate; *HF*, heart failure; *IV*, intravenous.

- Currently, two vasopressin antagonists are available for clinical use: conivaptan and tolvaptan.
- It may be reasonable to consider a vasopressin antagonist to treat symptomatic hypervolemic or normovolemic hyponatremia in patients with HF.

Ultrafiltration

- Conventional ultrafiltration (UF) requires central venous access and the typical volume removed per session is 3 to 4 L, accompanied by decreases in right atrial and pulmonary venous pressures.
- In the Ultrafiltration versus Intravenous Diuretics for Patients Hospitalized for Acute Decompensated Congestive Heart Failure (UNLOAD) trial, the weight loss was more sustained than with furosemide treatment.
- However, the enthusiasm has waned after the results of the Cardiorenal Rescue Study in Acute Decompensated Heart Failure (CARRESS-HF) trial, which demonstrated that a stepped pharmacologic therapy algorithm was superior to a strategy of UF for the preservation of renal function at 96 hours, with a similar amount of weight loss.
  - UF was associated with a higher rate of adverse events.
- Recent guidelines indicate that in patients for whom diuretic strategies have been unsuccessful or with severe renal dysfunction and/or refractory fluid retention, UF may be necessary.

CIRCULATORY SUPPORT

Inotropic Agents (see Chapter 17)

- These agents are indicated in the presence of hypotension and end-organ hypoperfusion with or without congestion refractory to diuretics and vasodilators at optimal doses.
- Because their use is potentially harmful because they increase oxygen demand and calcium loading, they should be used with caution.
- More recent data do not support the routine intravenous use of these agents as an adjunct to standard therapy in the treatment of patients hospitalized for ADHF.
- The choice of agent depends on the predominant hemodynamic abnormality.
- Inotropes are not indicated in patients with preserved systolic function.

Dopamine

Actions

- Physiologically, dopamine is the precursor of norepinephrine and releases norepinephrine from the stores of the nerve endings in the heart.
- Dopamine specifically increases renal blood flow by activating postjunctional dopaminergic receptors, observed at doses of 1 to 2 µg/kg/min and peaks at a dose of 7.5 µg/min.
- Because the inotropic effects of dopamine result primarily from its indirect effects, its use in advanced HF is limited by the neurotransmitter depletion present in the failing heart.

Use in ADHF

- Infusion with dopamine should be started at doses of 2 to 5 µg/kg/min and should not be increased beyond 5 µg/kg/min in patients with BPs of 100 mm Hg or greater.
- This agent may be deleterious in patients with ADHF because it may augment the LV afterload, pulmonary artery pressure, and pulmonary resistance.
- The addition of low-dose dopamine to diuretic therapy was not found to enhance decongestion or improve renal function.

- In patients markedly hypotensive with peripheral hypoperfusion, large doses of dopamine can be used to support systemic BP.
- Recent data, however, showed no significant difference in the rate of death between patients with shock who were treated with either dopamine or norepinephrine as the first-line vasopressor agent.

Dobutamine

Actions

- Dobutamine is a β-adrenergic agonist that stimulates β_1-adrenergic, β_2-adrenergic, and α_1-adrenergic receptors.
- Cardiac contractility is increased by virtue of its β_1 and α_1 effects, but because the α_1-adrenergic effects are generally counterbalanced by the β_2 actions, there is generally little change in BP.
- Dobutamine markedly increases C,O but produces only modest changes in LV filling pressures and virtually no increase in BP.
- Heart rate generally increases only when doses greater than 10 µg/kg/min are used.
- Compared with dobutamine, dopamine is a better vasoconstrictor and milrinone is a better vasodilator.

Use in ADHF

- The usual dose of dobutamine is 2.5 to 20 µg/kg/min.
- Short-term infusions are often extremely effective in the treatment of unstable ADHF, especially when systolic pressures are preserved.
- Long-term infusion should be avoided because of the development of hemodynamic tolerance.
- Dobutamine is likely to increase myocardial oxygen consumption and can cause serious arrhythmias.
- There are no controlled trials on dobutamine in patients with ADHF.

Milrinone

Actions

- Milrinone is a type III phosphodiesterase inhibitor that produces dose-dependent increases in CO and decreases in LV filling pressures as a result of the interaction of its positive inotropic, positive lusitropic, and peripheral vasodilator actions.
- The net result is a hemodynamic profile similar to that of the combination of nitroprusside and dobutamine.
- However, myocardial ischemia has been provoked by these agents, and marked hypotensive episodes have been observed.

Use in ADHF

- Milrinone requires a loading dose of 25 to 75 µg/kg over 10 minutes followed by a maintenance infusion of 0.375 to 0.75 ng/kg/min.
- The dose should be adjusted in patients with decreased renal clearance.
- The data regarding the effects of milrinone administration on the outcome of patients with ADHF are insufficient but raise concerns about safety.
- The routine administration of milrinone in ADHF is to be discouraged owing to its adverse effects on heart failure, arrhythmias, and BP.

Vasopressors

- Norepinephrine is an endogenous α_1-adrenergic vasoconstrictor and a β_1-adrenergic agonist that is stored in the sympathetic nerve terminal.
- This agonist is now more commonly used as the preferred vasopressor over dopamine to support patients with ADHF with refractory hypotension.

MECHANICAL SUPPORT

- The only mechanical modality evaluated by a randomized trial is the use of an intraaortic balloon pump to treat cardiogenic shock caused by MI.
- However, the IABP-Shock-II trial showed that this intervention did not reduce mortality among patients with an acute MI who were destined for percutaneous coronary intervention.
- Several other percutaneous and surgical LV and RV assist devices are now available at many hospitals to stabilize patients as either a bridge to recovery or bridge to decision.
- These advanced interventions are discussed in detail in chapters 24 and 25.
- The chest radiograph can be helpful for the diagnosis of acute HF (Fig. 7.6), but up to 20% of patients with ADHF may have normal chest radiographs.

CHAPTER 8

Acute Fulminant Myocarditis

Common Misconceptions

- Myocarditis is a rare cause of acute nonischemic cardiomyopathy.
- Corticosteroids are of benefit in mild to moderately severe acute myocarditis.
- All patients with eosinophilic myocarditis will have a peripheral eosinophilia.

Clinical Presentation

- Myocarditis is defined as inflammation of the myocardium owing to infection, ischemia, or trauma.
- Approximately 2.5 million cases of myocarditis and cardiomyopathy were diagnosed globally in 2015.
- Most cases of acute myocarditis present with chest pain or mild left ventricular systolic dysfunction
- Fulminant myocarditis (FM), a specific form of myocarditis requiring circulatory support to maintain tissue perfusion, accounts for less than 10% of cases.

ETIOLOGY

- Most commonly, FM is caused by a viral infection.
  - Enteroviruses were previously the most common cause, but more recently parvovirus B19 has superseded them.
    - In 2020, the SARS-CoV-2 (COVID-19) virus, causing a pandemic affecting much of the world, has been cited in numerous case reports as causing FM.
- Giant cell and necrotizing eosinophilic myocarditis are also rapidly fatal forms of myocarditis.
- Immune checkpoint inhibitors, used in numerous cancers, have recently been recognized as a cause of myocarditis.

Pathophysiology

- Pathogens, such as viruses, cause direct cytotoxicity to the myocardium, whereas cytokines released during the immune response, such as tumor necrosis factor α (TNF-α), lead to further myocyte death.
- T effector cells and proinflammatory macrophages contribute to myocardial depression.
- Within weeks, the regulatory immune elements increase and downregulate the acute response.
- The hypothesis that a robust immune response can clear viral infection at the price of short-term myocardial depression followed within weeks by recovery is supported by clinical data from those patients with FM who can frequently be bridged to recovery with mechanical circulatory support (MCS).

Investigations

LABORATORY TESTS

- Myocarditis should be suspected in all cases of acute nonischemic cardiomyopathy (Table 8.1).
- Cardiac troponins and creatine kinase levels are elevated in many cases of acute myocarditis, and the current American Heart Association (AHA) scientific statement and European

TABLE 8.1 ▪ Etiologies of Myocarditis

Infectious Myocarditis	
Bacterial	*Staphylococcus*, *Streptococcus*, *Pneumococcus*, *Meningococcus*, *Gonococcus*, *Salmonella*, *Corynebacterium diphtheriae*, *Haemophilus influenzae*, *Mycobacterium* (tuberculosis), *Mycoplasma pneumoniae*, *Brucella*
Spirochaetal	*Borrelia* (Lyme disease), *Leptospira* (Weil disease)
Fungal	*Aspergillus*, *Actinomyces*, *Blastomyces*, *Candida*, *Coccidioides*, *Cryptococcus*, *Histoplasma*, *Mucormycoses*, *Nocardia*, *Sporothrix*
Protozoal	*Trypanosoma cruzi*, *Toxoplasma gondii*, *Entamoeba*, *Leishmania*
Parasitic	*Trichinella spiralis*, *Echinococcus granulosus*, *Taenia solium*
Rickettsial	*Coxiella burnetii* (Q fever), *R. rickettsii* (Rocky Mountain spotted fever), *R. tsutsugamushi*
Viral	RNA viruses: coxsackieviruses A and B, echoviruses, polioviruses, influenza A and B viruses, respiratory syncytial virus, mumps virus, measles virus, rubella virus, hepatitis C virus, dengue virus, yellow fever virus, Chikungunya virus, Junin virus, Lassa fever virus, rabies virus, human immunodeficiency virus–1
	DNA viruses: adenoviruses, parvovirus B19, cytomegalovirus, human herpes virus–6, Epstein-Barr virus, varicella-zoster virus, herpes simplex virus, variola virus, vaccinia virus
Immune-Mediated Myocarditis	
Allergens	Tetanus toxoid, vaccines, serum sickness
	Drugs: penicillin, cefaclor, colchicine, furosemide, isoniazid, lidocaine, tetracycline, sulfonamides, phenytoin, phenylbutazone, methyldopa, thiazide diuretics, amitriptyline
Alloantigens	Heart transplant rejection
Autoantigens	Infection-negative lymphocytic, infection-negative giant cell
	Associated with autoimmune or immune-oriented disorders: systemic lupus erythematosus, rheumatoid arthritis, Churg-Strauss syndrome, Kawasaki disease, inflammatory bowel disease, scleroderma, polymyositis, myasthenia gravis, insulin-dependent diabetes mellitus, thyrotoxicosis, sarcoidosis, Wegener granulomatosis, rheumatic heart disease (rheumatic fever)
Toxic Myocarditis	
Drugs	Amphetamines, anthracyclines, cocaine, cyclophosphamide, ethanol, fluorouracil, lithium, catecholamines, hemetine, interleukin-2, trastuzumab, clozapine
Heavy metals	Copper, iron, lead (rare, more commonly cause intramyocyte accumulation)
Miscellaneous	Scorpion sting, snake, and spider bites; bee and wasp stings; carbon monoxide; inhalants; phosphorus, arsenic, sodium azide
Hormones	Pheochromocytoma, vitamins: beri-beri
Physical agents	Radiation, electric shock

From Caforio AL, Pankuweit S, Arbustini E, et al. Current state of knowledge on aetiology, diagnosis, management, and therapy of myocarditis: a position statement of the European Society of Cardiology Working Group on Myocardial and Pericardial Diseases. *Eur Heart J.* 2013;34:2636–2648.

Society of Cardiology (ESC) position statements recommend that such biomarkers be measured.

■ Natriuretic peptides and soluble ST2 can be useful to assess heart failure (HF) in patients with myocarditis.

ELECTROCARDIOGRAPHIC FINDINGS

■ The current AHA scientific statement and ESC position statements recommend an electrocardiogram be obtained because diffuse concave ST-T segment elevations without reciprocal changes are suggestive of myocarditis.

■ Conduction disturbances with left ventricular systolic dysfunction should raise suspicion for Lyme disease, cardiac sarcoidosis, or giant cell myocarditis.

ECHOCARDIOGRAPHY

■ Echocardiography is useful to exclude other causes of HF and to define cardiac function.

■ Myocarditis may present with dilated, hypertrophic, or restrictive cardiomyopathy.

■ A thicker left ventricle with diminished systolic function is more typical of FM.

INDICATIONS FOR ENDOMYOCARDIAL BIOPSY (EMB)

■ EMB should be performed in patients with new onset of unexplained cardiomyopathy with:
  ■ HF requiring inotropic or MCS
  ■ Mobitz type 2 second-degree or higher heart block
  ■ Sustained or symptomatic ventricular tachycardia
  ■ Failure to respond to medical management within 1 to 2 weeks.

■ If these are absent, further diagnostic evaluation may be pursued with magnetic resonance imaging.

MAGNETIC RESONANCE IMAGING

■ The AHA scientific statement asserts that in patients with suspected myocarditis, MRI may be useful.

■ If patients also meet criteria for EMB, cardiac MRI prior to biopsy may help target specific areas of the myocardium.

■ Non–contrast-enhanced T2-weighted sequences and early post-gadolinium T1-weighted sequences have been used separately and in combination to diagnose myocarditis.

■ An international consensus group for cardiovascular MRI in myocarditis has established the Lake Louise criteria to define the diagnosis of myocarditis on MRI.

■ Delayed gadolinium enhancement can evolve from a focal to a diffuse pattern (Fig. 8.1) and resolve over 2 to 4 weeks.

Management

■ FM should be managed in accordance with the current guidelines for systolic HF, as outlined by the AHA/American College of Cardiology (ACC) and the ESC.

■ Patients with FM require hemodynamic support or MCS, so early transfer to a tertiary care center with expertise in heart transplantation and destination MCS is essential.

■ Intravenous amiodarone has been shown to be effective for the management of ventricular arrhythmias.

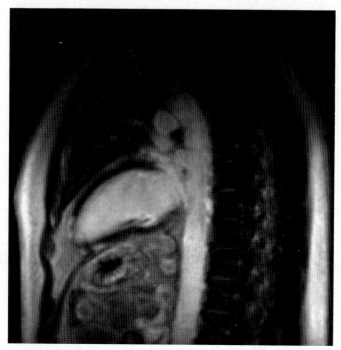

Fig. 8.1 T1-weighted magnetic resonance imaging of patient with myocarditis. Apical and inferior late gadolinium enhancement are consistent with myocarditis (1.5 T scan). (Courtesy Robert Manka, MD, University Hospital Zurich.)

- Digoxin is contraindicated, as the risk for atrioventricular block is increased.
- Temporary pacing may be required if complete atrioventricular block develops.
- Some patients may require a Lifevest during the acute phase if ventricular tachyarrhythmias persist, but implantable cardioverter defibrillator therapy should be deferred, because there is a significant rate of LV recovery.
- In myocarditis related to systemic autoimmune disease, treatment is based on the underlying disorder and often includes immunosuppression.
- Treatment of mild to moderately severe acute myocarditis with immunosuppression with prednisone and either azathioprine or cyclosporine is no more effective than placebo.
- Two randomized trials in chronic idiopathic inflammatory cardiomyopathy showed favorable results with prednisone alone or with azathioprine or cyclosporine.
- Nonsteroidal antiinflammatory drugs should be avoided because of the risk of increased inflammation and mortality in experimental models.
- Interferon, high-dose immunoglobulin, and immunoadsorption are currently not recommended.
- Giant cell myocarditis can deteriorate rapidly into cardiogenic shock and multiorgan failure, with a rate of death or cardiac transplantation of 89% and the recurrence rate is 20% to 25% in the allograft.
- Eosinophilic myocarditis can be a manifestation of hypersensitivity to certain medications, such as sumatriptans, which responds well to high-dose steroid therapy and guideline-directed medical management.

- A lack of evidence, other than that for guideline-directed medical management, has been highlighted in a recent meta-summary case review for coronavirus-induced myocarditis.
- The clinical trajectory of myocarditis is variable.
  - Approximately 50% of patients improve within 2 to 4 weeks
  - 25% develop persistent cardiac dysfunction
  - 12% to 25% potentially will require a transplant or long-term MCS.
  - The average rate of survival after cardiac transplantation is similar to other types of cardiomyopathy.
- Competitive sport participation should be avoided for a minimum of 3 months after diagnosis.

CHAPTER 9

Stress (Takotsubo) Cardiomyopathy

Common Misconceptions

- The presence of bystander coronary artery disease invalidates a diagnosis of stress cardiomyopathy.
- Stress cardiomyopathy affects both sexes equally.
- Uniformly a preceding trigger leads to stress cardiomyopathy.

Presentation

- Stress cardiomyopathy (SCM) is a generally reversible acute cardiac syndrome that was originally described in the Japanese population over 30 years ago.
  - Hence, the term *takotsubo* (an octopus trap with a narrow neck and round bottom) cardiomyopathy (Fig. 9.1).
  - SCM is also known as apical ballooning syndrome (ABS) and broken heart syndrome.
- The clinical features mimic acute coronary syndrome (ACS).
- The typical patient is a postmenopausal woman with symptoms of myocardial ischemia following a stressful event, with positive cardiac biomarkers and/or an electrocardiogram (ECG) demonstrating ischemia.
- SCM is the final diagnosis in approximately 1% to 2% of all patients initially suspected of ACS, and in up to 12% in women with ST elevation myocardial infarction (STEMI) and in 8% of patients with cardiogenic shock.
- Approximately 90% of all cases are in postmenopausal women.
- Patients who are conscious typically have symptoms that are similar to those associated with MI, with angina-like chest pain, present in approximately 50% of cases; less common symptoms include dyspnea, syncope, or loss of consciousness from cardiac arrest.
- Typically, the ejection fraction is reduced to 30% to 40%, which may be accompanied by significant diastolic dysfunction and elevated left ventricular end-diastolic pressure (LVEDP).
- Acute heart failure is a frequent complication, and cardiogenic shock may develop in approximately 10% to 15% of patients.
- Atrial fibrillation occurs in 5% of cases, whereas ventricular tachyarrhythmias have been reported in 3% to 4% of patients and asystole in 0.5%.
- Rare complications include LV thrombus, thromboembolism, and cardiac rupture.
- Hypotension may be owing to the reduction in stroke volume and, in some cases, dynamic left ventricular outflow tract obstruction (LVOTO).
- The ventricular dysfunction usually resolves over days to weeks, with complete recovery by 4 to 8 weeks.
- The prognosis of SCM is good in the absence of significant underlying comorbid conditions.
- In-hospital mortality is approximately 3% to 5%.
- The subgroup of patients in whom there is a physical trigger—such as major surgery, malignancy, and fractures—appears to have a worse prognosis.
- The recurrence rate is approximately 1% to 2% per year.

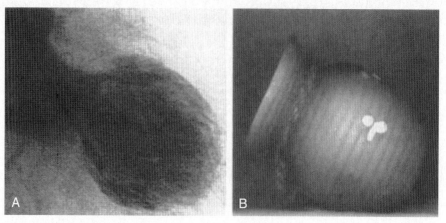

Fig. 9.1 **(A)** Ventriculogram. **(B)** An octopus pot ("takotsubo"). (Courtesy #FOAMed Medical Education Resources, LITFL.)

Pathophysiology

- A preceding stressful trigger is present in over two-thirds of patients, but the precise pathophysiology of SCM remains to be established.
- Clinical observations suggest that the sympathetic nervous system plays an important role.
    - These include the temporal relationship with emotional or physical stress, hyperadrenergic states, such as pheochromocytoma and subarachnoid hemorrhage causing a cardiomyopathy similar to SCM, with high levels of catecholamines.
- Microvascular dysfunction can be detected in at least two-thirds of the patients and its severity correlates with the troponin elevation and ECG abnormalities.

Investigations

- The characteristic features of the syndrome have been incorporated into several proposed diagnostic criteria.
- Table 9.1 lists the Mayo Clinic criteria that can be applied at the time of presentation.
    - All four criteria must be present.

ELECTROCARDIOGRAM

- Between 30% and 50% of patients have ST segment elevation at presentation, but ECG findings do not reliably distinguish SCM from ACS.
- Q waves, T-wave inversion, or nonspecific T-wave abnormality may be present or the ECG may be normal.
- Characteristic evolutionary changes during hospitalization include resolution of ST segment elevation and diffuse deep T-wave inversion associated with QT prolongation (Fig. 9.2).

CARDIAC BIOMARKERS

- Troponin levels are invariably elevated on admission and peak within 24 to 48 hours.
- Troponin levels are lower than with STEMI but similar to non-STEMI.
- Blood level of natriuretic peptides are elevated in the majority of patients and may correlate with LVEDP.

TABLE 9.1 ■ Proposed Mayo Clinic Criteria for Apical Ballooning Syndrome

1. Transient hypokinesis, akinesis, or dyskinesis of the left ventricular mid-segments with or without apical involvement. The regional wall motion abnormalities extend beyond a single epicardial vascular distribution. A stressful trigger is often present, but not always.[a]
2. Absence of obstructive coronary disease or angiographic evidence of acute plaque rupture.[b]
3. New electrocardiographic abnormalities (either ST segment elevation and/or T-wave inversion) or modest elevation in cardiac troponin.
4. Absence of pheochromocytoma, myocarditis.

From Prasad A, Lerman A, Rihal CS. Apical ballooning syndrome (takotsubo or stress cardiomyopathy): a mimic of acute myocardial infarction. *Am Heart J.* 2008;155:408–417.

[a] There are rare exceptions to these criteria, such as those patients in whom the regional wall motion abnormality is limited to a single coronary territory.

[b] It is possible that a patient with obstructive coronary atherosclerosis may also develop apical ballooning syndrome (ABS). However, this is very rare in our experience and in the published literature, perhaps because such cases are misdiagnosed as an acute coronary syndrome. syndrome.

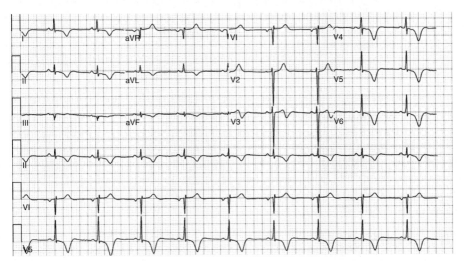

Fig. 9.2 Twelve-lead electrocardiogram with T-wave inversion in the precordial and limb leads associated with prolongation of the QT interval.

LEFT VENTRICULAR IMAGING AND CORONARY ANGIOGRAPHY

■ Transthoracic echocardiography demonstrates preservation of left ventricular function, but there is hypokinesis or akinesis of the mid to apical segments leading to the "ballooning" appearance (Fig. 9.3).

   ■ The regional wall motion abnormality (RWMA) extends beyond the distribution of a single coronary artery.

   ■ In a significant proportion of patients, apical contraction is preserved and the wall motion abnormality is restricted to the mid segments (apical-sparing variant).

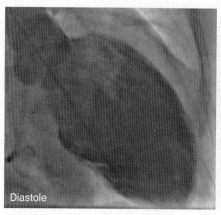 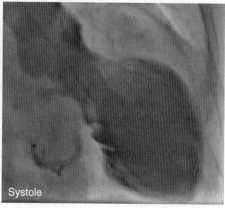

Fig. 9.3 Left ventriculogram in diastole and systole of a patient with stress cardiomyopathy with hyperdynamic basal contraction and akinesis of the mid- and apical segments.

- ◾ The least common variant is inverted or reverse takotsubo with hypokinesis of the basal segment of the LV but preserved apical function.
- ◾ The variant forms of SCM have similar clinical characteristics and prognosis as the typical form.
- ◾ The right ventricle also develops a similar pattern of RWMA in approximately one-third of cases.
- ◾ Cardiac magnetic resonance may be a useful imaging modality for documenting the extent of RMWA and differentiating SCM (absence of late gadolinium enhancement) from myocarditis and MI with late gadolinium enhancement.
- ◾ Coronary angiography should be performed in order to exclude an ACS, but patients with SCM either have angiographically normal coronary arteries or mild atherosclerosis.
  - ◾ When present, obstructive plaque is generally insufficient to account for the widespread RWMA.

Management

- ◾ The recommendations for SCM management are based on expert opinion, as clinical trials have not been conducted owing, in part, to the low incidence and the fact that supportive therapy leads to spontaneous recovery in the great majority of patients.
- ◾ The initial therapy is frequently directed toward treating myocardial ischemia with aspirin, anticoagulants, statins, and β-blockers because ACS is usually the working diagnosis.
- ◾ Aspirin, anticoagulants, and statins can be discontinued once the diagnosis of SCM has been made unless coexisting coronary atherosclerosis is documented.
- ◾ In the absence of contraindications, a β-blocker should be initiated because excess catecholamines have been implicated in the pathogenesis.
- ◾ Initiation of angiotensin-converting enzyme inhibitor or angiotensin receptor blocker therapy for acute LV dysfunction is recommended.
- ◾ Mild to moderate acute heart failure responds to diuretic therapy, but severe cases with pulmonary edema may require intubation and mechanical ventilation.
- ◾ If present, LVOTO may be treated with phenylephrine with the goal of increasing afterload and left ventricular cavity size.

- Inotropes are often used with good effect in cardiogenic shock, although there are theoretic reasons for avoiding them because of the potential role of catecholamine toxicity in precipitating the syndrome.
  - Intraaortic balloon pump counterpulsation or other mechanical support devices may be preferable in the absence of LVOTO.
- Although torsade de pointes is rare, patients should be on continuous ECG monitoring until the QTc is less than or equal to 500 msec.
  - If pause-dependent torsade de pointes occurs, β-blocker therapy should be withheld and temporary pacing considered.
- Implantable cardioverter-defibrillator therapy is not routinely indicated for ventricular tachycardia or fibrillation because the cardiomyopathy is reversible.

Cardiorenal Syndrome Type 1

Definition and Classification

- Combined disorders of the heart and kidney are referred to as cardiorenal syndromes (CRS); they are defined as a complex pathophysiologic disorder of the heart and the kidneys whereby acute or chronic dysfunction in one organ may induce acute or chronic dysfunction in the other organ.
- The CRSs are classified into five subtypes based on the primary organ that is dysfunctional (Table 10.1).
- The temporal sequence of the organ dysfunction and which problem predominates can also be used to distinguish types 1 or 2 (cardiac first) from types 3 or 4 (renal first).
- In the Cardiac Intensive Care Unit (CICU) environment, the most commonly encountered CRS is type 1.
- CRS type 1 is characterized by an acute deterioration in cardiac function that then leads to a reduction in glomerular filtration rate (GFR) and acute kidney injury (AKI).
- The most common precipitants of acute cardiac dysfunction in the CICU that result in AKI are cardiogenic shock, acute decompensated heart failure (ADHF), acute myocardial infarction (MI), acute mitral or aortic regurgitation, pericardial tamponade, constrictive pericarditis, or prolonged arrhythmias with associated hypotension or cardiogenic shock.
- There are four patterns of CRS type 1: (1) *de novo* cardiac injury leading to *de novo* kidney injury; (2) *de novo* cardiac injury leading to acute-on-chronic kidney injury; (3) acute on chronic cardiac decompensation leading to *de novo* kidney injury; and (4) acute-on-chronic cardiac decompensation leading to acute-on-chronic kidney injury.

Prevalence

- CRS type 1 has been found in 27% to 45% of hospitalized patients with ADHF and in 9% to 54% of patients with acute coronary syndromes.
- Of patients with preexisting chronic kidney disease who present with ADHF, approximately 60% will develop AKI.

TABLE 10.1 ■ **Classification of the Cardiorenal Syndromes**

Class	Type	Description	Examples
1	Acute cardiorenal syndrome	Acute worsening of cardiac function resulting in AKI	ADHF Cardiac surgery Acute coronary syndromes CIN
2	Chronic cardiorenal syndrome	Chronic abnormalities of cardiac function leading to CKD	Hypertension CHF
3	Acute renocardiac syndrome	Abrupt worsening of renal function leading to acute cardiac dysfunction	Acute pulmonary edema in AKI Arrhythmia owing to acidosis or electrolyte abnormalities or volume overload CIN leading to CHF
4	Chronic renocardiac syndrome	CKD leading to chronic cardiac dysfunction	Left ventricular hypertrophy in CKD
5	Secondary cardiorenal syndrome	Systemic disorders causing cardiac and renal dysfunction	Sepsis Systemic lupus erythematosus Diabetes

ADHF, Acute decompensated heart failure; *AKI*, acute kidney injury; *CHF*, congestive heart failure; *CIN*, contrast-induced nephropathy; *CKD*, chronic kidney disease.
Modified from Cruz DN. Cardiorenal syndrome in critical care: the acute cardiorenal and renocardiac syndromes. *Adv Chronic Kidney Dis*. 2013;20:56–66.

Prognosis

- The development of CRS type 1 is associated with worse clinical outcomes, more rehospitalizations, and greater health care expenditures.
- The mortality risk associated with CRS type 1 is most pronounced early, but an increased risk of death has been observed 10 years after the index hospitalization for acute MI in patients who develop AKI.

Risk Factors

- Nonmodifiable risk factors include a history of diabetes, prior admissions for ADHF or MI, and more severe cardiac dysfunction at the time of presentation (pulmonary edema, tachyarrhythmias, worse Killip class, or lower ejection fraction).
- Impaired kidney function on admission has consistently been associated with higher risk for CRS type 1.
- Modifiable risk factors include high doses of diuretics (e.g., daily furosemide dose > 100 mg/day or in-hospital use of thiazides) and/or vasodilator therapy as well as higher contrast volumes during imaging studies, cardiac catheterization, and coronary intervention.

Diagnosis

- The diagnosis of CRS type 1 is made retrospectively after treatment to improve cardiac performance results in improvement in renal function.

Pathophysiology

- ADHF may reduce GFR by several mechanisms, including neurohumoral adaptations, reduced renal perfusion, increased renal venous pressure, and right ventricular dysfunction (Fig. 10.1).
- In addition, exposure to nephrotoxins may precipitate CRS type 1.
- The pathophysiology of CRS type 1 may vary at different time points during a single hospitalization.
- Early in a CICU admission, AKI may be related to a low cardiac output state and/or a marked increase in central venous pressure.
- There are multiple iatrogenic causes of CRS type 1 (Fig. 10.2).

Prevention

- CRS type 1 is a result of the interaction between complex pathogenic factors; once it becomes clinically apparent, it is difficult to abort and is often irreversible.
- Prevention of CRS is paramount in clinical practice, with an aim to identify and avoid precipitating factors, as well as to use measures to maintain optimal functioning of the heart and kidneys.

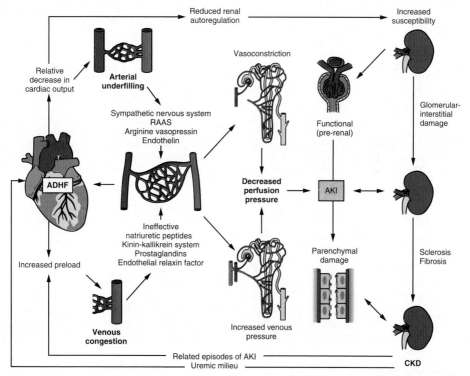

Fig. 10.1 Pathogenesis of CRS type 1. Acute decompensated heart failure (ADHF) via arterial underfilling and venous congestion sets off a series of changes in neurohormonal and hemodynamic factors that culminate in acute kidney injury (AKI). *CKD*, Chronic kidney disease; *CRS*, cardiorenal syndrome; *RAAS*, renin-angiotensin-aldosterone system. (Modified from Ronco C, Cicoira M, McCullough PA. Cardiorenal syndrome type 1. Pathophysiological crosstalk leading to combined heart and kidney dysfunction in the setting of acute decompensated heart failure. J Am Coll Cardiol. 2012;60:1031–1042.)

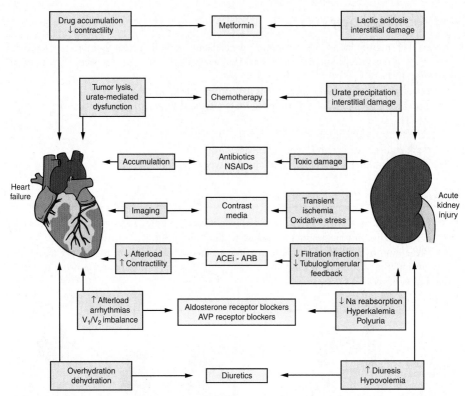

Fig. 10.2 Iatrogenic causes of CRS type 1. Multiple sources of iatrogenic injury, some of which may be unavoidable, can result in either cardiac, renal, or cardiorenal impairment and kidney damage in patients with acutely decompensated heart failure (ADHF). ACEi, Angiotensin-converting enzyme inhibitor; ARB, angiotensin receptor blocker; AVP, arginine vasopressin; NSAIDs, nonsteroidal anti-inflammatory drugs. (Modified from Ronco C, Cicoira M, McCullough PA. Cardiorenal syndrome type 1. Pathophysiological crosstalk leading to combined heart and kidney dysfunction in the setting of acute decompensated heart failure. J Am Coll Cardiol. 2012;60:1031–1042.)

- There are no guideline recommendations for the management of CRS type 1.
- The multitude of pathophysiologic interactions and their complexity render the management of CRS challenging.
- Improving the natural history of heart failure and avoiding acute decompensation are the cornerstones of prevention of CRS type 1.
- Another mainstay of prevention is to recognize patients at risk for CRS.
- Patients at risk for CRS type 1 have a narrow window for blood pressure and volume status. Extremes in either parameter can result in worse renal function (Fig. 10.3).
- Renoprotective measures can then be selectively instituted in those patients at high risk to reduce the risk of acute CRS (Table 10.2).

Management

- No medical therapies directly increase the GFR (manifested clinically by a decline in serum creatinine) in patients with heart failure.
- On the other hand, improving cardiac function can result in increases in GFR, indicating that CRS type 1 has substantial reversible components.

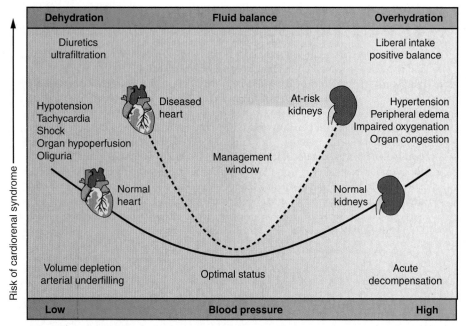

Fig. 10.3 Volume and blood pressure management window. Patients at risk for cardiorenal syndrome type 1 have a narrow window for management of both blood pressure and volume; extremes in either parameter can be associated with worsened renal function. (Modified from Ronco C, Cicoira M, McCullough PA. Cardiorenal syndrome type 1. Pathophysiological crosstalk leading to combined heart and kidney dysfunction in the setting of acute decompensated heart failure. *J Am Coll Cardiol.* 2012;60:1031–1042.)

TABLE 10.2 ■ **Renoprotective Strategies in the Cardiac Intensive Care Unit**

■ Regular monitoring of fluid intake/output, urine output, renal function, blood pressure
■ Accurate and frequent monitoring of volume status
■ Hold ACE inhibitors/ARBs in patients with worsening renal function
■ Optimize volume status
■ Adjust diuretic doses based on volume status
■ Pharmacovigilance (drug monitoring, avoid nephrotoxins, attention to drug interactions)
■ Initial use of vasodilators (nitrates, hydralazine) in ADHF if blood pressure is adequate
■ Avoid unnecessary use of iodinated contrast agents
■ Optimize volume status before use of iodinated contrast agents
■ Minimize volume of iodinated contrast agents

ACE, Angiotensin-converting enzyme; *ADHF*, acute decompensated heart failure; *ARBs*, angiotensin receptor blockers.
Modified from Cruz DN. Cardiorenal syndrome in critical care: the acute cardiorenal and renocardiac syndromes. *Adv Chronic Kidney Dis*. 2013;20:56–66.

■ AKI induced by primary cardiac dysfunction implies inadequate renal perfusion until proven otherwise.
■ Inadequate perfusion may be a consequence of a low cardiac output state, increased central venous pressure leading to renal congestion, or both.
■ A careful history and physical examination can usually differentiate a volume-depleted patient from one who is severely volume overloaded.

- Diuretics, typically beginning with a loop diuretic, are first-line therapy for managing volume overload in patients with ADHF as manifested by peripheral and/or pulmonary edema.
- The goal of diuretic therapy is to eliminate fluid retention even if this leads to asymptomatic mild to moderate reductions in blood pressure or renal function.
- The optimal diuretic regimen has not been determined in randomized, controlled trials. Continuous intravenous infusion of diuretics traditionally has been considered more effective than bolus in severe ADHF.
- The role of inotropes in patients with CRS is uncertain and the routine use of inotropes is not recommended, given their lack of proven efficacy and their association with adverse events when used in patients other than those with cardiogenic shock or ADHF.
- Ultrafiltration is an alternative to loop diuretics for the management of fluid overload in patients with ADHF and worsening kidney function.
- Although ultrafiltration may be helpful for fluid removal in ADHF in patients unresponsive to diuretic therapy, the available evidence does not establish ultrafiltration as first-line therapy for ADHF or as an effective therapy for CRS type 1.

CHAPTER 11

Sudden Cardiac Death

Common Misconceptions

- Survival following in-hospital cardiac arrest is significantly better than out-of-hospital cardiac arrest.
- In aortic stenosis, the risk of sudden cardiac death is eliminated following aortic valve replacement.
- In patients post-myocardial infarction (MI) with severe left ventricular dysfunction, an implantable cardioverter defibrillator (ICD) must be placed prior to discharge to reduce early mortality.

Presentation

- Cardiovascular disease accounts for approximately 1 of every 2.9 deaths in the United States and approximately 17 million deaths worldwide each year.
- More than 50% occur suddenly, making sudden cardiac death (SCD) one of the most common causes of death.
- SCD is defined as the sudden cessation of cardiac activity with hemodynamic collapse within 1 hour of the onset of symptoms in the absence of an extracardiac cause, whereas sudden cardiac arrest (SCA) is used to describe a nonfatal event.
- Estimates of the incidence of SCD vary widely, ranging from 180,000 to 450,000 annually.
- Owing to the rarity of autopsies, the true incidence and mechanism of out-of-hospital cardiac arrests (OHCA) is difficult to establish.
- In monitored victims, ventricular fibrillation (VF) or ventricular tachycardia (VT) is the most common initial rhythm (75% to 80%).
- With advances in the treatment of coronary artery disease (CAD) and an increase in implantable cardioverter defibrillators, VT/VF now accounts for less than 30% of the initial rhythms.
- Pulseless electrical activity (PEA) is increasingly identified as the initial rhythm (25% of the time) owing to patients being older, sicker, and with more acute triggers for PEA (i.e., metabolic, respiratory) and less able to sustain VT/VF until emergency medical services arrival.
- The initial rhythm correlates with the duration of the event as VF is seen early and degenerates to asystole over time (Fig. 11.1).
- Recent advances in cardiopulmonary resuscitation (CPR) and postresuscitation care have improved survival rates, from 5.7% in 2005 to 8.3% in 2012.
- Survival rates are higher for individuals in whom VF is the initial rhythm, with 30% surviving to hospital discharge.
- Nonshockable rhythms have been associated with poor long-term survival rates (8% for PEA).

6:02 A.M.

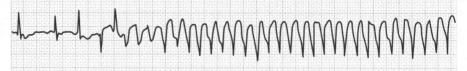

6:05

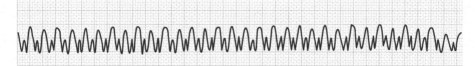

6:07

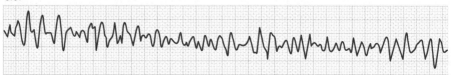

6:11

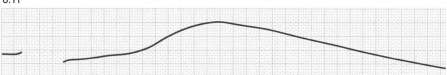

Fig. 11.1 Fortuitous Holter recording from a patient who experienced sudden cardiac death outside the hospital documents the usual and typical sequence of events. The initial rapid ventricular tachycardia continues into the second panel with widening of the QRS, probably owing to myocardial metabolic changes. Subsequent degeneration to ventricular fibrillation is shown in the third panel, followed by asystole in the fourth panel. The prognosis depends on the initial documented rhythm and how soon emergency personnel arrive to treat the individual. (Modified from National Heart, Lung, and Blood Institute. What Is An Implantable Cardioverter Defibrillator? https://www.nhlbi.nih.gov/health/health-topics/topics/icd.)

- The risk of suffering an SCA increases with age, with only 1% occurring in individuals younger than age 35 years.
- The presence of underlying structural heart disease (SHD) results in a 6- to 10-fold increase in the risk of SCA.
- Studies suggest that 21% to 45% of victims of SCD have a normal cardiac postmortem examination.
- Men are two to three times more likely to experience an SCA than women.
- Women who experience a cardiac arrest are more likely to be at home, be older, and present with PEA.
- Women have increased rates of successful resuscitation and survival from shockable rhythms.
- African Americans have been documented to have higher rates of SCD and worse survival from SCA, owing to their increased likelihood of an unwitnessed event or PEA as the initial rhythm.

- The rate of survival to hospital discharge in African-American SCA victims with VT/VF documented as the initial rhythm is 27% lower than in Caucasian patients.
- Possible contributing factors include receiving treatment at hospitals with worse outcomes and a decreased likelihood of receiving bystander CPR.
■ Approximately half of all SCD victims will have usually transient warning symptoms 4 weeks preceding their SCA event.
■ Of the symptoms experienced, 46% complain of chest pain and 20% report dyspnea.

Pathophysiology

■ SCD is the outcome of an interaction between an abnormal cardiac substrate and a transient functional disturbance that triggers the arrhythmia.

Abnormal Cardiac Substrate

■ To predict SCA, it is important to recognize the etiologies that can potentially lead to abrupt cessation of cardiac output.
■ Figure 11.2 shows data derived from various studies demonstrating the predominant pathologic substrates of SCD.
■ The relative risk of SCD is dependent on the underlying substrate and is graphically demonstrated for various populations in Figure 11.3.

CORONARY ARTERY DISEASE

■ CAD is the most common underlying substrate, accounting for 60% to 75% of all cases.
■ The majority (40% to 75%) of SCA events attributed to CAD occur in individuals with evidence of a prior MI.
■ Approximately 15% of SCA victims initially present during a new ST elevation myocardial infarction (STEMI).

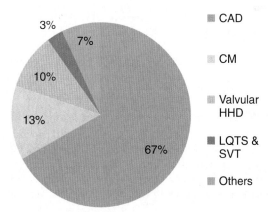

Fig. 11.2 Prevalence of underlying heart disease in adult patients who have experienced sudden cardiac death, based on data derived from several studies. The predominant substrates are coronary artery disease (CAD), cardiomyopathies (CM), valvular and hypertensive heart disease (HHD), and inheritable arrhythmia syndromes. *LQTS,* Long QT syndrome; *SVT,* supraventricular tachycardia. (Modified from Deshpande S, Vora A, Axtell K, Akhtar M. Sudden cardiac death. In Brown DL, editor. Cardiac Intensive Care. Philadelphia: Saunders, 1998, 391–404.)

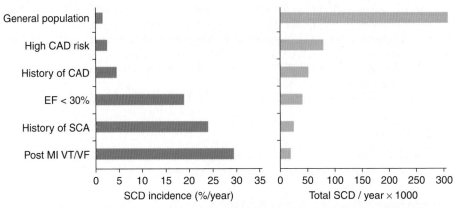

Fig. 11.3 The incidence and number of patients with sudden cardiac death (SCD) in various subgroups of patients. *Left*, SCD incidence percent per year in each subgroup. *Right*, Total number of SCDs per year (*n*×1000). *CAD*, Coronary artery disease; *EF*, ejection fraction; *MI*, myocardial infarction; *SCA*, sudden cardiac arrest; *VT/VF*, ventricular tachycardia/ventricular fibrillation. (Modified from Myerburg RJ, Kessler KM, Castellanos A. Sudden cardiac death: structure, function and time-dependence of risk. Circulation. 1992;85[Suppl I]:I-2–I-10.)

Coronary Artery Anomalies

- Although significant coronary artery anomalies are uncommon (0.21% to 5.79% prevalence), they are the second most common cause of SCD in young adults.
- The anomaly most commonly associated with SCD occurs when an anomalous coronary artery originates from the opposite sinus of Valsalva and traverses between the aorta and pulmonary trunk.
- Such SCD events typically occur during or shortly after vigorous exercise, owing to compression of the coronary artery when the great vessels dilate.

Vasculitis

- During the acute phase of Kawasaki disease, coronary artery aneurysms and ectasia develop in 10% to 25% of patients.
- In later years, shrinkage of the aneurysm, intimal proliferation, and coronary calcification contribute to stenosis, which may result in SCD from cardiac arrhythmia and acute MI.
- Polyarteritis nodosa and syphilitic aortitis can affect the coronary circulation and SCA may be a sequela.

Myocardial Bridging

- Myocardial bridging is a rare (0.5% to 4.5% of the general population) congenital variant in which an epicardial coronary artery traverses through the myocardium during a portion of its course, typically the left anterior descending coronary artery.
- During exertion, a critical degree of systolic compression that extended into diastole on the tunneled segment may occur, resulting in myocardial ischemia and occasionally SCA.

Coronary Artery Spasm

- Coronary artery vasospasm is a sudden narrowing of the coronary artery caused by the contraction of smooth muscle tissue in the vessel wall.
- Coronary artery spasm can occasionally trigger ventricular arrhythmias and SCA.
- Vasospastic angina may also occur as a result of cocaine abuse.

Coronary Artery Dissection

- Spontaneous dissection of the coronary arteries results from separation of the media layer of the artery wall by hemorrhage.
- It is associated with Marfan syndrome, pregnancy, type I aortic dissection, or rupture of a sinus of Valsalva aneurysm, all of which can potentially cause SCA.

MYOCARDIAL DISEASE

Hypertrophic Cardiomyopathy (HCM)

- HCM is the most common cause of SCD in young adults and the second leading cause of SCD overall, with an annual mortality rate ranging from less than 1% in asymptomatic patients to 6% in patients with multiple risk factors.
- Unlike most other heart diseases, the risk of SCA in HCM declines with age.
- HCM is inherited as an autosomal dominant condition.
- Patients with HCM have asymmetric, diffuse left ventricular (LV) hypertrophy without compensatory dilatation of the LV chamber and in the absence of any known cardiac or systemic cause.
- On histologic examination, there is gross disorganization of muscle bundles and myofibrillar architecture, altered gap junctions, increased basal membrane thickness, and interstitial fibrosis.
- Possible mechanisms for SCA include malignant ventricular arrhythmias, syncope from LV outflow tract (LVOT) obstruction, and ischemia, most commonly manifested as VT/VF.

Nonischemic Dilated Cardiomyopathy (NIDCM)

- NIDCM is defined by the presence of LV or biventricular dilatation and impaired systolic function in the absence of any ischemia or abnormal loading conditions.
- Primary causes include familial cardiomyopathies, infections, autoimmune disorders, metabolic conditions, or toxins.
- Genetic mutations are identified in up to 40% of patients, with genes encoding titin (TTN), myosin heavy chain (MYH7), cardiac troponin T (TNNT2), and lamin A/C (LMNA) the most common.
- A distinct form is defined by noncompaction of the ventricular myocardium, caused by the arrest of normal embryogenesis of the endocardium and myocardium.
  - Manifestations include heart failure, embolic events, and arrhythmias.
  - SCD accounted for 50% of deaths in reported series.
- Following a diagnosis of NIDCM there is a 70% survival at 1 year and 50% survival at 2 years, with the majority of deaths being sudden.
- NIDCM is responsible for 10% of all adult SCD cases and can be the initial presentation.

Arrhythmogenic Right Ventricular Cardiomyopathy (ARVC)

- ARVC is an inherited cardiomyopathy with the replacement of right ventricular (RV) myocytes by adipose and fibrous tissue.
- The hallmark on electrocardiogram (ECG) is the presence of epsilon (ε) waves (Fig. 11.4).
- Often, the signal-averaged ECG is markedly abnormal, with late potentials being commonly seen.
- Diagnostic findings on imaging include regional RV akinesia, dyskinesia, or aneurysmal dilatation.

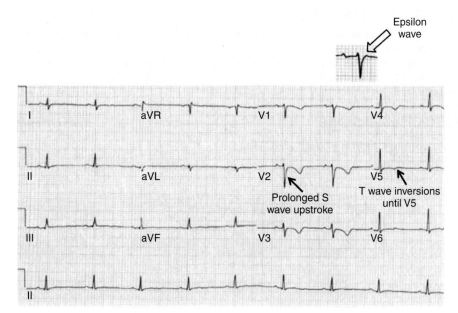

Fig. 11.4 Electrocardiograph morphology of arrhythmogenic right ventricular dysplasia with inverted T waves, ε waves, notched S wave, and widening of QRS (>110 ms) in the right precordial leads (V₁–V₃). (From Nasir K, Bomma C, Tandri H, et al. Electrocardiographic features of arrhythmogenic right ventricular dysplasia/cardiomyopathy according to disease severity: a need to broaden diagnostic criteria. Circulation. 2004;110:1527–1534.)

- Intramyocardial fat, RV wall thinning, and delayed enhancement on cardiac magnetic resonance imaging are complementary findings, but are not diagnostic.
- The estimated prevalence of ARVC is 1 in 2000 to 5000 and it is inherited in an autosomal dominant fashion, although owing to incomplete penetrance the disease occurs in only 30% to 50% of offspring.
- More than 60% of mutations occur in genes encoding desmosomal proteins, which anchor intermediate filaments to the cytoplasmic membrane in adjoining cells in the gap junction.
- Although, patients are generally asymptomatic, unexplained syncope or SCD may be the initial clinical manifestation in up to 50% of cases.

Valvular Heart Disease

- In 1% to 5% of victims of SCD, the cause of death is attributed to valvular heart disease (VHD).
- Rheumatic VHD, in rare cases, can result in SCD owing to arrhythmias, ball valve thrombosis in the left atrium, embolization to the coronary arteries, or acute low output circulatory failure.
- In aortic stenosis (AS), hypertension and low cardiac output with left ventricular hypertrophy (LVH) provoke coronary hypotension and contribute to VT.
- Prior to aortic valve replacement, asymptomatic patients with severe AS have an annual SCD rate of 13%.

- SCD is one of the most common modes of death in patients with AS **even after aortic valve replacement**, attributable to arrhythmias and thromboembolism.
- Although mitral valve prolapse is typically benign, certain characteristics—such as leaflet thickness, redundancy, fibrosis of the papillary muscles and inferobasal wall, and LV dilation—are associated with increased ventricular tachyarrhythmias.
- Although VT is associated with these characteristics, this may not contribute to SCD risk.

Inflammatory and Infiltrative Disorders

- Myocarditis is defined by inflammation of the myocardium that has an infectious origin.
  - Patients are typically asymptomatic, and SCD can be the only presenting sign in up to 12% of adult patients with myocarditis.
  - Initially, direct myocardial injury produces edema, necrosis, and contractile dysfunction.
  - Scarring after the acute myocarditis has resolved may contribute to SCA.
- Noninfectious inflammatory conditions such as collagen vascular diseases, systemic sclerosis, and granulomatous also can cause SCA.
  - Cardiac sarcoidosis is defined by the development of sarcoid granulomas in the heart muscle that can affect the conduction system, causing complete heart block; create granulomatous scar, contributing to the development of macro-reentrant ventricular arrhythmias; or impair myocardial contractility, resulting in heart failure.
    - Compared with other patients with NIDCM, patients with cardiac sarcoidosis appear to receive more frequent appropriate ICD therapies.
- Infiltrative diseases, such as hemochromatosis and amyloidosis, also can increase the risk of SCA.
  - Amyloidosis cardiomyopathy results from the deposition of amyloid protein in the myocardial interstitium, contributing to diffuse myocardial thickening with ventricular systolic and/or diastolic dysfunction.
    - SCD can result from pump failure, ventricular tachyarrhythmias, or thrombus. Prognosis for patients with cardiac amyloidosis and symptomatic heart failure is extremely poor, with a median survival of 4 to 6 months.
    - Finally, appropriate ICD therapies for ventricular arrhythmias are common (27% in one series).

Congenital Heart Disease

- SCD is a major cause of mortality in adults with congenital heart disease (ACHD), affecting 7% to 19% of the population.
- Arrhythmias are the most common cause of SCD in the ACHD population. Factors that were associated with SCD in ACHD include supraventricular tachycardia, moderate to severe dysfunction of the systemic ventricle, and increased QRS duration.
- Congenital aortic stenosis can predispose to SCA.
  - The risk for SCA correlates with the severity of the stenosis.
- Both cyanotic and noncyanotic Eisenmenger syndrome can predispose to SCA.
- Patients who have undergone surgical procedures to correct transposition of the great arteries may be at an increased risk for SCA resulting from bradycardia and tachycardias.
  - Long-standing right ventricular strain, abnormal electrophysiologic architecture secondary to general and physical stress, and sequelae of the surgical corrective procedure all contribute to the increased risk of SCD in patients who have had correction of transposition of their great arteries.
  - The incidence of late SCD is approximately 50%, but has been reduced with the arterial switch operation.

- Up to 5% of patients with surgically repaired tetralogy of Fallot may experience potentially fatal arrhythmias as a late complication.
  - The mechanism for sustained monomorphic VT in patients with ACHD is generally macro-reentrant with a critical isthmus located within an extensively scarred right ventricular outflow tract (RVOT) or ventriculotomy incision.

Wolff-Parkinson-White (WPW) Syndrome

- Although the prevalence of WPW syndrome is 0.1% to 0.3% of the general population, the incidence of sudden death in asymptomatic individuals is as high as 1 per 100 patient years.
- In symptomatic patients, the estimated lifetime risk of SCD is approximately 3% to 4%.
- SCA occurs as a result of atrial fibrillation with a very rapid ventricular response over an accessory pathway with short refractory periods, leading to VF.
- Patients with preexcited R-R intervals of less than or equal to 250 ms during induced atrial fibrillation are at increased risk of SCD.
- Patients with multiple accessory pathways, a family history of WPW syndrome with SCD, and those with concomitant heart disease are at a higher risk for SCA.

Cardiac Conduction System Abnormalities

- Patients with congenital atrioventricular block or nonprogressive intraventricular block have a lower risk for SCA, which is usually noted in young, otherwise healthy individuals without a prior history of arrhythmia.
- Both acquired atrioventricular nodal and His-Purkinje disease, owing to CAD and primary fibrosis, can also uncommonly cause SCA.

INHERITED ARRHYTHMIC DISORDERS

- In individuals younger than age 35 years who suffered SCD, an autopsy fails to demonstrate a cause in 27% to 29% of cases, although this percentage decreases when detailed histologic examination is performed.
- Approximately 50% of such patients will have an inherited arrhythmic syndrome, such as long QT syndrome, short QT syndrome, Brugada syndrome, or catecholaminergic polymorphic VT.
- Table 11.1 describes the known mutation, chromosome locus, mode of inheritance, and effect on the ion channel.

Long QT Syndrome

- Long QT syndrome (LQTS) is an inherited channelopathy, with a prevalence of 1 to 2 per 10,000; it results in delayed myocardial repolarization and prolongation of the QT interval.
- Patients with LQTS are predisposed to torsades de pointes, which may degenerate into VF.
- Clinically, patients with LQTS may present with syncope, aborted cardiac arrest, or SCD, with SCD being the initial and only symptom in 10% to 15%.
- The young are primarily affected, with 50% experiencing their first cardiac event before the age of 12 years.
- Approximately 60% of patients will have a pathogenic mutation identified on genetic testing, but there may be incomplete penetrance and/or variable expressivity and 90% of the mutations are found in three genes: *KCNQ1*, *KCNH2*, and *SCN5A*, causing LQT1, LQT2, and LQT3, respectively, characterized by their ECG appearance (Fig. 11.5) and specific triggers (Fig. 11.6). The remaining pathogenic mutations are rarer (see Table 11.1).
- Exercise should be restricted in all such patients to prevent cardiac events.

TABLE 11.1 ■ Characteristics of Ion Channelopathies

Type	Gene Mutation	Mode of Inheritance	Locus	Effect on Ion Current	Frequency	Arrhythmia Trigger	Syndrome
Long QT							
LQT1	KCNQ1	AD/AR	11p15.5	↓ IKs	30%	Exercise or emotion	Jervell and Lange-Nielsen type I (AR)
LQT2	KCNH2	AD	7q35-q36	↓ IKr	46%	Auditory, emotion, or rest/sleep	
LQT3	SCN5A	AD	3P21	↑ INa	42%	Rest/sleep	
LQT4	ANK2	AD	4q25-q27	↓ Coordination of Ncx, Na/K ATPase	Rare	Exercise	Severe SB and episodes of AF
LQT5	KCNE1	AD/AR	21q22.1-q22.2	↓ IKs	2%–3%		Jervell and Lange-Nielsen type II
LQT6	KCNE2	AD	21q22.1	↓ IKr	Very rare		
LQT7	KCNJ2	AD	17q23.1–24.2	↓ IK1	Rare		Andersen-Tawil
LQT8	CACNA1C	AD	12p13.3	↑ ICa-L	Rare		Timothy
LQT9	CAV3	AD	3p25	↑ INa	Rare		
LQT10	SCN4B	AD	11q23	↑ INa	Rare		
LQT11	AKAP9	AD	7q21-q22	↓ IKs	Very rare		
LQT12	SNTA1	AD	20q11.2	↑ INa	Very rare		
LQT13	KCNJ5	AD	11q24	↓ IK1	Very rare		
Short QT							
SQT1	KCNH2	AD	7q35-q36	↑ IKr			
SQT2	KCNQ1	AD	11p15.5	↑ IKs			
SQT3	KCNJ2	AD	17q23.1–24.2	↑ IK1			
Brugada							
BrS1	SCN5A	AD	3p21	↓ INa	25%–30%		
BrS2	GPD1L	AD	3p24	↓ INa			

TABLE 11.1 ■ Characteristics of Ion Channelopathies—cont'd

Type	Gene Mutation	Mode of Inheritance	Locus	Effect on Ion Current	Frequency	Arrhythmia Trigger	Syndrome
BrS3	CACNA1C	AD	12p13.3	↓ICa-L			
BrS4	CACNB2b	AD	10p12.33	↓ICa-L			
BrS5	SCN1B	AD	19q13.1	↓INa			
BrS6	KCNE3	AD	11q13-q14	↑IKs/Ito			
BrS7	SCN3B	AD	11q23.3	↓INa			
BrS8	KCNJ8	AD	12p11.23	↑Ik-ATP			
BrS9	HCN4	AD	15q24.1	—			
BrS10	RANGRF	AD	17p13.1	↓INa			
BrS11	KCNE5	AD	Xq23	—			
BrS12	KCND3	AD	1p13.2	↑Ito			
BrS13	CACNA2D1	AD	7q21.11	↓ICa			
BrS14	SLMAP	AD	3p14.3	—			
BrS15	TRPM4	AD	19q13.33	—			
BrS16	SCN2B	AD	11p23.3	↓INa			
BrS17	SCN10A	AD	3p22.2	—			
CPVT							
CPVT1	RYR2	AD	1q42.1-q43	↑ SR Ca²⁺ release	60%	Exercise or emotion	
CPVT2	CASQ2	AR	1p13.3-p11	↑ SR Ca²⁺ release	~3%		
CPVT3	KCNJ2	AD	17q23.1-24.2	↓IK1	Rare		
CPVT4	TRDN	AR	6q22-q23	↓ SR Ca²⁺ release	Rare		
CPVT5	CALM1	AD	14q31-q32	↓ SR Ca²⁺ release	Rare		

Characteristics include gene mutation, mode of inheritance, chromosomal location, the effect on the ion current, the frequency of the mutation in patients, triggers for arrhythmia, and the name of the syndrome if present.

AD, Autosomal-dominant; *AF,* atrial fibrillation; *AR,* autosomal recessive; *BrS,* Brugada syndrome; *CPVT,* catecholaminergic polymorphic ventricular tachycardia; *LQT,* long QT; *Ncx,* sodium-calcium exchanger; *SB,* sinus bradycardia; *SQT,* short QT; ↑, gain of function; ↓, loss of function.

- The development of early afterdepolarization-induced triggered activity underlies the substrate and acts as a trigger for the development of life-threatening ventricular arrhythmias.
- Acquired QT prolongation is more commonly encountered than congenital long QT (see Fig. 11.5) and up to one third of patients with acquired long QT carry a mutation for a gene causing congenital long QT.
- Some of the triggers include ischemia, hypokalemia, hypomagnesemia, hypothermia, bulimia/anorexia nervosa, antiarrhythmic agents, antibiotics, psychotropic medications, and methadone.

Short QT Syndrome

- Short QT syndrome (SQTS) is a rare condition inherited as an autosomal-dominant syndrome characterized by a QTc of 330 ms or less in the absence of tachycardia or bradycardia and tall peaked symmetric T waves on ECG (see Fig. 11.5).
- Patients are at increased risk of atrial fibrillation, VF, and SCD.

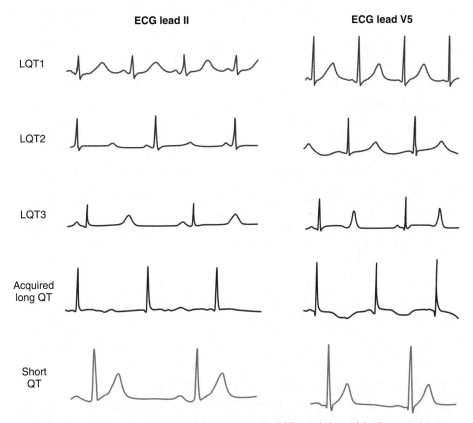

Fig. 11.5 Electrocardiographs (ECGs) demonstrating the typical QT morphology of the three most common long QT syndromes as well as an ECG characteristic of acquired long QT and an ECG characteristic of short QT syndrome. *LQT*, Long QT syndrome. (Modified from Mortada ME, Akhtar M. Sudden cardiac death. In Jeremias A, Brown DL, editors. Cardiac Intensive Care. Philadelphia: Saunders, 1998; and Giustetto C, Di Monte F, Wolpert C, et al. Short QT syndrome: clinical findings and diagnostic-therapeutic implications. Eur Heart J. 2006;27:2440–2447.)

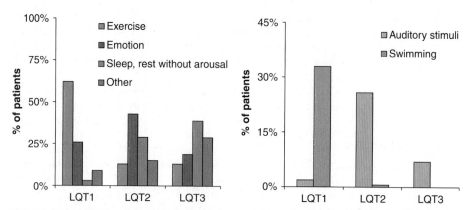

Fig. 11.6 Gene-specific triggers for life-threatening arrhythmias in the three most common long QT (LQT) syndromes. *Left*, Exercise, emotion, sleep, or other triggers. *Right*, Swimming versus auditory stimulus as a trigger for cardiac events in patients with the most common LQT syndromes. (Modified from Schwartz PJ, Priori SG, Spazzolini C, et al. Genotype-phenotype correlation in the long-QT syndrome: gene-specific triggers for life-threatening arrhythmias. Circulation. 2001;103:89–95.)

Brugada Syndrome

- Brugada syndrome (BrS) is a rare condition in which symptomatic patients have syncope or SCA owing to VT or VF.
- The characteristic type 1 Brugada ECG has a coved-type ST segment with at least 2 mm J-point elevation in the right precordial leads (V_1 to V_3), typically followed by negative T waves.
- Arrhythmias typically occur while at rest, during sleep, or after large meals, possibly owing to a high vagal tone.
- Fever is an additional risk factor for inducing a Brugada pattern leading to arrhythmic events and febrile illnesses should be aggressively treated with antipyretics.
- The mean age of patients with BrS and arrhythmic events is 41 years, with a male predominance (70% to 95%).
- A spontaneous type 1 pattern is sufficient for the diagnosis of BrS.
- The type 1 ECG pattern is dynamic; up to 50% of patients with Brugada syndrome may have a transient normalization of the ECG or a saddleback-type ST elevation, that is, a type 2 ECG pattern (Fig. 11.7).
- A causal mutation is identified in up to 35% of patients with BrS, with the most common mutation involving the *SCN5A* gene.

Catecholaminergic Polymorphic Ventricular Tachycardia (CPVT)

- CPVT is a rare inherited disorder (prevalence 1 in 10,000) characterized by physical or emotional stress-induced bidirectional or polymorphic VT.
- Affected individuals usually develop arrhythmic events (syncope, aborted SCA, or SCD) during sympathetic stimulation in the first or second decade of life.
- Two mutations account for the majority of cases; a mutation in the cardiac ryanodine receptor 2 (*RYR2*) results in a gain of function in ryanodine release and is identified in approximately 65% of cases and a loss-of-function mutation in calsequestrin 2 (*CASQ2*).

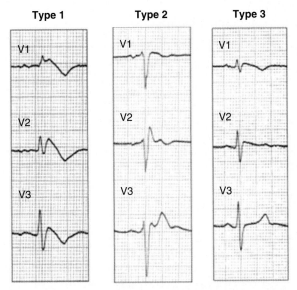

Fig. 11.7 Types of electrocardiographic (ECG) morphology for Brugada syndrome. A spontaneous type I appearance *(left)* with coved-type ST segment elevation in right precordial leads followed by inverted T waves is diagnostic for Brugada syndrome. If the saddleback-type ST elevations as noted in type 2 ECG appearance *(middle)* or type 3 ECG *(right)* appearance is noted in a patient with clinical suspicion of Brugada syndrome, a drug challenge with a sodium channel blocker may be performed to observe for conversion to type 1 ECG pattern. (From Napolitano C, Priori SG. Brugada syndrome. Orphanet J Rare Dis. 2006;1:35.)

FUNCTIONAL MODULATORS

- A fatal arrhythmia is the result of the interaction between the structural abnormality and a functional modulator converting stable abnormalities in electrical conduction to an unstable state.
- Functional modulators, such as ischemia or long QT, can even initiate a fatal arrhythmia without SHD, particularly in the setting of an intense stimulus.

Transient Ischemia

- Ischemia contributes to heterogeneity in the myocardium by preferentially opening the ATP-sensitive K^+ channels in the epicardial cells as opposed to the endocardial cells.
- The resulting refractoriness increases the susceptibility of the myocardium to arrhythmias.

Hemodynamic Deterioration

- In the setting of hemodynamic deterioration, cardiac arrest carries a high short-term mortality rate.
- Hypoxemia can also result in ischemia and alteration of metabolic substrates contributing to SCD.
- Furthermore, a hypoxemic event often precedes a bradycardic and/or asystolic arrest.

Metabolic Disturbances

- Hypokalemia and hyperkalemia have been implicated in SCD.
- Both hypokalemia and hypomagnesemia play a role in the genesis of polymorphic VT.
- Similarly, acidosis has been shown to be a contributing factor to SCD.

Altered Systemic Autonomic Balance

- Structural abnormalities, particularly those resulting in cardiomyopathy and systolic heart failure, affect the neurohormonal milieu generating autonomic disturbances which manifest as a loss of heart rate variability, a marker for risk of SCA.

Drug Toxicity

- Both cardiac (antiarrhythmic) and noncardiac drugs, particularly those resulting in QT prolongation are documented as cause of SCA.
- Recent reports have demonstrated an increased risk of SCA with concomitant use of cocaine and alcohol.

Investigations

Electrocardiogram

- Repolarization abnormalities after cardiac arrest are common, transient, and nonspecific, caused by cardioversion, electrolyte abnormalities, or hypothermia.
- Thus, it is recommended that the ECG be repeated as the patient stabilizes following return of spontaneous circulation (ROSC).

Laboratory Testing

- Immediate laboratory evaluation is aimed at determining the presence of triggering agents (electrolyte abnormalities, ischemia, acidosis, metabolic disturbances) and screening for toxic substances.

Cardiac Catheterization

- A complete cardiac catheterization—including coronary angiography, left and right heart hemodynamics, and left ventriculography—is usually performed early in the evaluation of cases of SCA.
- Patients with a STEMI after ROSC following SCA should also undergo revascularization, as appropriate.
- In the absence of an acute coronary syndrome, coronary angiography is often still performed to exclude CAD.
- Long-term outcomes appear to be improved in individuals who have successful urgent revascularization coronary lesions even if the initial ECG did not demonstrate ST elevation.
- If myocarditis or a cardiomyopathy is suspected, a right ventricular endomyocardial biopsy performed may provide additional diagnostic information.

Echocardiography

- Evaluation of LV function is critical because it is the strongest independent predictor for recurrence and long-term survival following OHCA.
- Because global LV dysfunction from myocardial stunning can be seen following cardiac arrest, evaluation of left ventricular ejection fraction (LVEF) is recommended to be performed at least 48 hours after ROSC.
- Potential etiologies that can be identified include CAD, HCM, ARVC, AS, NIDCM, and cardiac amyloidosis.

Cardiac Magnetic Resonance Imaging (CMR)

- When standard evaluation fails to elucidate a diagnosis, CMR imaging can be useful in the evaluation of possible SHD.
- In HCM, delayed enhancement is a risk factor for SCD and wall thickness may be more accurately quantified, given the limitations of echocardiography.
- Diagnostic features of myocarditis include myocardial edema in T2-weighted images, hyperemia/capillary leak in T1-weighted sequences, and necrosis/fibrosis in delayed enhanced sequences.
- In patients with ARVC, CMR imaging may allow for more accurate assessment of RV dysfunction and evaluation of intramyocardial fat and myocardial fibrosis.

Signal-Averaged Electrocardiography (SAECG)

- Signal-averaged electrocardiography is an excellent negative predictor for SCA in patients with CAD (negative predictive value, 89% to 99%), but is less well defined in patients with nonischemic heart disease, except for ARVC and HCM.
- In ARVC, the presence of late potentials on an SAECG is a minor Task Force criterion for diagnosis.

Exercise Stress Testing

- The provocation of ischemia with exercise is useful because VT/VF provoked during exercise predicts a higher recurrence rate of SCA.
- In patients without SHD, exercise testing can be used in the diagnosis of LQTS or CPVT. In LQTS, evidence of QT prolongation with sympathetic stimulation and increased heart rate is suggestive of LQT1.
- In patients with CPVT, the pathognomonic finding of bidirectional VT may be seen rarely during exercise testing, but provoked polymorphic VT may be suggestive of CPVT.
- Finally, it can also be useful in patients with WPW syndrome, because resolution of the delta wave with increased heart rate correlates with decreased likelihood of preexcited atrial fibrillation.

Pharmacologic Challenge

- In patients with a normal resting ECG, echocardiogram, coronary angiogram, and CMR, a drug challenge can be used to elicit diagnostic ECG changes suggestive of inherited arrhythmia disorders.
- Infusion of epinephrine (0.025 to 0.3 µg/kg/min) is used to induce polymorphic VT suggestive of CPVT.
- Challenge with low-dose epinephrine can also be used to assess for LQTS (specifically, LQT1) owing to the paradoxic increase of the QT interval with increased heart rate and sympathetic stimulation; the negative predictive value of low-dose epinephrine for LQT1 is 96%.
- Procainamide challenge (10 mg/kg IV over 10 minutes) can also be used to induce BrS.

Electrophysiology Study (EPS)

- Electrophysiologic testing is not usually performed in patients with an established etiology for their SCD.
- In patients with specific high-risk conditions (e.g., ischemic cardiomyopathy, NIDCM, BrS, HCM, and ARVC) who are not candidates for an ICD implantation, EPS may be useful.

- The likelihood of inducing a sustained ventricular arrhythmia depends on the underlying heart disease.
- Aggressive stimulation protocols can induce polymorphic VT or VF in some individuals without cardiac disease and, although VF may occasionally be induced, it may be irrelevant.
- However, evidence indicates that inducible VF, particularly when induced repeatedly with nonaggressive protocols, suggests the diagnosis of idiopathic VF and recurrent events.

Genetic Testing

- Performance of genetic testing in survivors or postmortem (a "molecular autopsy") results in identification of an inheritable arrhythmic syndrome in up to 35% of cases of SCD.

Management

- Survivors of SCA are usually cared for in a cardiac intensive care unit (CICU) with continuous rhythm monitoring.
- A significant proportion of these patients succumb to cardiogenic shock, congestive heart failure, respiratory complications, and sepsis, accounting for an in-hospital mortality of up to 60%.
- The most immediate threat after resuscitation is recurrent cardiovascular collapse because myocardial function in the early phase post-ROSC is usually depressed and many patients require transient interventions for hemodynamic stabilization to prevent secondary injury from hypotension.

PHARMACOLOGIC THERAPY

- All post-MI trials and LV dysfunction trials show significant survival benefit associated with the use of a β-blocker.
- In addition, angiotensin-converting enzyme inhibitors, angiotensin-receptor blockers, and HMG-CoA reductase inhibitors are essential in patients after MI to reduce the risk for future acute coronary syndrome and mortality.
- In general, β-blockers are first-line therapy in the management of ventricular arrhythmias in the prevention of SCD.
- Amiodarone has a broad spectrum of antiarrhythmic activity that may inhibit or terminate ventricular arrhythmias, making it useful as an adjunct therapy to an ICD.
  - Although a survival benefit compared with placebo has not been demonstrated for the use of amiodarone in patients with reduced LVEF, it can be used without increasing mortality in patients with heart failure.
- Antiarrhythmic medications, such as sotalol, dofetilide, mexiletine, ranolazine, or quinidine (alone or in combination), may also be useful as an adjunct in reducing the frequency of ventricular arrhythmia.
- In survivors of SCA with normal heart structure, pharmacologic therapy may be helpful in reducing the risk of VT/VF and recurrence of SCA.
  - β-Blockers, calcium channel blockers, sotalol, and flecainide have been used in RVOT tachycardias.
  - The β-blocker sotalol is the drug of choice in ARVC to treat frequent ventricular ectopy or nonsustained VT.
  - However, recent registry data suggest that amiodarone may be superior in preventing ventricular arrhythmias in patients with ARVC.

- In patients with LQTS (and some carriers of a causative LQTS mutation with normal QT interval) β-blockers are the drug of choice to prevent dysrhythmia.
- In patients with LQT3, sodium channel blockers may be considered as add-on therapy to shorten the QT interval to less than 500 ms.
  - In contrast, sodium channel blockers increase the risk of arrhythmia and SCA in BrS.
  - Quinidine is highly effective in reducing the frequency of VF in BrS, especially in VT storm.
    - Quinidine and disopyramide are effective in reducing the frequency of VT/VF in patients with LSQTS type 1.
  - Either disopyramide or β-blockers may be used in patients with HCM.
  - In CPVT, β-blockers, but not calcium channel blockers, are recommended in all patients.
- Correcting the secondary causes of SCA may be accomplished with a pharmacologic approach or with oxygen supplementation (e.g., hypoxia).
- Drug toxicity can be managed by stopping the medication.
- Electrolyte imbalance can be addressed by electrolyte supplementation or dialysis in extreme cases.

MYOCARDIAL REVASCULARIZATION AND ARRHYTHMIA SURGERY

- It is assumed that the prevention or reduction of myocardial ischemia can consequently decrease the incidence of SCA in patients with CAD and myocardial ischemia.
- In addition, myocardial revascularization has been shown to reduce the incidence of SCA in patients who have been successfully resuscitated from a previous episode related to an acute MI.
- Furthermore, early revascularization for survivors of SCA in the setting of STEMI and/or SCA survivors with no evidence of ischemia on ECG but suspicion for acute ischemia has been shown to improve survival and neurologic outcomes.
- Revascularization alone is unlikely to eliminate clinical or inducible monomorphic VT, especially in patients with a fixed anatomic substrate (myocardial scar/ventricular aneurysm).
- Thus, an ICD will be indicated, with the possible need for an EPS-guided excision or ablation.

CATHETER ABLATION

- Catheter ablation is potentially curative for VT and as adjunctive therapy to an ICD. In a minority of patients, the underlying etiology for SCA may be supraventricular in origin (e.g., WPW syndrome) and for WPW, radio-frequency (RF) ablation is safe and successful.
- Patients with bundle branch reentry, idiopathic, or fascicular VT may also have SCA.
- The utility of performing a detailed EPS in an SCA survivor is highlighted by the fact that the majority of idiopathic VTs can be cured by ablation.
- The outcomes for ablation in patients with SHD remain poor, with less than a 50% success rate and excess risk of stroke and death.
- Nonetheless, catheter ablation has an important role in controlling VT and reducing ICD shocks.
- Catheter ablation of scar-related VT involves the identification of potential reentry circuit isthmi and exit sites.
- Substrate ablation has been used in the setting of unmappable VT to create scar homogenization by RF ablation of all sites with abnormal electrograms and has been shown to increase freedom from VT in patients with SHD.

- Most of these sites can be approached endocardially or, if that fails, an epicardial approach may be used.

IMPLANTABLE CARDIOVERTER DEFIBRILLATOR

- The basic premise behind the ICD is that the majority of SCDs result from malignant ventricular tachyarrhythmias.
- Furthermore, survivors of arrhythmic SCA are at increased risk of recurrent VT/VF with rates of recurrent arrhythmia nearing 43% at 5 years.
- Currently, ICD implantation utilizes transvenous lead(s) inserted into the right ventricle heart for both pacing and for defibrillation with a defibrillation vector between an intracavitary right heart coil and the implanted defibrillator located in the pectoral region (Fig. 11.8).
- Periprocedural mortality is less than 1%.
- Long-term studies have demonstrated the efficacy of ICDs over a mean follow up of 8 years and also complications including an approximate 6% rate of infection and 17% rate of lead failure over 12 years.
- The therapeutic options for treatment of ventricular tachyarrhythmias include antitachycardia pacing, low-energy synchronized cardioversion, and high-energy cardioversion/defibrillation.
- A detection algorithm allows differentiation of sinus tachycardia or supraventricular arrhythmias from ventricular tachyarrhythmias to obviate unnecessary delivery of therapy.
- However, inappropriate shocks may still occur in up to 20% of delivered therapies.
- The majority of ICDs are now capable of remote patient monitoring (RPM) as well as wireless RPM.

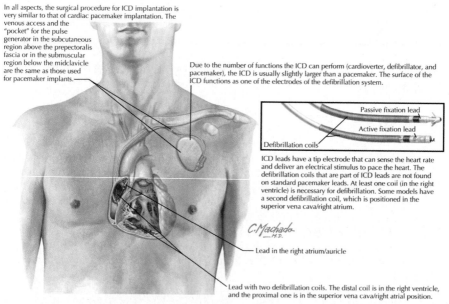

In all aspects, the surgical procedure for ICD implantation is very similar to that of cardiac pacemaker implantation. The venous access and the "pocket" for the pulse generator in the subcutaneous region above the prepectoralis fascia or in the submuscular region below the midclavicle are the same as those used for pacemaker implants.

Due to the number of functions the ICD can perform (cardioverter, defibrillator, and pacemaker), the ICD is usually slightly larger than a pacemaker. The surface of the ICD functions as one of the electrodes of the defibrillation system.

Passive fixation lead

Active fixation lead

Defibrillation coils

ICD leads have a tip electrode that can sense the heart rate and deliver an electrical stimulus to pace the heart. The defibrillation coils that are part of ICD leads are not found on standard pacemaker leads. At least one coil (in the right ventricle) is necessary for defibrillation. Some models have a second defibrillation coil, which is positioned in the superior vena cava/right atrium.

C. Machado
_M.D.

Lead in the right atrium/auricle

Lead with two defibrillation coils. The distal coil is in the right ventricle, and the proximal one is in the superior vena cava/right atrial position.

Fig. 11.8 Implantable Cardiac Defibrillator (Dual-Chamber Leads) From: Gehi AK, Mounsey JP. Chapter 44: Cardiac Pacemakers and Defibrillators. In: Stouffer GA, Runge MS, Patterson C, Rossi JS, eds. *Netter's Cardiology*, 3rd edn. Elsevier; 2019:302-308. Netter illustration used with permission of Elsevier Inc. All rights reserved. www.netterimages.com

- Evidence suggests that RPM is associated with a significantly lower risk of mortality and rehospitalization.
- In addition to the conventional transvenous ICD system, an entirely subcutaneous ICD (SICD) system is now available for patients who do not require bradycardia pacing as shown in Figure 11.9.
  - Advantages include decreased risk for lead-related complications, easier reintervention, lack of systemic dissemination in the case of device infection, and obviating the need for intravascular access.
  - Available data suggest that the SICD is safe and effective at preventing sudden death (with a rate of inappropriate shock of ~11% at 3 years).
- The ICD effectively terminates VT/VF regardless of its mechanism (Fig. 11.10).
- In this regard, it provides unsurpassed protection against arrhythmic SCD because it does not attempt to modulate the structural or functional abnormalities as antiarrhythmic drugs do.

Indications for ICD

- Clinical trials consistently support the implantation of an ICD in all patients surviving an SCA that was not owing to transient or reversible causes.
- A meta-analysis of these trials has demonstrated that ICD therapy is associated with a 50% relative risk reduction in arrhythmic mortality and a 28% relative risk reduction for overall mortality.

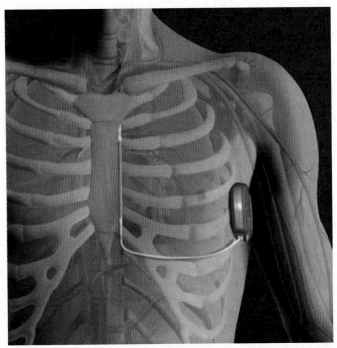

Fig. 11.9 Schematic representation of a current subcutaneous implantable cardioverter defibrillator (S-ICD) and lead system. The electrodes on the lead system are tunneled from the pocket in the midaxillary line to an incision at the xiphoid process and then tunneled to the superior incision along the left sternal border. This lead is connected to a pulse generator overlying the serratus muscle in the vicinity of the fifth to sixth intercostal spaces along the midaxillary line. (From Hauser RG. The subcutaneous implantable cardioverter-defibrillator—should patients want one? J Am Coll Cardiol. 2013;61[1]:20–22.)

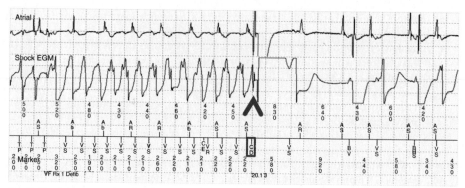

Fig. 11.10 Dual-chamber intracardiac electrograms (EGM) showing polymorphic VT with AV dissociation treated with shock. The atrial EGM, high-voltage ("shock") EGM, and dual-chamber marker channel are shown. The red arrowhead denotes shock, designated by CD (charge delivered) on the marker channel. After the shock, the atrial rhythm is sinus with premature atrial complexes; the ventricular rhythm is biventricular (BV) paced with premature ventricular complexes (PVCs) in the sinus rate zone (VS). From Peter Libby, Braunwald's Heart Disease: A Textbook of Cardiovascular Medicine. 12 ed. Philadelphia: Elsevier, 2022.

- Furthermore, recent studies and updated guidelines consider an ICD essential in the primary prevention of SCD in patients at high risk.
- All patients with ischemic or nonischemic LV dysfunction (EF < 35%) and heart failure despite optimized medical therapy are considered at high risk for SCD.
- LV function must be reevaluated after 90 days of optimal medical therapy and revascularization (if performed); if the EF remains 35% or less, the risk for SCD still exists and an ICD is recommended.
- In medically treated patients with acute MI with LV dysfunction, an ICD must be deferred for at least 40 days after the MI because studies have shown no difference in outcome between patients with or without ICD during this period.
- An exception to the 90- or 40-day waiting period would be made if the patient developed nonsustained VT and had inducible sustained VT on EPS.
- Some patients with LV dysfunction are candidates for cardiac transplantation; the ICD may also be used as a "bridge to cardiac transplantation" for SCD prevention in selected individuals.
- Indications for an ICD in patients with HCM include a history of prior resuscitation from VT/VF, presence of a very thick intraventricular septum (>3 cm), failure to raise blood pressure on exercise testing, nonsustained VT or inducible sustained VT on an EPS, and a strong family history of SCD.
- ICD implantation is recommended for patients with congenital heart disease who are survivors of an aborted SCA, have symptomatic sustained VT, have an EF less than 35% in the systemic ventricle, have syncope with advanced ventricular dysfunction or inducible sustained VT/VF on EPS, have tetralogy of Fallot with multiple risk factors, or have advanced single or systemic RV dysfunction and multiple risk factors.
- Patients with a structurally normal heart can also be at high risk for SCA if they have an inherited arrhythmia disorder, although these cases are rare.
- An ICD is recommended in the following high-risk subgroups:
  - ARVC: Patients who have a history of aborted SCA or sustained VT that is not hemodynamically tolerated or with depressed LV function or inducible sustained VT on EPS
  - LQTS: Survivors of SCA, syncope, and/or VT while receiving an adequate dose of β-blockers

- Brugada: Survivors of an aborted SCA or have documented sustained spontaneous VT or a spontaneous type 1 ECG and a history of syncope
- SQTS: Survivors of an aborted SCA or sustained spontaneous VT
- CPVT: Survivors of SCA, recurrent syncope, or polymorphic/bidirectional VT despite optimal therapy
- There are a few conditions for which ICD implantation is contraindicated. They include the following:
    - VT/VF resulting from arrhythmias amenable to ablation (e.g., WPW syndrome, RVOT VT)
    - VT/VF owing to a transient reversible disorder (e.g., acute MI, stress cardiomyopathy, electrolyte imbalance, drugs)
    - Terminal illnesses with life expectancy of less than 6 months (e.g., metastatic cancer)
    - Noninducible VT on EPS in cases for which a complex EPS is indicated
    - Psychiatric illness that may be aggravated by device implantation or may preclude follow up
    - Incessant VT or VF

WEARABLE AUTOMATIC DEFIBRILLATOR

- An external defibrillator attached to a wearable vest has been shown to identify and terminate VT/VF successfully.
- It has been approved by the US Food and Drug Administration for patients with a transient, high risk for VT/VF, such as those awaiting cardiac transplantation, as a bridge until an ICD is implanted, or in patients who are candidates for ICD, but who have or at high risk for infection.
- Registry data has demonstrated that the rate of sustained VT/VF within 3 months was 3% in patients with ischemic cardiomyopathy and congenital/inherited disease and 1% among nonischemic cardiomyopathy patients; the rate of inappropriate therapy was 0.5%.

CHAPTER 12

Ventricular Tachycardia

Common Misconceptions

- A wide-complex tachycardia that is hemodynamically well tolerated is most likely to be supraventricular tachycardia.
- It cannot hurt to give a stable patient with a wide-complex tachycardia adenosine or a calcium channel blocker to assess the response of the rhythm.
- Left ventricular dysfunction is always the cause rather than the consequence of incessant ventricular tachycardia.

Ventricular tachycardia (VT) accounts for 5% to 10% of admissions to the Cardiac Intensive Care Unit (CICU). Many of these admissions are for VT storm or incessant VT.

Definition

- *VT storm* is usually defined by three or more episodes of VT, ventricular fibrillation (VF), or appropriate implantable cardioverter defibrillator (ICD) shocks in a 24-hour period.
- This definition does not capture those patients with an ICD who have had multiple episodes of VT slower than the programmed detection rate of the device or VT terminated by antitachycardia pacing.
- Causes of VT storm (Table 12.1)
- Incessant VT is defined as hemodynamically stable VT that lasts for more than 1 hour.

Triggers

- Correctable triggers should be considered in all patients presenting with VT storm or incessant VT (Table 12.2).

Clinical Presentation

- The clinical presentation of patients with *VT storm* is variable and depends on the ventricular rate, presence and degree of underlying heart disease, left ventricular (LV) function, and the presence or absence of an ICD or left ventricular assist device (LVAD).
- Patients without an ICD may present without any symptoms, palpitations, presyncope, or syncope if the ventricular arrhythmia is hemodynamically well tolerated.
- When the arrhythmia is not hemodynamically tolerated, patients without an ICD may develop cardiac arrest.
- Patients with an ICD usually present with multiple ICD therapies, including antitachycardia pacing or ICD shocks.
- Patients with *incessant VT* may present with chest pain, new or worsening dyspnea, palpitations, presyncope, or syncope, depending on the VT rate and their hemodynamic tolerance of it.

TABLE 12.1 ▓ Causes of Ventricular Tachycardia Storm/Incessant Ventricular Tachycardia

Structural heart disease
Ischemic heart disease
Acute or recent myocardial infarction/acute coronary syndrome
Prior myocardial infarction
Nonischemic heart disease
Dilated cardiomyopathy
Hypertrophic cardiomyopathy
Arrhythmogenic right ventricular dysplasia/cardiomyopathy
Valvular heart disease
Corrected congenital heart disease
Myocarditis
Cardiac sarcoidosis
Chagas disease
Metastatic cardiac tumor
Structurally normal hearts (abnormal electrical substrate)
Primary causes
Idiopathic
Brugada syndrome
Early repolarization syndrome
Long QT syndrome
Short QT syndrome
Catecholaminergic polymorphic ventricular tachycardia
Secondary causes
Electrolyte abnormalities
Toxic/drug related
Endocrinologic
Perioperative
Iatrogenic (T-wave pacing)

From Maruyama M. Management of electrical storm: the mechanism matters. *J Arrhythmia*. 2014;30:242–249.

TABLE 12.2 ▓ Reversible Triggers of Ventricular Tachycardia Storm/Incessant Ventricular Tachycardia

Acute myocardial ischemia
Electrolyte abnormalities (hypokalemia and hypomagnesemia)
Decompensated heart failure
Hyperthyroidism
Infections, fever
QT prolongation
Drug toxicity
Electrolyte imbalance

- Patients with hemodynamically well-tolerated VT may present days after its onset complaining of new heart failure symptoms from the development of a tachycardia-mediated cardiomyopathy.
- The 12-lead electrocardiogram (ECG) may give important clues to the predisposing substrate, including evidence of acute or prior myocardial infarction (MI), myocardial ischemia, conduction abnormalities, and prolonged or shortened QT intervals.
- Assessment of the QT interval is especially important for patients with VT storm from polymorphic VT, as the approach to patients with prolonged QT interval is different than from patients with a normal QT interval.

- In cases in which the initial ECG or telemetry monitoring demonstrates a regular wide-complex tachycardia, VT must be distinguished from ventricular preexcitation, rate-related aberrancy, or preexisting bundle branch block in the setting of supraventricular tachycardia (SVT).
- The hemodynamic tolerance of the arrhythmia is not helpful in making the distinction.
- The administration of treatments for SVT, such as adenosine or calcium channel blockers, can precipitate cardiac arrest in patients with VT who were otherwise hemodynamically tolerating the arrhythmia.
- The only finding with 100% positive predictive value for the diagnosis of VT is the demonstration of atrioventricular dissociation manifested by fusion or capture beats.
- In the absence of fusion or capture beats, various algorithms are available to help differentiate VT from SVT, but because no algorithm is perfect, a wide-complex tachycardia in patients with underlying structural heart disease should be assumed to be VT until proven otherwise (Fig. 12.1).
- Patients with electrical storm/incessant VT can be further divided into those with and without structural heart disease to facilitate diagnosis and treatment (Fig. 12.2). On interrogation of ICDs of patients with VT storm, 86% to 97% have monomorphic VT, 1% to 21% have primary VF, 3% to 14% have combined VT/VF, and 2% to 8% have polymorphic VT.
- Monomorphic VT storm is usually associated with structural heart disease and is caused by electrical wavefront reentry around a fixed anatomic barrier, most commonly scar tissue following a prior MI, fibrosis in nonischemic cardiomyopathies, arrhythmogenic right ventricular cardiomyopathy/dysplasia, sarcoidosis, amyloidosis, Chagas disease, or a prior surgical incision (Fig. 12.3).

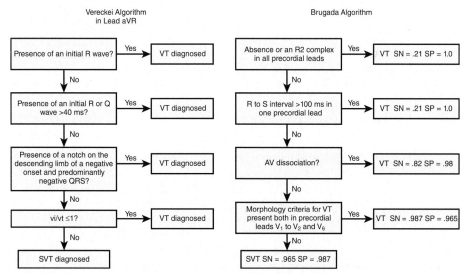

Fig. 12.1 The Vereckei and Brugada algorithms for differentiation of ventricular tachycardia from supraventricular tachycardia. *SN*, Sensitivity; *SP*, specificity; *SVT*, supraventricular tachycardia with aberrancy; *vi/vt*, initial (vi) and terminal (vt) ventricular activation velocity ratio; *VT*, ventricular tachycardia. (From Baxi RP, Hart KW, Vereckei A, et al. Vereckei criteria as a diagnostic tool amongst emergency medicine residents to distinguish between ventricular tachycardia and supra-ventricular tachycardia with aberrancy. J Cardiol. 2012;59:307–312.)

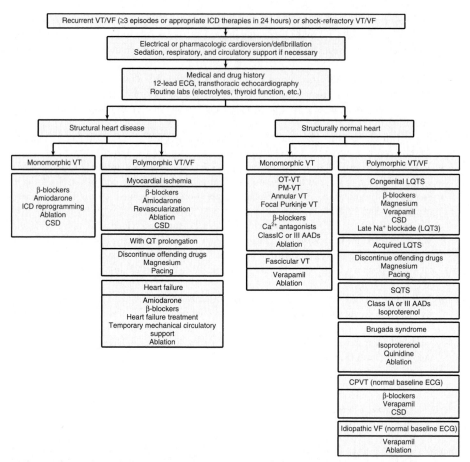

Fig. 12.2 Management of electrical storm. *ADDs*, Antidysrhythmic drugs; *CPVT*, catecholaminergic polymorphic ventricular tachycardia; *CSD*, cardiac sympathetic denervation; *ICD*, implantable cardioverter defibrillator; *LQTS*, long QT syndrome; *OT-VT*, outflow ventricular tachycardia; *PM-VT*, papillary muscle ventricular tachycardia; *SQTS*, short QT syndrome; *VF*, ventricular fibrillation; *VT*, ventricular tachycardia. (Modified from Maruyama M. Management of electrical storm: the mechanism matters. J Arrhythmia. 2014;30:242–249.)

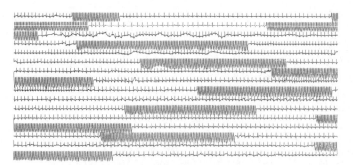

Fig. 12.3 Monomorphic ventricular tachycardia storm. Continuous electrocardiographic strips in a patient with recurrent syncopal episodes are shown. (From Maruyama M. Management of electrical storm: the mechanism matters. J Arrhythmia. 2014;30:242–249.)

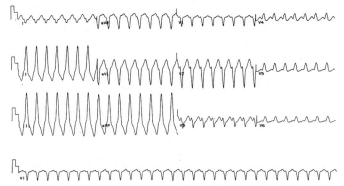

Fig. 12.4   A 12-lead electrocardiogram (ECG) of right ventricular outflow tract (RVOT) ventricular tachycardia demonstrating a left bundle branch block pattern in the precordial leads with transition from a small r wave to a large R wave at V_3 to V_4 consistent with a right-sided site of origin. Also consistent with the outflow tract site is the inferior ECG axis. (From Prystowsky EN, Padanilam BJ, Joshi S, Fogel RI. Ventricular arrhythmias in the absence of structural heart disease. J Am Coll Cardiol. 2012;59:1733–1744.)

- When monomorphic VT occurs in structurally normal hearts, it is referred to as idiopathic VT. The characteristics of idiopathic VT depend on the origin of the VT.
- VT arising from the outflow tract is the most common form of idiopathic VT; characteristically, it will present with a left bundle branch block and inferior axis (Fig. 12.4).
- Fascicular (or idiopathic) VT is the second most common cause of monomorphic VT in the absence of structural heart disease.
- The mechanism is thought to involve macro-reentry involving the Purkinje fiber network, which connects to the left fascicle.
- Fascicular VT is classified according to the ECG morphology (right bundle branch pattern and superior or inferior QRS axis) and corresponding fascicle coupled to the reentrant circuit:
  - Left posterior fascicular VT
  - Left anterior fascicular VT
  - Left upper septal VT
- The fascicular VTs have characteristic ECGs demonstrating a relatively narrow QRS that results from rapid spread of depolarization using the specialized conduction system.
- Left posterior fascicular VT is the most common fascicular VT (Fig. 12.5).
- Other, less common causes of monomorphic VT storm in structurally normal hearts include non-reentrant focal Purkinje VT, papillary muscle VT, and mitral/tricuspid annular VT.
- It is important to realize that these patients may have depressed LV function when they come to medical attention that is owing to the detrimental impact of incessant VT on LV function rather than an indication of structural heart disease.
- The LV dysfunction in such situations tends to be global as opposed to segmental and usually recovers after the VT is terminated.
- VF is fatal if not treated immediately.
- Following defibrillation, VF may recur repeatedly (VF storm) with mortality rates of 85% to 97%.
- Because ischemia is the primary mechanism of VF storm, patients should be emergently triaged to coronary angiography and revascularization.
- Patients with a structurally normal heart can develop VF storm triggered by closely coupled monomorphic premature ventricular contractions (PVCs).

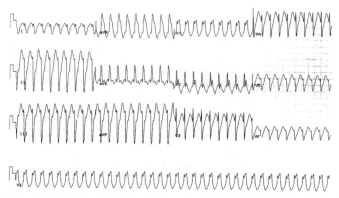

Fig. 12.5 A 12-lead electrocardiogram of left posterior fascicular ventricular tachycardia demonstrating a right bundle branch block pattern with a superior axis. This type of tachycardia has a site of origin near the left posterior fascicle. (From Prystowsky EN, Padanilam BJ, Joshi S, Fogel RI. Ventricular arrhythmias in the absence of structural heart disease. J Am Coll Cardiol. 2012;59:1733–1744.)

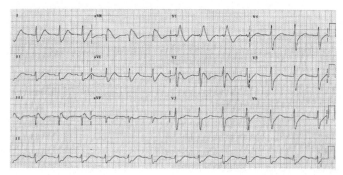

Fig. 12.6 A 12-lead electrocardiogram of Brugada syndrome demonstrating coving of the ST segment in the early precordial leads and right bundle branch block pattern. (From Prystowsky EN, Padanilam BJ, Joshi S, Fogel RI. Ventricular arrhythmias in the absence of structural heart disease. J Am Coll Cardiol. 2012;59:1733–1744.)

- Brugada syndrome, an inherited arrhythmia syndrome caused by mutations in the cardiac sodium channel gene, can present as recurrent VF or VF/VT storm and a characteristic ECG pattern of right bundle branch block and ST segment elevation in leads V1 to V3 (Fig. 12.6). Polymorphic and monomorphic VT reflect different arrhythmogenic mechanisms.
- Polymorphic VT can occur with a normal or prolonged QT interval and is most often encountered in patients with acute coronary syndromes (Fig. 12.7).
- VT storm can be the initial manifestation of acute ischemia.
- In acute MI, polymorphic VT can be caused by ischemia, altered membrane potentials, triggered activity, necrosis, or scar formation.
- Ischemia may cause dispersion of electrical refractory periods between the endocardium and epicardium, which is required for multiple waves of reentry.
- Patients without acute ischemia, such as those with acute myocarditis or hypertrophic cardiomyopathy, can also develop polymorphic VT storm.
- Polymorphic VT storm is rare in structurally normal hearts, but can occur in patients with primary genetic abnormalities, owing to secondary causes or with no discernible cause, referred to as idiopathic VF.

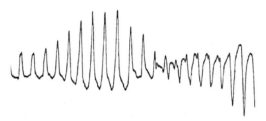

Fig. 12.7 Drug-induced torsades de pointes following quinidine treatment. (From Schwartz PF, Woosley RL. Predicting the unpredictable. Drug-induced QT prolongation and torsades de pointes. J Am Coll Cardiol. 2016;67:1639–1650.)

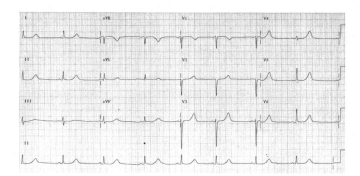

Fig. 12.8 A 12-lead electrocardiogram of long QT syndrome demonstrating a QT interval of 580 ms and a corrected QT interval of 513 ms. Genetic testing revealed an LQT1 syndrome. (From Prystowsky EN, Padanilam BJ, Joshi S, Fogel RI. Ventricular arrhythmias in the absence of structural heart disease. J Am Coll Cardiol. 2012;59:1733–1744.)

- Treatment strategies differ greatly among patients with polymorphic VT storm.
- The baseline ECG is of critical importance in making the diagnosis.
  - If the QT interval is markedly prolonged, the polymorphic VT is most likely torsades de pointes owing to congenital or acquired long QT syndrome (LQTS).
  - The congenital LQTS is an ion channel disorder characterized by abnormally prolonged QT intervals (corrected QT interval > 440 ms in men and > 460 ms in women) with or without morphologic abnormalities of the T waves Fig. 12.8.
  - At least 15 different genes involved in inherited LQTS have been described. The first 3—LQT1, LQT2, and LQT3—account for 60% to 75% of the genotyped LQTS cases.
  - Approximately 25% of affected patients have no identifiable gene mutations.
  - Acquired LQTS is caused by QT-prolonging drugs.
  - A list of drugs that have a risk of QT prolongation and/or torsades des pointes can be found on the CredibleMeds website (https://www.crediblemeds.org/).
  - Electrolyte abnormalities or drugs that induce hypokalemia, hypocalcemia, or hypomagnesemia can also lead to torsades de pointes in patients with or without genetic susceptibility.
- Brugada syndrome—which is characterized by a distinct ECG pattern, the absence of structural heart disease, and a high risk of polymorphic VT/VF and sudden death—can present as electrical storm.
  - Hypokalemia, high vagal tone, and fever are predisposing factors for VT storm.
  - Three different types of ECG changes have been associated with Brugada syndrome based on the morphology in V1 and V2.

- Type 1 ECG is characterized by a 2 mm or greater J-point elevation, coved type ST-T segment elevation, and inverted T wave in leads V1 and V2 (see Fig. 12.6).
- Type 2 ECG is characterized by a 2 mm or greater J-point elevation, 1 mm or greater ST segment elevation, saddleback ST-T segment, and a positive or biphasic T wave.
- Type 3 ECG is the same as type 2, except that the ST segment elevation is less than 1 mm.
- Among these three types of ECGs, only type 1 is diagnostic of Brugada syndrome.
- In patients with a normal ECG and a structurally normal heart who present with polymorphic VT/VF storm, the possible diagnoses include catecholaminergic polymorphic VT (CPVT) and idiopathic VF.
  - CPVT is an inherited abnormality of intracellular calcium handling and is commonly seen in young patients with stress- or exertion-induced syncope.
  - The hallmark of CPVT is alternating left bundle branch and right bundle branch QRS complexes.
  - Idiopathic VF presents as syncope or aborted sudden cardiac death in young people with normal hearts and no identifiable genetic syndrome.
  - The events are typically unrelated to stress or activity, but may occur in clusters characterized by frequent ventricular ectopy and short episodes of VF or polymorphic VT.
  - The spontaneous VF or polymorphic VT events are triggered by premature ventricular contractions (PVCs), generally with a short coupling interval, often referred to as short coupled torsade.
  - The PVCs triggering the events may arise from the Purkinje fibers or the myocardium; the former generally has shorter coupling intervals.
  - Isoproterenol may be effective in suppressing VF storms in the acute setting.

Management of VT Storm/Incessant VT

- Patients with VT storm or incessant VT should be rapidly assessed for hemodynamic instability.
- Pulseless patients or those with clinical evidence of hemodynamic compromise manifested by hypotension, chest pain, dyspnea, or altered mental status should be immediately treated according to advanced cardiac life support protocols with electrical cardioversion.

Pharmacologic Therapy

- In hemodynamically stable patients with VT storm or incessant VT, urgent pharmacologic therapy is indicated both to terminate the ventricular arrhythmia and to interrupt the detrimental effect of the associated intense adrenergic stimulation on the heart.
  - Intravenous amiodarone is the most commonly used agent to treat patients with VT storm or incessant VT in patients with structural heart disease (see Fig. 12.2).
  - The usual dose is 150 mg by intravenous (IV) bolus followed by 1 mg/min IV infusion for 6 hours, followed by 0.5 mg/min for an additional 18 hours.
  - Amiodarone has minimal negative inotropic effects and is therefore safe in patients with depressed left ventricular ejection fraction.
  - In addition, despite the potential for causing QT prolongation, the incidence of torsades de pointes is low. About 60% of patients will have their electrical storm terminated by intravenous amiodarone.
  - Because of the adrenergic stimulation associated with VT storm, incessant VT, or ICD shocks, β-blockers should be administered along with amiodarone.
  - Although metoprolol is the more commonly used agent, propranolol may suppress electrical storm that is refractory to metoprolol.

- In patients with congestive heart failure, propranolol decreases sympathetic outflow more than metoprolol.
- The lipophilic nature of propranolol enables penetration of the central nervous system, allowing blockade of central and prejunctional receptors in addition to peripheral β receptors.
- The dose of intravenous propranolol is 1 to 3 mg every 5 minutes to a total of 5 mg.
- The dose of intravenous metoprolol is 2.5 to 5 mg over 5 minutes, which can be repeated to a maximum dose of 15 mg over 15 minutes.
- Oral amiodarone and β-blockers should be initiated once the patient is stable.
- Outside of the setting of ischemia, lidocaine has relatively weak antiarrhythmic properties.
- Conversion rates from VT are 8% to 30%; a randomized trial has demonstrated that survival is significantly greater with amiodarone than lidocaine for treatment of out-of-hospital, shock-resistant VT or VF.
- Thus, amiodarone has replaced lidocaine as first-line therapy for refractory VT and VF.
- If lidocaine is used, it is administered as an IV bolus of 1 to 1.5 mg/kg followed by an initial bolus of 0.5 to 0.75 mg/kg that can be repeated every 5 to 10 minutes as needed to a total dose of 3 mg/kg. A continuous IV infusion of 1 to 4 mg/min is used to maintain therapeutic levels.
- In patients without structural heart disease, the treatment should be tailored to the specific underlying cause.
  - Outflow tract VT can be suppressed by β-blockers.
  - Alternatively, nondihydropyridine calcium channel blockers, such as verapamil or diltiazem, may be effective at suppressing outflow tract VT.
  - The distinctive feature of fascicular VT is its sensitivity to intravenous verapamil, which is the preferred therapy.
- The initial treatment of polymorphic VT storm in patients with LQTS is discontinuation of QT-prolonging medications and/or rapid correction of electrolyte abnormalities.
  - β-Blockers are primary pharmacologic therapy for congenital long QT syndromes types 1 and 2.
  - Intravenous verapamil effectively suppresses polymorphic VT in patients who are refractory to β-blockers.
  - Intravenous magnesium may facilitate termination of polymorphic VT associated with LQTS.
  - If the long QT syndrome genotype is known to be type 3, drugs with late sodium current blocking effects—such as mexiletine, ranolazine, and propranolol—are helpful.
  - In patients with acquired LQTS, β-blockers may promote VT by inducing bradycardia.
  - Temporary pacing is the treatment of choice in patients with bradycardia-dependent polymorphic VT in LQTS.
  - Isoproterenol can be used while awaiting pacemaker insertion.
  - In patients with short QT syndrome, class I and class III antidysrhythmic drugs—such as quinidine, disopyramide, and amiodarone—are effective at prolonging the QT interval.
  - Isoproterenol suppresses VT storm in Brugada syndrome.
  - Quinidine may also prevent VT/VF in Brugada syndrome.
- The trauma that patients with electrical storm or incessant VT experience from multiple electrical cardioversions can have short-term and long-term physical and emotional consequences.
  - Thus, all patients with electrical storm should be sedated.
  - Short-acting agents—such as propofol, benzodiazepines, and some general anesthetics—have been shown to convert or suppress VT.

- Left stellate ganglion blockade and thoracic epidural anesthesia have been reported to suppress VT storm that was refractory to multiple antidysrhythmic therapies.
- General anesthesia may also be helpful.

Nonpharmacologic Therapies

- For patients with VT storm and incessant VT in whom acute myocardial ischemia is thought to be an inciting factor, coronary angiography and percutaneous revascularization should be urgently performed because restoration of coronary perfusion may terminate arrhythmias.
- An intraaortic balloon pump or other temporary percutaneous LV mechanical support device may also be placed while in the catheterization laboratory.
- These devices may suppress ventricular arrhythmias by increasing coronary perfusion pressure or unloading a failing LV.
- Balloon counterpulsation has been reported to terminate VT storm even in the absence of ischemia, presumably by reducing afterload, LV size, and wall tension.
- In extreme cases of refractory arrhythmias, extracorporeal membrane oxygenation can be considered, but should be implemented early in the course before irreversible end-organ damage has occurred.
- Ultimately, recurrent refractory ventricular arrhythmias may be an indication to place an LVAD or list a patient for cardiac transplantation.
- Catheter ablation is effective therapy for many patients with VT storm or incessant VT refractory to or intolerant of medical therapy.
  - In one series, radiofrequency (RF) ablation completely suppressed drug-refractory electrical storm in 95 of 95 patients, many of whom were hypotensive and required hemodynamic support. Long-term suppression of electrical storm was achieved in 92% of patients, and 66% were free of VT at 22 months.
  - RF ablation is also indicated in recurrent polymorphic VT when specific triggers, such as monomorphic PVCs, can be identified and targeted.
  - This approach has been successful in suppressing electrical storm in patients with both ischemic and nonischemic cardiomyopathies.
  - Antiarrhythmic therapy should be continued in patients in the CICU who have undergone RF ablation.
  - Withdrawal of antidysrhythmic medications may be considered later.

Diagnosis and Treatment of Unstable Supraventricular Tachycardia

Common Misconceptions

- Sinus tachycardia requires treatment to slow the heart rate.
- Hemodynamic stability is useful in differentiating ventricular tachycardia from supraventricular tachycardia (SVT).
- Adenosine is the first treatment of choice for hemodynamically stable SVT.

Presentation

- Supraventricular tachycardias occurs in up to 10% to 20% of critically ill patients and are associated with increased morbidity and mortality.
- An immediate exact diagnosis is not necessary, and initial management should focus on ensuring hemodynamic stability.

Investigations

- A differential, rather than a precise, diagnosis can be generated initially by assessing the QRS width, rate, regularity, and onset, ideally on a 12-lead electrocardiogram (ECG) (Table 13.1).

Pathophysiology

- Sinus tachycardia is a regular tachycardia of gradual onset that reaches a maximum rate of 220 beats/min minus the patient's age (Fig. 13.1).
    - Sinus tachycardia is not pathologic and is addressed by treating the underlying condition.
- Atrial fibrillation (AF) is the most common tachyarrhythmia in critically ill patients (Fig. 13.2), owing to simultaneous depolarization of multiple wavelets within the atria, with variable conduction to the ventricle.
    - Acute AF is characterized by a rapid rise in ventricular rate and an irregular ventricular response.
    - Without severe left ventricular systolic or diastolic dysfunction, AF rarely causes hemodynamic instability.
    - The ECG shows an absence of discernable P waves and an irregular ventricular rhythm.
- Atrial flutter (Fig. 13.3) is the second most common pathologic SVT and, in its typical form, involves a reentry circuit around the tricuspid valve.
    - The flutter rate is usually around 300 beats/min, with the ventricular rate determined by the degree of atrioventricular node (AVN) block.
    - Acute atrial flutter presents with a rapid rise in ventricular rate to about 150 beats/min, consistent with 2:1 AVN block.

TABLE 13.1 ■ Differential Diagnosis of the Supraventricular Tachycardias (SVTs), Arranged by Regularity

SVT	Underlying Conditions	Regularity	Rate (beats/min)	Onset	P:QRS Ratio	Adenosine Response	ECG
Atrial fibrillation (AF)	Cardiac disease, pulmonary disease, pulmonary embolism, hyperthyroidism, postoperative	Irregular	100–220	Acute gradual (if in chronic AF)	None	Transient slowing of ventricular rate	
Multifocal atrial tachycardia (MAT)	Pulmonary disease, theophylline	Irregular	100–150	Gradual	Changing P morphology prior to QRS	None	
Frequent atrial premature contractions (APC)	Caffeine stimulants	Irregular	100–150	Gradual	P prior to QRS	None	
Sinus tachycardia (ST)	Sepsis, hypovolemia, anemia, pulmonary embolism, pain, fear, fright, exertion, myocardial ischemia, hyperthyroidism, heart failure	Regular	Up to 220 – Age	Gradual	P prior to QRS	Transient slowing	
Atrial flutter (Aflutter)	Cardiac disease	Regular (occasionally irregular if variable AV conduction)	150	Acute	Flutter waves	Transient slowing of ventricular rate	

Atrioventricular (AV) nodal reentrant tachycardia (AVNRT)	None	Regular	150–250	Acute	No apparent atrial activity or R' at termination of QRS	Terminate	
AV reentrant tachycardia (AVRT)	Rarely, Epstein anomaly	Regular	150–250	Acute	Orthodromic AVRT: retrograde P wave. Antidromic AVRT: P wave usually not seen. AF with WPW: no P waves present	Terminate	Orthodromic AVRT Antidromic AVRT AFib with WPW
Atrial tachycardia (AT)	Cardiac disease, pulmonary disease	Regular	150–250	Acute	P prior to QRS	Terminates 60%–80%	

ECG, Electrocardiogram; WPW, Wolff-Parkinson-White syndrome.

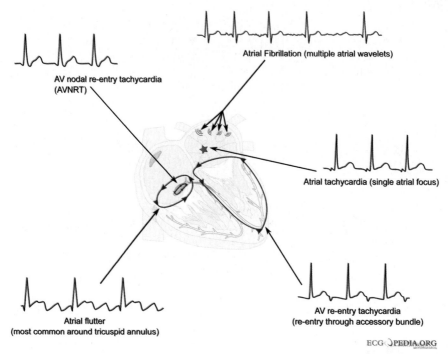

AV nodal re-entry tachycardia
(AVNRT)

Atrial Fibrillation (multiple atrial wavelets)

Atrial tachycardia (single atrial focus)

Atrial flutter
(most common around tricuspid annulus)

AV re-entry tachycardia
(re-entry through accessory bundle)

ECG PEDIA.ORG

Fig. 13.1 Basic mechanisms of supraventricular tachycardia (SVT). Typical atrial flutter (Aflutter) is a reentrant circuit around the tricuspid valve in the right atrium. Atrioventricular nodal reentry tachycardia (AVNRT) is reentry within the atrioventricular node (AVN) and perinodal tissue. Orthodromic AVNRT is a reentry circuit that traverses down the AVN and up a bypass tract, leading to a narrow QRS. In antidromic atrioventricular reentry tachycardia *(AVRT)*, conduction is first down the bypass tract and then up the AVN, leading to a wide QRS complex. Atrial tachycardia *(AT)* is an ectopic focus of atrial activity at a faster rate than the sinus node. Atrial fibrillation *(AFib)* is several simultaneous wavelets in the atrium with variable conduction through the AVN. Multifocal atrial tachycardia *(MAT)* involves at least three distinct ectopic atrial foci. (ECGPEDIA.ORG, https:// en.ecgpedia.org/index.php?title=File:SVT_overview.svg. Clinical practice: evaluation and initial treatment of supraventricular tachycardia. N Engl J Med. 2012;367[15]:1438–1448.)

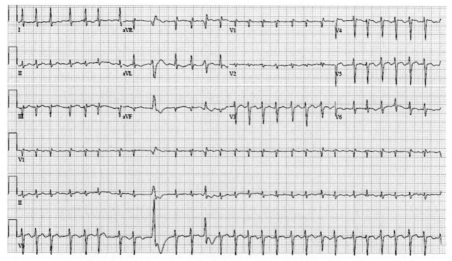

Fig. 13.2 Atrial fibrillation with rapid ventricular response.

- ◾ The ventricular rate can be irregular with variable AVN block. Typical sawtooth-appearing flutter waves can be seen on the ECG.
- ◾ Atrioventricular nodal reentry tachycardia (AVNRT; Fig. 13.4) is a reentry circuit within the AVN characterized by a rapid-onset, regular tachycardia with a rate between 150 and 250 beats/min.

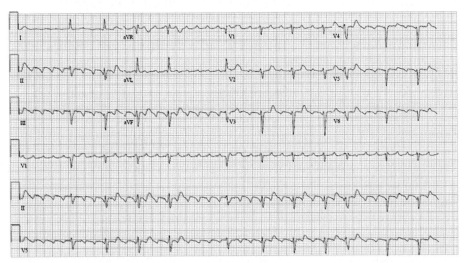

Fig. 13.3 Typical atrial flutter with variable conduction. Typical negatively deflected flutter waves are seen in the inferior leads with positive flutter waves in V_1. 2:1 atrial flutter can sometimes be difficult to distinguish from atrioventricular nodal reentry tachycardia; adenosine can be used to increase the degree of atrioventricular block and unmask the flutter waves.

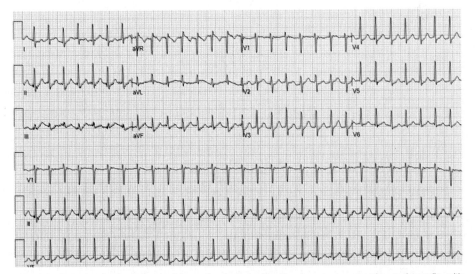

Fig. 13.4 Typical atrioventricular nodal reentry tachycardia. Regular narrow complex tachycardia with pseudo–S wave pattern seen in inferior leads and retrograde P wave seen shortly after the QRS in lead V_1.

- ■ There are two pathways within the AVN with different conduction properties, allowing for a premature atrial contraction (PAC) or premature ventricular contraction (PVC) to conduct down one pathway while the other is refractory.
  - ■ Conduction can then propagate retrograde up the previously refractory pathway, initiating a continuous circuit within the AVN.
  - ■ Conduction of the atria (retrograde) and ventricle (anterograde) occur simultaneously, with the P wave buried in the QRS or occurring shortly after (pseudo S wave).
- ■ Atrioventricular reentry tachycardia (AVRT) is a reentry circuit involving the AVN and an atrioventricular tract distant from the AVN.
  - ■ It is also precipitated by a PAC or PVC and is characterized by a rapid onset with a ventricular rate between 150 and 250 beats/min.
  - ■ If conduction occurs initially down the AVN and then retrograde up the bypass tract, the QRS complex is narrow (orthodromic AVRT).
  - ■ If conduction occurs down the bypass tract first, there is slow ventricular depolarization with retrograde conduction through the AVN, leading to a wide QRS complex (antidromic AVRT).
  - ■ A prior ECG may identify preexcitation down a bypass tract characterized by a short PR interval with a delta wave.
  - ■ AF with conduction down an accessory pathway (Fig. 13.5) can lead to ventricular fibrillation.
- ■ Atrial tachycardia (Fig. 13.6) involves an ectopic atrial pacemaker, characterized by an acute-onset, regular tachycardia with a ventricular rate generally less than 220 beats/min.
  - ■ There is often a slow increase in rate over the first 5 to 10 seconds, and it generally occurs in frequent short bursts.
  - ■ The ECG is characterized by a regular ventricular rate and P wave morphology variably distinct from the P wave in sinus rhythm, depending on the distance of the ectopic focus from the sinoatrial node.
- ■ Multifocal atrial tachycardia (MAT) involves the presence of multiple ectopic atrial pacemakers with a faster rate than the sinus node.

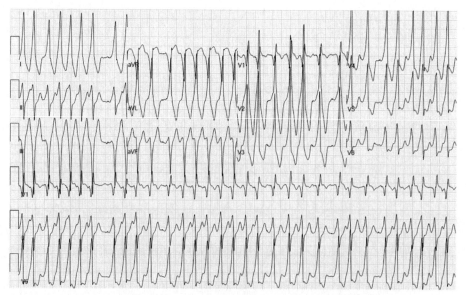

Fig. 13.5 Preexcited atrial fibrillation characterized by a bizarre, wide complex irregular tachycardia.

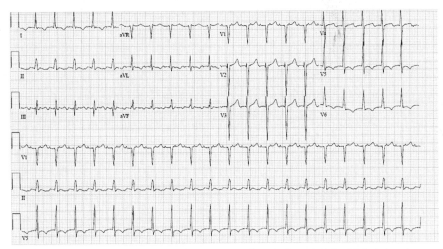

Fig. 13.6 Atrial tachycardia with 2:1 atrioventricular block. Note the P waves in lead III that do not appear to be sinus P waves. The 2:1 atrioventricular pattern is most clearly seen in lead V_1.

- The ECG shows an irregular ventricular rhythm with at least three distinct P wave morphologies and variable PR intervals.

Treatment

- The therapy for SVT is consistent with the 2015 American Heart Association (AHA) Advanced Cardiac Life Support (ACLS) guidelines and the 2015 American College of Cardiology (ACC)/AHA/Heart Rhythm Society (HRS) SVT guidelines.
- If the SVT is causing hemodynamic instability, it should immediately be treated with synchronized direct current cardioversion (DCCV).
  - Adequate sedation should be provided during the procedure.
  - Pads should be placed on the chest with the heart in between.
- For patients who have a symptomatic SVT but are hemodynamically stable, vagal maneuvers should be performed to temporarily block AVN conduction, which can terminate 20% to 40% of AVN–dependent reentrant arrhythmias (AVNRT, AVRT).
- For AF, atrial tachycardia, atrial flutter, or MAT, vagal maneuvers may temporarily block AVN conduction to unmask atrial activity (e.g., flutter waves).
- For patients who do not respond to vagal maneuvers, adenosine, which transiently blocks the AVN, should be administered rapidly via a large-bore intravenous catheter immediately followed by flushing with saline.
  - Adenosine is useful therapeutically and diagnostically because it can terminate AVN–dependent reentry SVT or unmask atrial activity with increased AVN block.
  - In the presence of significant reactive airway disease, it can cause bronchospasm.
  - Adenosine can also precipitate AF in up to 10% to 15% of patients.
- β-blockers and nondihydropyridine calcium channel blockers (diltiazem, verapamil) can also be used to block the AVN and suppress reentrant tachycardias.
- An anti-arrhythmic drug (AAD) can be administered to cardiovert patients with SVT, facilitate DCCV, or maintain sinus rhythm.
  - The most commonly used AAD in this setting is amiodarone.
- Unlike most other SVTs, preexcited AF frequently causes hemodynamic instability.
  - Prompt DCCV or administration of procainamide or ibutilide is a reasonable initial management option.

CHAPTER 14

Acute Presentations of Valvular Heart Disease

Common Misconceptions

- A wide pulse pressure is a hallmark of acute aortic regurgitation.
- Inotropic agents are useful in acute aortic regurgitation.
- A widened mediastinum is pathognomonic for acute aortic dissection.
- In aortic stenosis, a softer murmur indicates less severe stenosis.

Aortic Regurgitation

CLINICAL PRESENTATION

- Aortic regurgitation (AR) occurs as a result of either dilation of the aortic root or disruption of the valve leaflets.
- The most common etiologies are infective endocarditis (IE) and aortic dissection (AD).
    - IE is more likely in a prediseased valve and AR occurs through endothelial damage, nonbacterial thrombotic vegetation, adherence of organisms, proliferation of infection, and valve destruction.
    - Acute, type A, AD is complicated by AR in 50% of cases.
        - AD can lead to AR by direct extension of the dissection to the base of the aortic valve (AoV) leaflets, dilation of the sinuses with leaflets, incomplete coaptation, involvement of a valve commissure, and/or prolapse of the dissection flap across the AoV.
    - Other etiologies are listed in Table 14.1.
- The clinical features of AR are profoundly different in the acute setting, including a markedly elevated left ventricular end-diastolic pressure (LVEDP), but absent wide pulse pressure.
- Acute AR on the unprepared left ventricle (LV) may lead to the rapid onset of acute heart failure (HF) or cardiogenic shock.
- Patients typically present with dyspnea, weakness, or hypotension and are often misdiagnosed with sepsis, pneumonia, or nonvalvular heart disease.
    - They are often tachycardic.
    - The LV impulse may be normal in both location and duration.
    - The first heart sound is often soft or inaudible.
    - Occasionally, mitral valve (MV) closure may be heard during diastole and accompanied by mitral regurgitation (MR).
    - The Austin-Flint murmur, which is thought to represent turbulent flow from the left atrium (LA) to the LV because of partial MV closure from the AR jet, is either absent or brief.
    - An accentuated pulmonic closure sound suggests elevated pulmonary arterial pressure.
    - A third heart sound (S_3) is frequently heard.

- The acute AR murmur is characteristically short, early, and medium pitch.
- Edema and weight gain are not often seen because there is inadequate time for salt and water retention.
- The extremities may be cool and mottled owing to both poor cardiac output (CO) and elevated systemic vascular resistance (SVR).
- Clinical features seen in acute and chronic AR are listed in Table 14.2.

PATHOPHYSIOLOGY

- In acute, severe AR, increases in LV end-diastolic volume owing to regurgitant flow result in an abrupt rise in LVEDP (Fig. 14.1).

TABLE 14.1 ■ **Etiologies of Acute Aortic Regurgitation**

1.	**Infective endocarditis**	
2.	Aortic dissection—predisposing and associated conditions	Hypertension Marfan syndrome Bicuspid aortic valve Coarctation of aorta Ehler-Danlos syndrome Turner syndrome
3.	Chest trauma	
4.	Rupture of a myxomatous valve	
5.	Systemic connective tissue disorders	Ankylosing spondylitis Systemic lupus erythematosus
6.	Granulomatous diseases	Tertiary syphilis Giant cell arteritis Takayasu arteritis

TABLE 14.2 ■ **Clinical Features of Severe Aortic Regurgitation**

Feature	Acute	Chronic
Congestive heart failure	Rapid and sudden	Insidious
Rhythm	Sinus tachycardia	Regular rate
Point of maximal impulse	Not hyperdynamic and nondisplaced	Hyperdynamic and shifted inferolaterally
Pulse pressure	Normal	Widened
Heart sounds		
S_1	Soft or absent	Soft
S_2	Soft A2, accentuated P2	Normal P2
S_3	Present	Absent
S_4	Absent	Usually absent
Aortic regurgitation murmur	Soft, early	Holodiastolic
Cardiac output	Decreased	Normal
LVEDP	Increased	Normal
LV size	Normal	Increased

LV, Left ventricle; *LVEDP*, left ventricular end-diastolic pressure.

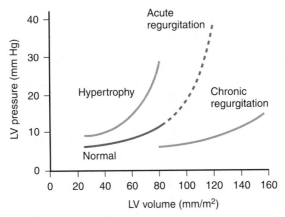

Fig. 14.1 Diastolic pressure-volume relationships in the left ventricle. *Acute regurgitation* is sudden volume loading of the left ventricle without the benefit of adaptive ventricular remodeling. It results in the left ventricle functioning on the steep portion of the normal curve *(dotted line)*. *Chronic regurgitation* is volume loading in the presence of a remodeled ventricle. It shifts the curve to the left and allows normalization of left ventricular (LV) filling pressure at significantly increased LV volumes. *Hypertrophy* (e.g., aortic stenosis) shifts the curve to the right and results in a noncompliant ventricle that is highly dependent on atrial booster pump function for LV filling. (From Hall RJ, Julian DG. Diseases of the Cardiac Valves. New York: Churchill Livingstone, 1989; 291.)

- Consequently, a rapid increase in the ventriculoatrial (VA) gradient can cause premature MV closure, preventing pulmonary edema.
- However, a further rise in the VA gradient reopens the MV in late diastole, leading to diastolic MR.
- Systolic MR can also manifest from the persistent VA gradient as a result of the high LVEDP level to the isovolumic contraction period during early systole.
- This MR is usually effective in lowering the LVEDP and the LA essentially serves as a reservoir.
- However, LA pressure may rise further, leading to pulmonary edema.
- Coronary ischemia can complicate acute AR because a reduction in coronary flow leads to a decrease in myocardial perfusion, whereas an elevated LVEDP and tachycardia increase myocardial oxygen demand.
- Diastolic coronary flow may be reduced by a reduction in diastolic blood pressure, elevation of LVEDP, and by the Venturi effect.
- The supply-demand mismatch is worsened if coronary artery disease (CAD) is present or when AD impairs coronary flow.
- To further complicate the picture, reflex sympathetic activation, in response to a reduction in CO and systemic blood pressure, produces tachycardia and increases SVR.
- This worsens regurgitant flow and impedes ejection of blood from the LV to the aorta so that a rise in aortic systolic pressure is inhibited.
- Aortic diastolic pressure usually does not fall significantly in the acute setting for two reasons:
  - The rapid increase in LVEDP reduces the driving gradient between the aorta and LV
  - Peripheral runoff is limited by an increase in SVR

INVESTIGATIONS

- Initial diagnostic testing includes an electrocardiogram (ECG), chest radiograph, blood cultures (if IE is suspected or if the patient has a prosthetic valve), and a transthoracic echocardiogram (TTE).
- An ECG is required in all patients with pulmonary edema, primarily to rule out acute myocardial infarction (MI).
  - The ECG in acute AR may be normal with left axis deviation. With early LV volume overload, there can be Q waves in leads I, aVL, and V_3 to V_6.
- The chest radiograph generally reveals a normal cardiac silhouette with evidence of pulmonary edema (Fig. 14.2).
  - A widened aortic root suggests the presence of dissection.
- TTE provides crucial information regarding the presence, severity, and etiology of the lesion.
  - With severe AR, in addition to visualizing the regurgitant jet, quantitative measurements, such as jet or vena contracta width, can be obtained (Fig. 14.3).
  - A jet width greater than 65% of the LV outflow tract and vena contracta greater than 0.6 cm are consistent with severe AR.
  - Continuous wave Doppler is used to calculate the pressure half-time, with acute, severe AR, the rapid equilibration of aortic and LV diastolic pressure results in a pressure half-time of less than 300 msec.

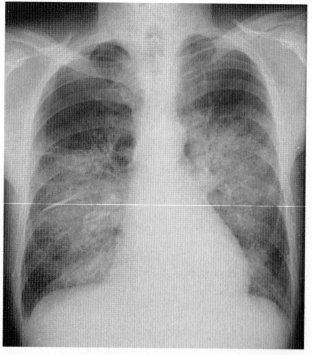

Fig. 14.2 Chest radiograph from a patient with acute aortic insufficiency secondary to pneumococcal endocarditis. Note the classic findings of acute pulmonary edema with a normal cardiac silhouette.

- Other supportive findings include premature MV closure and flow reversal in the descending aorta (Fig. 14.4).
- If TTE windows are limited, transesophageal echocardiography (TEE) may be required, which has increased sensitivity for evaluating the underlying etiology of AR, such as IE (vegetations or aortic root abscess; Fig. 14.5) or AD (dissection flap).
- AD should be considered in the differential diagnosis of any acute AR, confirmed by computed tomography (CT), TEE, or magnetic resonance imaging.
  - TTE can be a very useful and quick tool for identifying AoV dysfunction, abnormalities in the proximal ascending aorta and a short segment of the descending aorta.
    - The sensitivity for diagnosing AD with a TTE is higher for type A AD at 78% to 100%, but for type B it is only 31% to 55%.

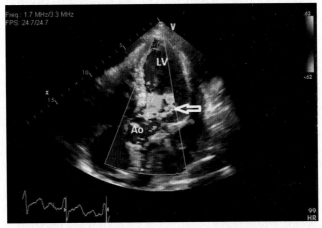

Fig. 14.3 Five-chamber transthoracic echocardiogram shows the presence of severe aortic regurgitation on color Doppler. *Ao,* Aorta; *LV,* left ventricle.

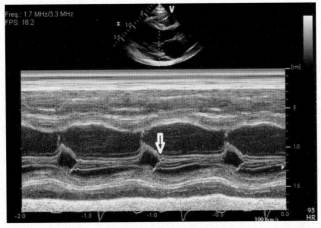

Fig. 14.4 M-mode transthoracic echocardiogram demonstrates the presystolic mitral valve closure *(arrow)* from the increased left ventricular pressure compared with left atrial pressure.

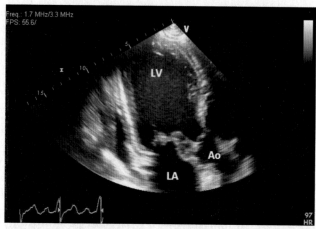

Fig. 14.5 Apical three-chamber transthoracic echocardiogram shows the presence of a mitral valve and aortic valve vegetation. *Ao*, Aorta; *LA*, left atrium; *LV*, left ventricle.

- Thus, TTE should be used to evaluate complications, not diagnosis, of acute aortic syndrome (AAS).
- TEE is highly accurate in detecting AAS owing to its ability to visualize both the ascending and descending aortas.
- A true dissection flap features random mobility, constant echo intensity, and margination of flow on color flow imaging.
- TEE can reach a sensitivity of 99% and a specificity of 89%.
- However, owing to its requirement for a skilled operator and adequate sedation, CT is the preferred modality for evaluation of AD in the emergency department (Fig. 14.6).
  - A contrast study is highly accurate, with a sensitivity and specificity of about 95% to 98%, and is able to provide the site and extent of the dissection.

MANAGEMENT

- The principles of management include reducing pulmonary venous pressure, maximizing CO, and initiating therapy for any underlying disorder.
- Invasive hemodynamic monitoring by placement of a Swan-Ganz pulmonary artery catheter is extremely helpful in that it allows the clinician to assess the response to therapy and gauge the tempo of the illness.
- Medical therapy for HF caused by acute AR includes both loop diuretics and intravenous vasodilators and the hemodynamic response to this determines the urgency of surgical intervention.
- In patients with acute AR, intravenous vasodilator therapy can significantly reduce pulmonary artery pressures and increase CO.
  - Nitroprusside is the vasodilator of choice.
    - The drug is started at 0.25 μg/kg/min intravenously and uptitrated by increments of 0.25 to 0.5 μg/kg/min with the goal of achieving optimal hemodynamics.
    - The speed of uptitration is dictated by the degree of hemodynamic compromise.
  - Intravenous diuretics should be initiated to induce a brisk sustained urine output.
- Inotropic agents do not play a significant role in acute AR because most cases occur in the setting of normal or accentuated LV function.

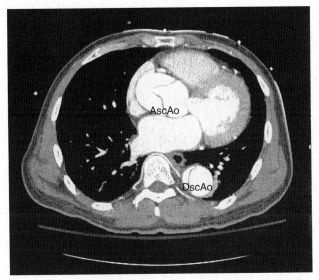

Fig. 14.6   Computed tomographic angiogram reveals a type A aortic dissection with the presence of an intimal flap in the ascending aorta *(AscAo)* and descending aorta *(DscAo)*. *LA,* Left atrium; *LV,* left ventricle.

- However, if preexisting myocardial dysfunction exists, agents, such as dobutamine, at a dose of 5 to 15 µg/kg/min may assist in maintaining CO.
- Intraaortic balloon pumps (IABPs) are contraindicated because balloon inflation during diastole would increase regurgitant flow.
- Additional medical therapy includes appropriate antibiotics in suspected IE.
- In the case of AD, intravenous β-blockers are thought to be useful in reducing the velocity of LV ejection, thereby minimizing aortic wall stress.
- However, when AD is complicated by acute AR, β-blockers should be used cautiously, because the compensatory tachycardia would be blunted, further reducing CO.
- If hemodynamic instability persists, emergent surgical valve repair or replacement represents the only curative option.
- Indications for surgery in the presence of IE are outlined in Table 14.3. Even in the presence of active IE, valve surgery should not be delayed.
- The International Registry of Acute Aortic Dissection (1995–2013) analysis, demonstrated a decline in overall mortality for AD type A from 31% to 22%, driven mostly by a reduction in surgical mortality from 25% to 18%.

Aortic Stenosis

CLINICAL PRESENTATION

- Aortic stenosis (AS) is a progressive disorder characterized by narrowing of the AoV orifice resulting in dyspnea, angina, or syncope.
- The etiology varies from an age-related degenerative process, chronic rheumatic heart disease, or congenital abnormalities in valve structure.
- Physical examination of the patient with AS reveals a small-volume, slowly rising pulse.

TABLE 14.3 ■ Indications for Surgery in Infective Endocarditis of Native or Prosthetic Valve

Early Surgery (During Initial Hospitalization Before Completion of Full Antibiotic Course)

Valve dysfunction causing heart failure symptoms (class I)

Left-sided infective endocarditis caused by highly resistant organism (Staphylococcus *aureus*, fungi) (class I)

Heart block, abscess, or destructive penetrating lesion (class I)

Persistent infection (persistent bacteremia or fevers lasting longer than 5 to 7 days despite appropriate therapy; class I)

Recurrent emboli and persistent vegetations despite appropriate antibiotic therapy (class IIa)

Large (>10 mm) mobile vegetation on native valve (class IIb)

Indication for surgery, but with complication of a stroke with no evidence of intracranial hemorrhage or extensive neurologic damage (class IIb)

Surgery

Relapsing prosthetic valve endocarditis (recurrence of bacteremia after completion of antibiotic course with subsequent negative blood cultures) (class I)

Complication of major ischemic stroke or intracranial hemorrhage and hemodynamically stable, delay surgery for at least 4 weeks (class IIb)

From Nishimura RA, Otto CM, Bonow RO, et al. 2017 AHA/ACC Focused Update of the 2014 AHA/ACC Guideline for the Management of Patients With Valvular Heart Disease. *J Am Coll Cardiol*. 2017;70:252–289.

■ The apical impulse of the heart may be displaced downward and to the left with a marked presystolic impulse or "a" wave.

■ The harsh ejection systolic murmur of AS is best heard at the base and is transmitted to the carotids.

■ In general, late peaking murmurs of longer duration signify more severe stenosis.

■ With decreasing CO, there is a fall in the gradient and in the intensity of the murmur.

Pathophysiology

■ Progressive valvular AS leads to increasing LV systolic pressure and so the LV hypertrophies to normalize wall stress.

■ But it also results in a shift of the LV pressure-volume curve upward and to the left; because of this, any diminution in preload will impair stroke volume (SV).

■ Therefore, acute volume reduction will result in a significant impairment of CO.

■ The altered LV pressure-volume relationship also makes LV preload critically dependent on atrial contraction.

■ Any impairment in the contribution of diastolic filling by atrial systole can lead to acute decompensation, increasing heart rate may impair LV filling simply by shortening diastole, and a markedly decreased heart rate will impair CO as it becomes heart rate dependent.

■ Any condition that further impairs LV relaxation (e.g., acute coronary ischemia) will also have a significant impact on diastolic filling.

■ Relative ischemia may also occur in the setting of normal coronary arteries or nonobstructive CAD when myocardial oxygen demands have exceeded coronary reserve.

TREATMENT

■ Atrial fibrillation should be treated with urgent synchronized cardioversion.

■ Atrioventricular (AV) conduction abnormalities should be managed with temporary pacing followed by a dual chamber permanent pacemaker if the disturbance persists.

- Once the patient is stabilized, urgent valve replacement should be undertaken.
- If there is a question of CAD, cardiac catheterization should be performed.
- Valve replacement for AS includes surgical or transcatheter aortic valve replacement (TAVR).
- Based on the updated 2020 American Heart Association/American College of Cardiology (AHA/ACC) guidelines for severe and symptomatic (stage D) aortic stenosis:
  - Surgical AVR is a class IA recommendation for patients less than 65 years of age.
  - TAVR is a class Ia recommendation for patients 65 to 80 years of age.
  - For patients at high surgical risk, TAVR are is a class IA recommendations.
- Mechanical circulatory support approaches have emerged as a rescue therapy in critical AS with or without cardiogenic shock or as a bridge to TAVR.

Post–Transcatheter Aortic Valve Replacement Aortic Regurgitation

- TAVR is now a well-established procedure performed for patients with surgically intermediate, high-risk, or inoperable severe AS.
- Because the valves are implanted without sutures and use oversizing to anchor the frame, incomplete apposition can lead to perivalvular aortic regurgitation (PAR) or leak.
  - Several studies have shown that up to 85% of all patients after TAVR have PAR after the procedure, with 12% graded moderate or severe.
  - After surgical AVR, the incidence of moderate or severe AR is 4%.
  - More than mild PAR has significant impact on prognosis after TAVR, with a two fold to four fold increased 1-year mortality risk compared with patients without PAR.
  - Based on the French Registry, the 1-year data demonstrated that the Edwards balloon-expandable valve (Edwards Lifesciences) is associated with moderate to severe PAR in 12.2% compared with 19.8% for the self-expandable CoreValve (Medtronic).
  - PAR develops by:
    - Suboptimal prosthesis placement leading to incomplete sealing of the annulus.
    - Incomplete apposition of the prosthesis owing to calcification of the annulus, native leaflets, or LV outflow tract.
    - Undersizing of the replacement AoV.
- Valve sizing is one of the strongest predictors of PAR.
- Appropriate sizing using multidetector CT is the gold standard and has been associated with reduced rates of significant PAR.
  - Intraprocedural imaging is important in establishing the diagnosis and severity of PAR and can be used to help guide the management of PAR when it occurs.
  - Corrective techniques include using balloon postdilation for underexpansion, valve-in-valve implantation for a malpositioned valve or central regurgitation, and snare technique for valves implanted too deeply.
  - In cases of properly placed valves with good expansion, transcatheter device closure can be attempted of the PAR.
- Acute circulatory collapse is a rare complication that may develop during or after TAVR.
  - Causes include:
    - Coronary ischemia
    - Severe AR
    - Cardiac tamponade
    - Valve embolization
    - LV failure.
  - For mild hemodynamic disturbances related to PAR, medical therapy may be sufficient.
  - However, for refractory cardiogenic shock owing to severe valvular regurgitation, mechanical support may be required, with the TandemHeart or Impella (Chapter 24).

Post–Left Ventricular Assist Device Aortic Regurgitation

- The use of mechanical circulatory support is increasingly used as a bridge to transplant, to a decision, or as a destination therapy.
- During implantation of LV assist devices (LVADs), an incompetent AoV is oversewn, repaired, or replaced to prevent a portion of the LVAD output immediately being returned to the pump.
- The development of *de novo* AoV disease, however, may occur in patients with an LVAD.
- Based on observational study, *de novo* development of AR is common and can occur early after LVAD placement.
- It is hypothesized that aortic blood flow dynamics and prolonged AoV closure contribute to AR, which contributes to changes in the sheer stress and diastolic luminal pressures experienced by the aorta, leading to aortic wall atrophy, dilation, and wall insufficiency, leading to valve malcoaptation and AR.
- Because the AoV remains closed during systole owing to the LVAD support, it is subjected to an unaccustomed high systolic pressure caused by the retrograde flow from the aortic outflow conduit and, because this is smaller in diameter than the aorta, a higher velocity is required to deliver the same volume.
- The valve trauma from high-velocity and pressure blood flow and intermittent AoV opening leading to progressive valve degeneration allows for *de novo* AR to develop.
- This appears to be associated with HF admissions and arrhythmias.
- Medical therapy targeting afterload and preload with vasodilators and diuretics to reduce volume overload is the mainstay of treatment.
- Inotropic support can be used when there is refractory HF or cardiogenic shock.
- There have been case reports regarding the use of TAVR to treat patients with impending hemodynamic collapse from progressive AR.

Acute Mitral Regurgitation

CLINICAL PRESENTATION

- A wide spectrum of clinical illness may be seen, ranging from complete papillary muscle rupture with cardiovascular collapse to mild dyspnea after chordal rupture.
  - A specific phenotype, such as Marfan or Ehlers-Danlos syndrome, may suggest chordal rupture.
  - Alternatively, peripheral manifestations of vascular (emboli, Janeway lesions) or immunologic (Osler nodes, Roth spots) findings consistent with IE may be present.
  - The presence of anginal-type chest pain leads one to suspect MI with papillary muscle disease as the underlying etiology.
- Most patients with acute MR demonstrate tachycardia, a compensatory mechanism to maintain CO with declining SV.
- The jugular venous pulse may be elevated, with 50% of patients having a prominent "a" wave.
- Precordial examination often reveals a hyperdynamic, nondisplaced apical impulse with a prominent presystolic expansion, suggesting LV overload with increased atrial systole.
- A left parasternal lift is common, as filling from the combination of pulmonary venous and regurgitant flow into the posterior LA lifts the entire organ anteriorly and is an indication of severe MR, often occurring with elevated right ventricular (RV) systolic pressures.
- A systolic apical thrill may be felt in up to 75% of patients with ruptured chordae tendineae, but is less common in papillary muscle dysfunction or rupture.

■ Cardiac auscultation reveals a normal S_1 because in most cases of acute MR the MV leaflets are normal, in contrast to chronic MR, in which S_1 is soft secondary to abnormal MV leaflets.

■ Accentuated pulmonary valve closure suggests pulmonary hypertension (PH) and, because the LV empties rapidly, the aortic component may close early, giving rise to a widened split of S_2.

■ Although an S_4 is common, an S_3 gallop is almost universal with severe MR owing to LV volume overload.

■ The murmur of acute MR differs in chronic MR according to the underlying pathophysiology.

■ In papillary muscle dysfunction, a crescendo-decrescendo murmur may be heard during mid-to-late systole, whereas papillary muscle rupture results in a pansystolic murmur.

■ Acute chordal rupture results in an ejection murmur that begins in the apex and radiates to the base of the heart.

■ Early termination of the murmur in acute MR results from rapid equalization of LA and LV pressures and suggests a greater degree of regurgitation.

■ Widely incompetent valves through which flow may be less turbulent or low flow owing to LV dysfunction may give rise to low-grade murmurs.

■ A summary of the differences in clinical presentation between acute and chronic MR is listed in Table 14.4.

TABLE 14.4 ■ **Clinical Features of Severe Mitral Regurgitation**

Feature	Acute	Chronic
Congestive heart failure	Rapid and sudden	Insidious
Rhythm	Sinus tachycardia	Atrial fibrillation
Point of maximal impulse	Hyperdynamic and nondisplaced	Hyperdynamic and shifted inferolaterally
Right ventricular lift	Present	Absent
Precordial thrill	Usually present	Absent
Jugular venous pressure	Prominent "a" wave	Normal tracing
Heart sounds		
S_1	Normal	Soft
S_2	Accentuated P2 with wide split	Normal P2 with wide split
S_3	Present	Present
S_4	Present	Absent
Mitral regurgitation murmur	Loud, decreasing in late systole	Blowing holosystolic
Radiation of mitral regurgitation murmur	Toward base	Toward axilla
Mitral diastolic flow murmur	Present	Absent
Cardiac output	Decreased	Normal
Ejection fraction	Normal to reduced	Normal to increased
LVEDP	Increased	Normal
LV size	Normal	Increased

LV, Left ventricle; *LVEDP*, left ventricular end-diastolic pressure.
From Depace NL, Nestico PF, Morganroth J. Acute severe mitral regurgitation: pathophysiology, clinical recognition and management. *Am J Med*. 1985;78:293.

PATHOPHYSIOLOGY

- The presentation of acute mitral regurgitation results in sudden, severe LV volume overload.
- The functional components of the mitral valve include the LA, mitral annulus, MV leaflets, chordae tendineae, papillary muscles, and the LV, and abnormalities of any can cause MR.
- Not surprisingly, therefore, there are numerous etiologies of acute MR, listed in Table 14.5.
- IE may cause acute MR by mechanisms that include leaflet perforation, abscess formation, or chordae tendineae rupture.
- CAD is another common cause of acute MR caused by:
  - Papillary muscle rupture after MI
  - Ischemic papillary muscle dysfunction
  - Papillary muscle fibrosis
  - Dyssynergy of the LV segment that anchors the functioning papillary muscle
  - Diffuse LV enlargement that causes mitral annular dilation.
- Other etiologies include myxomatous degeneration associated with MV prolapse or Marfan disease, spontaneous rupture, trauma, or rheumatic disease.
- With the increasing use of percutaneous balloon valvotomy for rheumatic mitral stenosis (MS), iatrogenic MR requiring valve replacement is more frequent as compared with closed surgical valvotomy.
- Finally, degeneration of a bioprosthetic valve, impaired closure of a mechanical MV by pannus, or perivalvular regurgitation from suture disruption may lead to acute prosthetic MR.
- The severity of MR depends on the volume of regurgitant flow, LA compliance, and LV function, which is a function of the size of the incompetent valve orifice and the LV to LA pressure gradient.
- In a relatively noncompliant LA, the abrupt increase in pressure is transmitted to the pulmonary circulation with resultant pulmonary edema.
- In the presence of MR, there are two outlets for LV ejection:
  - The high-impedance systemic circulation
  - The low-impedance LA
- In this setting, SV is highly dependent on SVR.
- As SVR increases, a greater proportion of the SV is directed to the LA and the regurgitant fraction increases.
- A reduction in CO increases SVR as neurohormonal systems that cause vasoconstriction are activated.
- The unwanted consequence of a rising SVR is worsening of MR.

TABLE 14.5 ■ Etiologies of Acute Mitral Regurgitation

1.	Myocardial infarction
2.	Chordal or papillary muscle rupture
3.	Myxomatous disease
4.	Infective endocarditis
5.	Rheumatic heart disease
6.	Acute cardiomyopathy
7.	Prosthetic valve dysfunction
8.	Trauma
9.	Iatrogenic

- As regurgitant flow increases further, CO declines and pulmonary congestion worsens.
- This leads to a vicious cycle with deleterious consequences on hemodynamics.

INVESTIGATIONS

- Initial noninvasive diagnostic tests include a chest radiograph, which typically reveals a normal cardiac silhouette with pulmonary venous congestion or edema.
  - However, with preexisting valvular or myocardial disease, there may be radiographic evidence of cardiac enlargement.
  - Occasionally, an unusual pattern of right upper lobe pulmonary edema can be confused with pneumonia (Fig. 14.7) as the MR jet is directed toward the right superior pulmonary vein.
- The ECG often reveals sinus tachycardia; however, atrial fibrillation with a rapid ventricular response is also common.
  - A large negative terminal deflection of the P wave in lead V_1 and broadened P wave in lead II suggest LA volume overload.
  - Nonspecific ST segment and T wave abnormalities are common; however, if acute MR occurs as a result of ischemia or infarction, careful analysis of the ECG becomes essential.
- Echocardiography is the most commonly used imaging modality in patients with acute MR.
  - Transthoracic imaging can be performed quickly and safely to determine accurately the etiology and severity.
    - In addition, overall LV function and wall motion abnormalities can be assessed.
    - Finally, structural cardiac disorders that mimic MR can be ruled out.
  - Depending on the etiology, a variety of echocardiographic abnormalities may be seen.
    - There may be an obvious flail leaflet, chordal rupture, or vegetation (Fig. 14.8).
    - Papillary muscle rupture is often directly visualized as a mass attached to the involved leaflet with discontinuity of the base of the muscle.
- TEE is a useful alternative modality for assessing acute MR, with superior resolution and a significant advantage in terms of visualizing the MV apparatus, especially when a prosthetic MV is present.

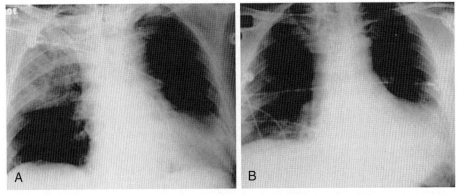

Fig. 14.7 Unusual radiographic appearance of acute mitral regurgitation mimicking lobar pneumonia. (**A**) Prominent right upper lobe alveolar infiltrate. (**B**) Rapid resolution occurred in 48 hours with diuretic therapy. (Courtesy Steve Primack, MD, Department of Radiology, Oregon Health Sciences University, Portland.)

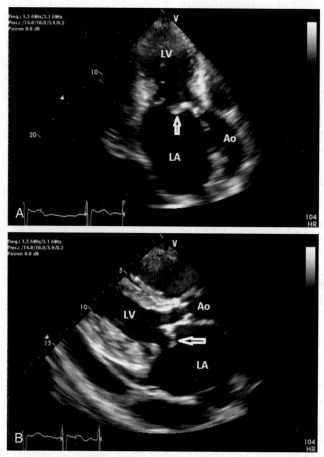

Fig. 14.8 **(A)** Apical three-chamber transthoracic echocardiogram shows a flail mitral valve leaflet *(arrow)*. **(B)** Parasternal long-axis transthoracic echocardiogram view of the flail mitral valve leaflet. *Ao,* Aorta; *LA,* left atrium; *LV,* left ventricle.

- Doppler imaging provides both qualitative and quantitative assessment of mitral regurgitation severity (Fig. 14.9).
- A color Doppler jet width at the vena contracta of more than 6 mm by multiplane TEE detects severe MR with a sensitivity and specificity of 95% and 98%, respectively.
- If systolic retrograde flow into the pulmonary veins is detected, MR is at least moderate (Fig. 14.10).
- Finally, echocardiography distinguishes acute MR from ventricular septal rupture, which can have a similar presentation (Fig. 14.11, Table 14.6).
  - If diagnostic studies suggest that ischemia or infarction is the underlying etiology of acute MR, urgent cardiac catheterization should be considered.

TREATMENT

- The principles of treatment focus on reducing LVEDP, decreasing aortic impedance, and initiating etiology-specific therapy.

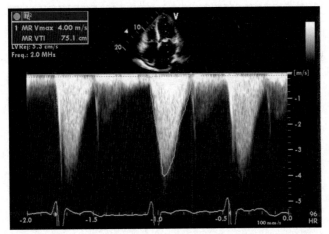

Fig. 14.9 Doppler image from a transthoracic echocardiogram shows the right-angle triangle appearance rather than the normal symmetric parabola owing to the transmitted left ventricular (LV) pressure to the left atrium (LA) from a wide-open mitral regurgitation and, consequently, the narrowed gradient between the LA and LV pressures.

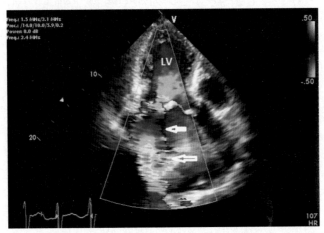

Fig. 14.10 Apical three-chamber transthoracic echocardiogram shows a flail mitral valve leaflet and Doppler demonstrating systolic retrograde flow into the pulmonary veins. *LV,* Left ventricle.

- The clinical severity of the regurgitation and the tempo of the illness, as evidenced by serial hemodynamic measurements via pulmonary artery catheter (Chapter 23), determine the urgency of valve surgery.
- In the case of papillary muscle rupture, which is the cause of death in 1% to 5% of fatal MIs, urgent surgical intervention is mandatory if the patient cannot be stabilized quickly with medical therapy.
- Vasodilator therapy is the key component of medical management and the preferred agent is intravenous nitroprusside (for dosage, see section on treatment for AR).
  - Its rapid onset and offset allow careful titration to response.

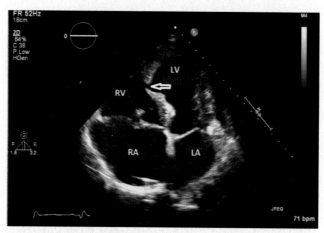

Fig. 14.11   Four-chamber transthoracic echocardiogram shows a ventricular septal defect *(arrow)*. *LA*, Left atrium; *LV*, left ventricle; *RA*, right atrium; *RV*, right ventricle.

TABLE 14.6 ▇ Differentiation of Papillary Muscle Rupture and Ventricular Septal Rupture

Feature	Papillary Muscle Rupture	Ventricular Septal Rupture
Age (mean, years)	65	63
Days after myocardial infarction	3–5	3–5
Anterior myocardial infarction	25%	66%
Murmur	Variable systolic	Pansystolic at lower sternal border
Palpable thrill	Rare	Yes
"v" wave in pulmonary capillary wedge tracing	++	++
Oxygen step-up from right atrium to pulmonary artery	±ᵃ	++
Echocardiographic findings	Flail or prolapsing leaflet	Visualize defect
Doppler	Regurgitant jet in LA	Detect shunt
Mortality rate		
Medical	90%	90%
Surgical	40% to 90%	50%

ᵃOxygen step-up may occasionally be seen in papillary muscle rupture as a result of the regurgitant "v" from the left atrium contaminating the mixed venous sample from the pulmonary artery.
+, occasionally present; ++, invariably present; ±, rarely present.
From Antman EM. ST-elevation myocardial infarction: management. In: Zipes DP, Libby P, Bonow RO, et al, eds. *Braunwald's Heart Disease: A Textbook of Cardiovascular Medicine.* 7th ed. Philadelphia: Elsevier; 2005:1204.

- Nitroprusside improves SV by decreasing aortic impedance and decreasing LV volume, which reduces the area of the incompetent MV orifice, thereby minimizing regurgitant flow.
- An additional degree of afterload reduction may be provided by placing an IABP.

- Improvement in diastolic coronary flow that occurs in response to an IABP may also have some salutary effects on LV function, especially in the presence of myocardial ischemia.
- If significant hypotension is present, dopamine (starting at 2.5 to 5 μg/kg/min to a maximum of 10 to 20 μg/kg/min) may be useful in stabilizing the patient and maintaining systemic blood pressure.
  - However, at doses greater than 5 μg/kg/min, α-adrenergic-induced peripheral vasoconstriction may actually worsen the degree of regurgitation by increasing afterload.
- If LV contractility is impaired and CO is significantly reduced, the addition of dobutamine (start at 2 to 5 μg/kg/min to a maximum 10 to 15 μg/kg/min) or milrinone (start at 0.25 μg/kg/min to a maximum of 1.0 μg/kg/min with or without a loading dose) can be beneficial.
- Finally, diuretics (as outlined in the section on treatment for AR) are useful to reduce pulmonary congestion.
- IE complicated by chordal rupture or leaflet perforation should be treated with appropriate antibiotics in addition to medical therapy.
- The decision to proceed with emergent valve surgery is based on the hemodynamic response to medical management. Indications for surgery are listed in Table 14.3.

ISCHEMIC MITRAL REGURGITATION

- Significant ischemic MR occurs in 3% of patients with an acute MI, 8% of those in cardiogenic shock, has a worse prognosis than other etiologies of MR, and 1-year mortality for patients with severe ischemic MR after an MI is 52% compared with 11% without MR.
- Papillary muscle rupture in the setting of MI represents the most dramatic presentation of ischemic MR and is a surgical emergency.
- Although this occurs in only 1% to 3% of patients with an acute MI, it accounts for up to 5% of infarct-related deaths, with an up to 70% mortality rate in the first 24 hours without surgical intervention.
- Acute MR occurs more frequently with inferior or posterior MIs and often leads to cardiogenic shock, but the longer-term outcomes if surgical correction is performed are similar to patients without papillary muscle rupture.
- Ischemic MR may also be secondary to papillary muscle dysfunction without rupture.
- The mechanism involves ischemic apical and posterior papillary muscle displacement and wall motion abnormalities, which result in tethering of MV leaflets and systolic tenting with incomplete valve closure.
- Intermittent papillary muscle dysfunction classically presents as recurrent episodes of dyspnea associated with pulmonary edema.
- A proposed algorithm for the management of patients with acute ischemic MR includes emergent surgery for acute ischemic MR with papillary muscle rupture, surgery or medical therapy for moderate to severe MR, and medical therapy for mild to moderate MR.

Acute Prosthetic Valve Dysfunction

CLINICAL PRESENTATION

- The clinical presentation is usually that of rapidly progressive HF with evidence of either prosthetic valvular regurgitation or stenosis.
- Acute prosthetic valve dysfunction related to thrombosis or endocarditis can manifest as thromboembolism (cerebral or peripheral).
- Normally functioning prosthetic valves are associated with various opening and closing clicks and systolic and, occasionally, diastolic flow murmurs.

■ A new or changing murmur may therefore signal a pathophysiologic alteration in function and, in addition, the absence or damping of normal characteristic valve clicks also suggests abnormalities.

PATHOPHYSIOLOGY

■ Acute prosthetic valve complications, may be classified as either structural or nonstructural leading to obstruction or regurgitation Table 14.7.
■ Mechanical valves have an extremely low risk of failure and usually last at least 20 to 30 years, but bioprosthetic valves have failed within 10 to 15 years.
■ Structural dysfunction owing to progressive tissue deterioration from cusp calcification is the main cause of bioprosthetic valve failure, which results in stenosis, abnormal coaption, or tears.
■ Progressive collagen deterioration is another common cause for prosthetic valve dysfunction. Mechanical prosthetic valves are more thrombogenic than bioprosthetic, with caged-ball valves having the highest thrombogenicity and bileaflet-tilting disk valves the lowest.
■ Formation of tissue overgrowth, thrombus, or perivalvular leaks contribute to nonstructural valve dysfunction in both bioprosthetic and mechanical valves (Fig. 14.12).

INVESTIGATIONS

■ As part of the initial evaluation, identification of the valve class, type, and model and the date of implantation is important.
■ The chest radiograph can be invaluable in assessing for the presence of HF and may provide evidence to the type of valvular prosthesis.
■ The ECG may show signs of LV overload, but these findings are not specific.

TABLE 14.7 ▧ Acute Complications of Prosthetic Valves

Structural Valve Dysfunction
Bioprosthesis
Valve degeneration: usually associated with leaflet calcification and tear
Mechanical Prosthesis
Ball or disk variance: change in ball or disk size and function owing to infiltration by lipid
Strut fracture (particularly with the older Bjork-Shiley valves)
Nonstructural Valve Dysfunction
Perivalvular leak
Thrombosis or pannus formation
Embolization
Hemolysis
Prosthetic valve endocarditis
Early (≤60 days postsurgery): occurs before endothelialization of valve, usually caused by *Staphylococcus epidermis* or *S. aureus;* occasionally gram-negative organisms or fungi may be implicated.
Late (≥60 days postsurgery): occurs after endothelialization of valve; caused by typical endocarditis organisms (*Viridans streptococci*, enterococci, and so forth)

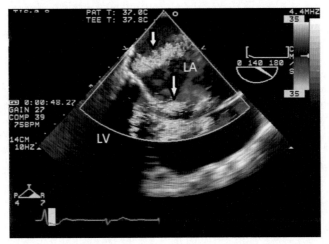

Fig. 14.12 Transesophageal echocardiogram shows a perivalvular jet of mitral regurgitation *(arrow)*. *LA*, Left atrium; *LV*, left ventricle.

- Anemia in association with an elevated serum lactic dehydrogenase level greater than 600 IU, suggesting hemolysis, is virtually never found in a normal functioning prosthesis and should raise the suspicion of perivalvular leak and hemolysis.
- Echocardiography is an essential tool in the evaluation of prosthetic valve dysfunction.
  - It serves the dual purpose of identifying the etiology of the valve abnormality and assessing LV function.
  - Doppler echocardiography to assess the color flow and pulsed wave, and continuous wave Doppler imaging should be performed to further interrogate the prosthesis.
  - Color Doppler flow mapping has several important applications in prosthetic valve disease:
    - Directing continuous-wave Doppler cursor parallel to the stenotic flow jet, allowing more accurate estimation of transprosthetic velocities and gradients
    - Semiquantitative evaluation of prosthetic valve regurgitation, which has been shown to correlate well with angiographically derived measurements
    - Differentiating valvular from perivalvular leaks
  - Expected values for different valve types can be found in the 2009 American Society of Echocardiography (ASE) Prosthetic Valve guidelines.
  - The transvalvular velocities measured by Doppler echocardiography correlate well with invasive measures in patients with native valve disease and after valve replacement.
  - When the valve orifice is smaller or more stenotic, the acceleration and velocity increase to maintain the same SV.
  - Using the Doppler-measured velocities proximal and distal to the valve, the pressure gradient or difference can be calculated.
  - Although transvalvular pressure differences are proportional to the degree of stenosis, variables, such as heart rate, contractility, CO, and the size and type of prosthesis, can alter the measured gradient.
- When transthoracic imaging is limited secondary to reverberatory artifacts caused by metallic components of a mechanical valve or technically difficult echocardiographic windows, TEE is a useful adjunctive tool.
  - Because imaging is performed without intervening cardiac structures, excellent delineation of valvular anatomy and function may be obtained.

- In addition, several studies have suggested that TEE may, in fact, be more sensitive and specific than TTE in the evaluation of partial valve thrombosis, aortic ring abscess, perivalvular leaks, and bioprosthetic valve degeneration.
- However, it should be emphasized that the combined approach of using TTE with TEE facilitates a more complete evaluation of LV function.
- In the case of acute prosthetic valve dysfunction with HF, pulmonary artery catheterization is essential for continuous hemodynamic monitoring and for helping to define therapeutic interventions.
- In some cases, simple fluoroscopy may be used to identify prosthetic valve dysfunction and assess the effects of thrombolytic therapy on abnormalities caused by clots that affect valve function.

TREATMENT

Congestive Heart Failure

- Medical management consists of reducing LA pressure and maximizing ventricular performance with a combination of vasodilators, diuretics, and inotropic support.
- Valve surgery is recommended in severe prosthetic valve stenosis and severe prosthetic valve or periprosthetic valve regurgitation with HF or intractable hemolysis.
- For high operative risk, yet symptomatic patients with bioprosthetic AoV stenosis or regurgitation, a transcatheter valve-in-valve procedure is now included as a class IIa recommendation in the AHA/ACC Valvular Heart Disease guidelines.
- Percutaneous repair is suggested for patients with severe perivalvular regurgitation with intractable hemolysis and New York Heart Association (NYHA) class III or IV HF who are at high risk from surgery.

Prosthetic Valve Endocarditis

- Specific management of prosthetic valve endocarditis (PVE) includes obtaining blood cultures and initiating empiric antibiotic therapy.
- In early infection within 2 months of implantation, the new valve apparatus has not endothelialized, allowing microorganisms direct access to the new structures from intraoperative contamination or hematogenous spread.
- In late infections, defined as 2 months or more after implantation, the valve apparatus has become endothelialized; thus, the pathogenesis is similar to that of native valve endocarditis.
- In addition to progressive HF, PVE may also be complicated by embolic phenomena or perivalvular leak (with or without hemolytic anemia).
- In the setting of aortic prosthetic valvular IE, the development of new AV conduction delay is specific for a valve ring abscess.
- The vast majority of patients with PVE will require valve replacement.
- Based on the 2015 AHA scientific statement regarding IE, early surgery during the initial hospitalization for antibiotic therapy is recommended for patients with PVE with one or more of the following:
  - Signs or symptoms of HF from valvular dysfunction
  - Heart block or valve abscess owing to perivalvular invasion
  - PVE caused by fungi or a highly resistant organism
  - Persistent bacteremia despite appropriate therapy
- Transcatheter heart valve endocarditis is an emerging complication of percutaneous valve replacement, at a rate of 0.3% to 0.4% per patient year.

- There is limited evidence regarding optimal treatment and surgical indications are made on an individual basis.

Prosthetic Valve Thrombosis (PVT)

- The incidence of PVT with currently available mechanical devices varies from 0.3% to 1.3%, with a rate of 6% with subtherapeutic anticoagulation.
- Mitral mechanical PVT is more common than aortic mechanical PVT.
- Although a major risk factor for PVT is inadequate anticoagulation, approximately 40% of patients have adequate prothrombin times at the time of presentation.
- This may be explained by the fact that PVT is a complex process that consists of a significant component of fibrous tissue ingrowth with associated secondary thrombosis.
- PVT may present acutely with HF or more indolently with slowly progressive symptoms of dyspnea and fatigue.
- A high level of suspicion must be maintained in any patient with a valvular prosthesis with nonspecific cardiac symptoms.
- TTE provides assessment of hemodynamic severity, whereas computed tomography (CT) imaging or fluoroscopy is often used to delineate valve motion and clot burden.
- TEE is useful in measuring thrombus size.
- Although the mortality rate for reoperation varies between reports, ranging from 4.5% to 35%, it tends to be high; there is a correlation between risk and advanced functional class.
- Options for the management of PVT include medical or surgical therapy.
  - The AHA/ACC valvular heart disease guidelines now include a class IIa recommendation for initiation of vitamin K antagonist agents in patients with suspected or confirmed bioprosthetic valve thrombosis who are hemodynamically stable based on case series data.
  - According to the AHA/ACC valvular heart disease guidelines, emergent surgery is a class I recommendation for patients with left-sided prosthetic valve thrombosis with NYHA class III to IV symptoms.
  - Surgery is a class IIa recommendation for left-sided prosthetic valve thrombosis that is mobile or large (>0.8 cm).
    - This is mostly based on a meta-analysis of seven observational studies that demonstrated that surgery for left-sided PVT with severe functional impairment was associated with significantly lower rates of thromboembolism, major bleeding, and recurrent PVT compared with fibrinolytic therapy.
    - Mortality rates and complete restoration of valve function did not differ significantly.
  - Fibrinolytic therapy (streptokinase or tissue plasminogen activator) for persistent valve thrombosis despite intravenous heparin therapy is a class IIa recommendation for right-sided prosthetic valve thrombosis or left-sided prosthetic valve thrombosis with:
    - Recent onset of symptoms (<14 days)
    - Stable thrombus (<0.8 cm^2)
    - NYHA class I/II symptoms.

Tricuspid Regurgitation (TR)

CLINICAL PRESENTATION

- The physical findings in acute TR are dependent, in part, on the severity of the RV volume overload.
- In the case of papillary muscle rupture or RV infarction, there may be hypotension and cardiovascular collapse.

- Most patients typically demonstrate findings consistent with right-sided HF.
- Usually a prominent "v" wave is visible in the jugular venous pulse and a holosystolic murmur along the left sternal border.
- The TR murmur increases in intensity with inspiration, a finding that differentiates it from MR.
- An S_3 gallop originating from the RV can be heard; abdominal examination may reveal a large and pulsatile liver.
- In general, peripheral stigmata of IE are absent when the tricuspid valve (TV) is affected and, if present, suggest paradoxic emboli or additional, left-sided valvular lesions.

PATHOPHYSIOLOGY

- Isolated, acute TR is a relatively uncommon medical emergency.
- The chronic form of TR, which predominates, usually results from annular dilation secondary to left-sided valvular pathology, severe LV dysfunction, or pulmonary hypertension (PH).
- In the current era, IE remains the most common cause of acute TR and is almost exclusively a disease of intravenous drug users.
- Despite antibiotic sterilization of the valve lesion, these individuals frequently develop ruptured chords or leaflet perforation.
- Occasionally, TR can be caused by a large, healed vegetation that impairs leaflet apposition.
- Rarer causes include nonpenetrating chest trauma and RV infarction.
- With the growing number of cardiac transplant recipients, an iatrogenic form of TR has been recognized, caused by damage from the bioptome during endomyocardial biopsy.

INVESTIGATIONS

- The ECG in cases of trauma may show right bundle branch block.
  - If the TR has been long-standing, there may be ECG criteria for RV hypertrophy.
  - RV infarction with acute TR rarely occurs in isolation and typically presents in conjunction with an inferior MI, which can be diagnosed by ST elevation in leads II, III, and aVF.
  - The presence of ST segment elevation in the right-sided lead V_4R confirms the diagnosis of an RV infarct and suggests that the patient may be at high risk for complications.
- The chest radiograph may show signs of cardiomegaly that represent RV and right atrium (RA) enlargement.
  - The presence of cavitary septic pulmonary emboli may also be seen with IE.
- As noted, blood cultures are an essential component of the diagnostic workup for patients with suspected IE.
- Pulmonary artery catheterization can be extremely helpful in confirming the diagnosis of pure TR and ruling out significant LV abnormalities.
  - The presence of a large "v" wave in the RA tracing with concomitant elevation in mean RA pressure usually signifies the presence of significant TR.
  - In addition, if the pulmonary artery and capillary wedge pressures are normal, the TR is likely to be related to primary dysfunction of the valvular apparatus and not secondary to left-sided heart dysfunction or PH.
- The diagnostic modality of choice for evaluating acute TR is two-dimensional and Doppler echocardiography.
  - The echocardiogram provides structural information about the TV, including detection of vegetations.
  - In addition, the severity of TR and RV dysfunction can be assessed and pulmonary artery pressures can be estimated using the modified Bernoulli equation.

- In general, TTE is satisfactory for assessing TV structure and RV function (Figs. 14.13 and 14.14).
- An important caveat, though, is that when the RV fails, flow directed into the pulmonary artery and backwards into the RA may be reduced so that the severity of PH or TR may be underestimated.
- TEE may not offer any significant diagnostic advantage over TTE.

TREATMENT

- The management strategy for acute TR should be focused primarily on medical therapy.
- Most patients can be treated effectively with a diuretic alone or in combination with an inotropic agent, such as dobutamine.

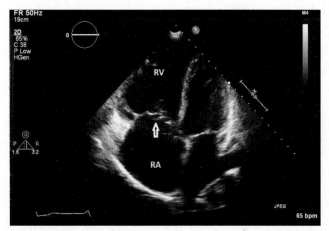

Fig. 14.13 Four-chamber transthoracic echocardiogram shows a flail tricuspid valve *(arrow)*. *RA*, Right atrium; *RV*, right ventricle.

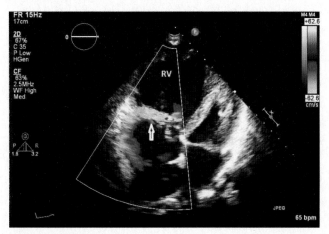

Fig. 14.14 Apical transthoracic echocardiogram with color Doppler, a flail tricuspid valve, and associated tricuspid regurgitation *(arrow)*. *RV*, Right ventricle.

- Milrinone, another inotropic agent, may be used as well, particularly in patients who have evidence of PH.
- In rare instances of acute massive TR, the patient who is refractory to medical therapy may require immediate surgical intervention.
- Whenever possible, TV repair, often with ring annuloplasty, is preferred over valve replacement.
- However, when valve replacement is required, a bioprosthetic valve is often used owing to a high incidence of valve thrombosis when mechanical valves are implanted in the tricuspid position.
- Other options include complete valve excision with no prosthetic replacement, valve repair after sterilization of the infection, and "vegectomy," which refers to isolated resection of the bacterial vegetation with preservation of the valvulochordal apparatus.
- Even with complete valve excision, many of these patients may continue to do well, with minimal symptoms of right-sided HF.
- The treatment of TR secondary to an inferior MI with RV involvement is revascularization.
- The type of revascularization procedure will depend on the nature of the coronary anatomy, extent of atherosclerotic disease, myocardial territory at risk, and LV function.

CHAPTER 15

Hypertensive Emergencies

Common Misconceptions

- Individuals with chronic hypertension are those most likely to develop a hypertensive emergency.
- The goal of treatment of hypertensive emergency is to achieve normal blood pressure as soon as possible.
- Nitroglycerin is a good choice for treatment of hypertension in the absence of ischemic chest pain or pulmonary edema.

Definition

- *Hypertensive emergencies* are characterized by elevations in blood pressure (BP) (>180/120 mm Hg) *with* organ dysfunction.
- Immediate BP reduction is essential.
- This contrasts with *hypertensive urgencies*, severe elevations *without* organ dysfunction, where a BP reduction over 24 to 48 hours is appropriate.
- Hypertensive emergencies and urgencies are referred to as *hypertensive crises*.
- Table 15.1 outlines definitions and management goals.

Incidence and Prevalence

- Approximately 1 billion individuals have hypertension worldwide.
- The prevalence is increasing, with 16% of the adults in sub-Saharan Africa and 27% in mainland China, owing to mass migration to urban settings and lifestyle changes.
- In the United States (US), the prevalence has increased from 24% to 29% from the 1990s to 2008.
- In France, Germany, Italy, Spain, and the United Kingdom, from 2010 to 2025, the prevalence of hypertension is anticipated to increase by 15% owing to population aging.
- Of patients presenting to the emergency department (ED), 1% to 6% will present with severe hypertension and one-third to one-half will have target organ damage, approximately 2 per 1000 ED visits.
- Risk factors include male sex, older age, and medication nonadherence.

Pathophysiology

- An abrupt rise in vascular resistance appears to be an initiating step and is accompanied by disruption of the arterial baroreflex.
- It is the rate of change, not the absolute degree of BP elevation, that increases the likelihood of target organ damage.
- Individuals with chronic hypertension have vascular changes that protect organs from BP changes, lowering the probability of a hypertensive emergency.

TABLE 15.1 ■ **Definitions of Hypertensive Emergency With Management Recommendations**

	2003 JNC 7 HTN Guideline	2013 ESH HTN Guideline	2013 ACCF/AHA STEMI Management Guidelines	2013 AHA/ASA Ischemic Stroke Guidelines	2010 ACCF/AHA Aortic Dissection Guidelines	2015 ACOG Acute, Severe HTN Guidelines in Pregnancy and the Postpartum Period
Definition	BP >180/120 mm Hg Associated with impending or progressive target organ damage	BP >180/120 mm Hg Associated with impending or progressive organ damage				SBP ≥ 160 or DBP ≥ 110 mm Hg In pregnancy or postpartum period
Management	Immediate BP reduction: <25% decrease in MAP within first hour. If stable, to 160/110–100 in the next 2–6 h; gradual reductions over next 24–48 h to a normal BP[a]	Prompt, but partial (<25%) BP reduction in the first few hours; proceed cautiously thereafter	Reduce BP to <180/110 mm Hg if fibrinolytic therapy is planned	Reduce BP if >220/120 mm Hg; If tPA planned, use IV antihypertensive medications to bring BP <185/110 mm Hg prior to tPA administration	Goals: heart rate <60 beats/min and SBP <120–100 mm Hg in acute abdominal or thoracic aortic dissection	Initiate fetal surveillance and if BPs remain severely elevated >15 min, begin intravenous antihypertensive therapy; delivery of the fetus may be necessary

[a]Exceptions include pregnant patients and patients with ischemic stroke or aortic dissection.
ACCF, American College of Cardiology Foundation; *ACOG*, American Congress of Obstetrics and Gynecology; *AHA*, American Heart Association; *ASA*, American Stroke Association; *BP*, blood pressure; *DBP*, diastolic blood pressure; *ESH*, European Society of Hypertension; *JNC 7*, The Seventh Report of the Joint National Committee on Prevention, Detection, Evaluation, and Treatment of High Blood Pressure 7; *MAP*, mean arterial pressure; *SBP*, systolic blood pressure; *STEMI*, ST elevation myocardial infarction; *tPA*, tissue plasminogen activator.

- Certain underlying conditions also predispose patients (Table 15.2).
- The causative mechanisms include endothelial injury, neurohormonal imbalance, and auto-regulatory dysfunction (Fig. 15.1).
- During the initial rise in BP, the endothelium maintains homeostasis through release of vasodilators such as nitric oxide and prostacyclin.
- When hypertension is sustained or severe, these are overwhelmed, leading to endothelial decompensation, rises in BP, and endothelial damage.

TABLE 15.2 ▓ **Underlying Causes of Hypertensive Emergencies**

Essential hypertension

Renal parenchymal disease

Acute glomerulonephritis

Vasculitis

Hemolytic-uremic syndrome

Thrombotic thrombocytopenic purpura

Polycystic kidney disease

Renovascular disease

Renal artery stenosis (atheromatous or fibromuscular dysplasia)

Pregnancy

Preeclampsia

Eclampsia

Endocrinopathy

Pheochromocytoma

Cushing syndrome

Renin-secreting tumors

Mineralocorticoid hypertension

Primary aldosteronism (adrenal aldosteronoma or adrenal hyperplasia)

Hypo- or hyperthyroidism

Hyperparathyroidism

Drugs

Sympathomimetics: cocaine, amphetamines, phencyclidine hydrochloride, lysergic acid diethylamide, diet pills, tricyclic antidepressants

Erythropoietin, cyclosporine, antihypertensive withdrawal

Monoamine-oxidase inhibitor interactions (tyramine pressor response)

Herbal supplements: ginseng, licorice, and ephedra (*ma huang*)

Lead intoxication

Autonomic hyperreactivity

Autonomic hyperactivity in presence of Guillain-Barré, Shy-Drager, or other spinal cord syndromes

Acute intermittent porphyria

Central nervous system disorders

Head trauma, cerebrovascular accident, brain tumors

Coarctation of aorta

Perioperative

Post coronary artery bypass grafting

Post carotid artery repair

Modified from Vaughan CJ, Delanty N. Hypertensive emergencies. *Lancet.* 2000;356:411–417.

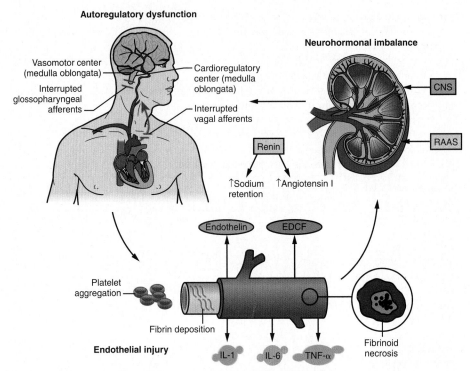

Fig. 15.1 Pathophysiology of hypertensive emergencies. Hypertensive emergencies are a complex consequence of biochemical vasoreactivity. Cerebral autoregulation is disrupted, as afferent feedback from the vagus and glossopharyngeal nerves to the medullary cardioregulatory and vasomotor centers is interrupted and vasomotor inhibition from descending general visceral efferents shifts toward sympathetic predominance. Endothelial control of vascular tone is overwhelmed as fibrin deposition and arteriolar fibrinoid necrosis contributes to increased endothelial permeability, platelet aggregation, and autocrine and paracrine release of vasoconstrictors. Endothelin-1, endothelium-derived contracting factor (EDCF), and inflammatory cytokines, including interleukin 1 (IL-1) and interleukin 6 (IL-6), and tumor necrosis factor-α (TNF-α) further compound systemic vasoconstriction and renal hypertensive damage. Acute changes in vascular resistance occur in response to excess aldosterone, antidiuretic hormone, and catecholaminergic influence on renal physiology, leading to increased renin production, sodium reuptake, and angiotensin II activity, causing potent vasoconstriction and further neurohormonal imbalance. *CNS*, Central nervous system; *RAAS*, renin-angiotensin-aldosterone system.

■ Local activation of the clotting cascade also ensues with platelet and fibrin deposition, and arteriolar necrosis leading to a vicious cycle of vascular injury, tissue ischemia, and release of vasoconstrictor substances.

■ Catecholamines, angiotensin II, vasopressin, and aldosterone also contribute to the pathophysiology of a hypertensive crisis.

■ Activation of the renin-angiotensin-aldosterone system (RAAS) leads to further vasoconstriction and induces expression of proinflammatory cytokines and vascular cell adhesion molecules, compounding vascular injury and vasoreactivity.

■ Aging, deconditioning, and chronic hypertension have all been implicated in baroreflex dysfunction.

■ Sympathetic inhibition (decreased peripheral resistance) and an increase in parasympathetic output (decreased heart rate and contractility) in response to BP rise never occur.

■ When coupled with acute endothelial damage, hypertensive emergencies ensue.

Evaluation and Management

- Patients with severely elevated BP (>180/120 mm Hg) should be screened for a hypertensive emergency. Up to 16% occur in patients without prior hypertension, such as children (acute renal disease), young women (eclampsia), and perioperative patients.
- The spectrum of hypertensive emergencies based on target organ damage is presented in Table 15.3.
- Evaluation should include duration, severity, and control of preexisting hypertension; antihypertensive drugs; and preexisting end-organ damage.
- The presence of concomitant illnesses (see Table 15.3) and other medications—including prescription drugs, over-the-counter preparations, immunosuppressive and recreational or illicit drugs—should be noted.
- Pregnancy status should be clarified along with family history predisposing to hypertensive crises.
- The most common presenting complaints are presented in Table 15.4; Table 15.5 provides additional guidance for history taking.
- The physical examination should start with serial BP measurements in both arms because BP differences between arms can result from aortic dissection (AD), coarctation, peripheral vascular disease, and neurologic or musculoskeletal abnormalities; a difference greater than 10 to 20 mm Hg is considered meaningful because each 10 mm Hg difference carries an increasing mortality hazard.
- Always treat the higher BP arm and repeat measurements on the same arm.
- The ocular fundi should be examined for acute hypertensive retinopathy.
- A third heart sound, elevated jugular venous pressure, and crackles on lung examination suggest pulmonary edema.
- An abdominal bruit suggests renal artery stenosis and an aortic aneurysm may be palpated.
- Discrepancies in peripheral pulses and the murmur of aortic regurgitation suggest AD.
- Focal neurologic findings, including visual field deficits and subtle cerebellar findings, are suggestive of a cerebrovascular accident or a mass lesion.
- Delirium or reduced consciousness is found in patients with hypertensive encephalopathy.
- The basic diagnostic evaluation includes a chemistry panel and complete blood count with a peripheral blood smear for microangiopathic anemia.
- A bedside glucose check should be done in patients with altered sensorium or neurologic deficits to exclude hypoglycemia or concomitant diabetes.
- Urine studies may reveal renal injury with proteinuria or hematuria.
- Additional studies include pregnancy testing and a urine drug screen.
- An electrocardiogram is needed to exclude acute myocardial ischemia and associated arrhythmias.
- A chest radiograph may demonstrate pulmonary edema from left ventricular failure or widening of the mediastinum caused by AD.
- Bedside ultrasound can be used to help identify acute AD, depressed myocardial function, and bladder outlet obstruction.
- Computed tomography (CT) or magnetic resonance imaging (MRI) may be needed to identify neurologic or vascular hypertensive emergencies.
- In select patients, measurement of plasma renin activity and aldosterone can be useful.
- Table 15.5 provides additional guidance for patient evaluation.
- Treatment of patients begins with appropriate monitoring—including serial BP assessments, cardiac telemetry, and intravenous access.
- BP reduction should not be deferred and an arterial line for continuous BP monitoring should be established.

TABLE 15.3 ■ Prevalence of Target Organ Damage in Patients With Hypertensive Emergency

Study	Inclusion Criteria: BP (mm Hg)	HTN Crisis, HTN Emergency, n (%)	MI/UA (%)	Acute Pulmonary Edema/Heart Failure (%)	Total CVA, Ischemic, Hemorrhagic (%)	Hypertensive Encephalopathy (%)	Acute Aortic Dissection (%)	Acute Renal Failure (%)	Eclampsia (%)
Pinna et al.,[a] 2014	≥ 220/120	1546 crisis 391 (25) emergency	70 (18) MI	121 (31)	86 (22) 60 (15) 26 (7)	19 (5)	31 (8)	23 (6)	–
Salkic et al., 2014	>180/120	85 crisis 14 (17) emergency	13 (93)	1 (7)	0	0	0	0	0
González et al., 2013	>180/120	538 crisis 412 (77) emergency	245 (60)	104 (25)	21 (5)	–	26 (6)	16 (4)	–
Martin et al., 2004	Diastolic ≥ 120	452 crisis 179 (40) emergency	14 (8) MI 9 (5) UA	45 (25)	104 (58) 70 (39) 34 (19)	0	0	0	7 (4)
Rodriguez et al., 2002	≥ 220/120	118 crisis 26 (22) emergency	15 (58)	4 (15)	5 (19) 4 (15) 1 (4)	2 (8)	0	0	0
Zampaglione et al., 1996	Diastolic ≥ 120	449 crisis 108 (24) emergency	13 (12) MI or UA	39 (36) 0	31 (29) 26 (24) 5 (5)	18 (17)	2 (2)	0	5 (5)
Total HTN emergencies[a,b]		1130 (100)	379/1130 UA	314/1130 (28)	247/1130 (22)	37/718 (5)	59/1130 (5)	39/1130 (4)	12/327 (4)

[a]In the Pinna et al. 2014 study, 391 patients were noted to have hypertensive emergencies, but only 350 are accounted for in their breakdown of target organ damage. This results in a shortfall of 10% in the sum of hypertensive emergencies (first row) and a shortfall of 5% in the sum of total hypertensive emergencies (last row).
[b]Studies that did not include these patients or target organ damage (denoted by –) were not included in the total HTN emergencies denominator.
CVA, Cerebrovascular accident; HTN, hypertension; MI, myocardial infarction; UA, unstable angina.

TABLE 15.4 ■ Presenting Signs and Symptoms in Patients With Hypertensive Emergency

Presenting signs or symptoms	N	%
Neurologic deficit	202/718	29
Chest pain	89/327	27
Dyspnea	81/327	25
Headache	65/327	20
Vertigo/dizziness	38/327	12
Nausea/vomiting	26/692	9
Syncope/faintness	16/287	6
Epistaxis	0/301	0

- The goal is a rapid but controlled reduction of the mean arterial pressure by 25% over several minutes to 1 hour.
- If the patient remains stable, then BP should be reduced to 160/100 to 110 mm Hg over the next 2 to 6 hours.
- If tolerated, further gradual reductions can be implemented in the next 24 to 48 hours.
- Exceptions to these include AD and hypertensive encephalopathy, which require more expeditious BP reductions.
- After BP has been controlled for 12 to 24 hours, oral agents may be initiated while intravenous agents are weaned.
- During hospitalization, patients should be evaluated for secondary hypertension (see Table 15.3), if indicated, and those noncompliant with medications should be interviewed for root causes and, if appropriate, alternatives should be offered along with lifestyle counseling and education.

Prognosis

- Untreated hypertensive emergency has a poor prognosis, with 1-year mortality rates as high as 79%.
- Mortality rates range between 2% and 4% in Europe and 5% and 10% in the US, but rates in developing countries are much higher.
- The major factor in prognosis is target organ damage.
- The most common cause of death is renal failure, followed by stroke, myocardial infarction (MI), or heart failure.

Specific Hypertensive Emergencies

CARDIOVASCULAR EMERGENCIES

Acute Coronary Syndrome

- BP goals for acute coronary syndrome (ACS) have not yet been established.
- There is an approximately 20% in-hospital mortality increase for every 10 mm Hg BP decrease at presentation.
- A systolic BP (SBP) of less than 100 mm Hg is associated with increased mortality risk, yet elevated BP (>140 mm Hg) is not.

TABLE 15.5 ▪ Pathogenesis, Presentation, and Evaluation of Hypertensive Emergencies

Condition	Pathophysiology/Risk Factors	Symptoms and Signs	Diagnostic Evaluation
Cardiovascular Emergencies			
Acute aortic dissection	Hypertension or congenital abnormality Intimal tear with dissection into media	Chest pain, back pain Unequal BPs (>20 mm Hg difference) in upper extremities	Widened mediastinum on chest radiograph Abnormal CT angiogram of chest and abdomen/pelvis or transesophageal echocardiogram of the aorta
Acute coronary syndrome/myocardial infarction	Thrombus or ruptured plaques in the coronary arteries leading to ischemia or infarction	Chest pain, nausea, vomiting, diaphoresis	Changes on ECG or elevated levels of cardiac biomarkers
Acute heart failure/pulmonary edema	Activation of the neurohormonal cascade, salt and water retention, increased vascular resistance, decreased cardiac output, increased pulmonary pressures	Dyspnea, chest pain or pressure Signs of heart failure on examination, including raised jugular venous pressure, crackles on chest auscultation, third heart sounds or gallop	Interstitial edema on chest radiograph
Neurologic Emergencies			
Hypertensive retinopathy	Vasoconstriction and choroidal ischemia results in optic disc edema Rupture of microaneurysms in retina (developed in response to chronic hypertension)	Blurred vision	Retinal hemorrhages and cotton wool spots (exudates), and sausage-shaped veins
Hypertensive encephalopathy/PRES	Hypertension leading to endothelial dysfunction, hydrostatic leakage across capillaries, and cerebral edema	Headache, altered mental status, nausea, vomiting, visual disturbance, altered level of consciousness, seizures (late)	May see papilledema, arteriolar hemorrhage, or exudates on funduscopic examination; may note cerebral edema with a predilection for the posterior white matter of the brain on MRI
Subarachnoid hemorrhage	Hypertension causing pseudoaneurysms and microbleeds	Headache, focal neurologic deficits	Abnormal CT of the brain; red blood cells on lumbar puncture
Intracerebral hemorrhage	Bleeding owing to autoregulatory dysfunction with excessive cerebral blood flow, aneurysm rupture, arteriopathy owing to chronic hypertension	Headache, new neurologic deficits	Abnormal CT of the brain
Acute ischemic stroke	Hypertension and atherosclerosis Thrombosis, embolism, or hypoperfusion	New neurologic deficits	Abnormal MRI or CT of the brain

Other Hypertensive Emergencies

Acute renal failure	Hypertension causing benign nephrosclerosis; Vascular, glomerular, and tubulointerstitial changes	Oliguria, hematuria (late); May have systolic or diastolic abdominal bruit	Urinalysis: proteinuria, microscopic hematuria, red blood cells, or hyaline casts; Chemistry panel: elevated BUN and creatinine, hyperkalemia or hypokalemia[a] hyperphosphatemia, acidosis, hypernatremia
Severe preeclampsia, HELLP syndrome, eclampsia	Primarily a disorder of first pregnancies; Possibly related to incomplete trophoblastic invasion and alterations in immune responses; Can occur up to 8 wk postpartum	Headache, visual disturbances, seizures, altered level of consciousness, congestive heart failure, right upper quadrant pain, oliguria	Proteinuria, normal or slightly elevated serum creatinine, thrombocytopenia, microangiopathic hemolytic anemia, elevated liver function tests
Acute perioperative hypertension	Sympathetic activation during induction of anesthesia; Exaggerated BP and heart rate response as anesthesia wears off (immediate postoperative period)	Bleeding unresponsive to direct pressure	Clinical diagnosis: manifestations of other hypertensive emergencies—such as myocardial ischemia, heart failure, renal insufficiency, and stroke
Sympathetic crisis[b]	Either direct or indirect effects on the sympathetic system	Anxiety, palpitations, tachycardia, diaphoresis, paresthesias	Clinical diagnosis in the setting of sympathomimetic drug use (e.g., cocaine, amphetamines) or pheochromocytoma (24-h urine assay for catecholamines and metanephrine or plasma fractionated metanephrines)

[a]Hyperaldosteronism (a secondary cause of hypertension) promotes renal potassium wasting.
[b]In this syndrome, acute end-organ dysfunction may not be measurable, but complications affecting the brain, heart, or kidneys may occur in the absence of acute treatment.
BUN, Blood urea nitrogen; CT, computed tomography; ECG, electrocardiogram; HELLP, hemolysis, elevated liver enzymes, low platelets; MRI, magnetic resonance imaging; PRES, posterior reversible encephalopathy syndrome.

- One trial even demonstrated a *protective* effect in patients with an SBP as high as 200 mm Hg.
- Thus, the only recommendation for BP control is for thrombolytic therapy to decrease the risk of intracerebral hemorrhage.
- Nitroglycerin should be given to patients with ongoing chest pain or pulmonary edema.
- For patients whose BP is refractory to nitroglycerin or who are experiencing ongoing ischemia or tachyarrhythmias (atrial fibrillation), intravenous β-blockers may be used.
- Of note, intravenous β-blockers are contraindicated in patients with hemodynamic instability owing to an increased risk of cardiogenic shock.
- Other agents with demonstrated risk reduction for patients with ACS, independent of BP lowering, include angiotensin-converting enzyme (ACE) inhibitors or angiotensin receptor blockers (ARB) and, in select patients, aldosterone antagonists (Tables 15.6 and 15.7).
- At discharge, a BP goal of less than 130/80 mm Hg is appropriate.

Aortic Dissection

Aortic dissection is discussed in Chapter 16. Management recommendations are given in Table 15.6.

Acute Pulmonary Edema

- Acute pulmonary edema in patients with severe hypertension may primarily be owing to transient diastolic dysfunction.
- Current recommendations include vasodilators and intravenous diuretics.
- Nitrates reduce BP, decrease myocardial oxygen consumption, and improve coronary flow.
- Diuretics improve symptoms but do not improve mortality.
- When hypertensive pulmonary edema is a result of ACS, nitrates are first-line agents.
- β-blockers should be reserved for atrial fibrillation with rapid ventricular response (see Table 15.6).

NEUROLOGIC EMERGENCIES

Hypertensive Encephalopathy/Posterior Reversible Encephalopathy Syndrome

- Headache, altered mental status, restlessness, and sometimes seizures and coma, in association with severely elevated BP, are recognized in the syndrome of hypertensive encephalopathy.
- Posterior reversible encephalopathy syndrome (PRES) is a disorder of reversible subcortical vasogenic edema, along the continuum of hypertensive encephalopathy.
- PRES is the consequence of disordered cerebral autoregulation leading to endothelial injury as well as the direct effects of cytokines on the endothelium.
- This leads to a breakdown of the blood–brain barrier, brain edema, and petechial hemorrhages (Fig. 15.2).
- The posterior regions are most susceptible to perfusion abnormalities owing to minimal sympathetic innervation.
- Manifestations include encephalopathy (50% to 80%), seizures (60% to 70%), headache (50%), visual disturbances (33%), and focal neurologic deficits.
- The onset is typically gradual, but some patients initially experience a seizure.
- At presentation, up to 20% of patients with PRES are normotensive or hypotensive, suggesting that proportional rise and rapidity of BP rise are important.

TABLE 15.6 ■ Hypertensive Emergencies: Specific Therapeutic Agents

Hypertensive Emergency	Agents to Use	Comments/Risks	Agents to Avoid
Cardiovascular Emergencies			
Acute coronary syndrome (ACS)	Nitroglycerin continuous IV infusion Metoprolol, bisoprolol, or labetalol IV bolus ACE I and ARBs IV bolus For cocaine-associated ACS, see hyperadrenergic states	Avoid nitrates in patients who have taken phosphodiesterase inhibitors for erectile dysfunction ≤ 24 h (48 h for tadalafil). Do not give β-antagonists in HF, low-output states, prolonged first-degree or high-grade AV block, or in patients with asthma/RAD or in those who use cocaine. ACE inhibitors may reduce infarct expansion/remodeling and chamber dilatation. Avoid ACE I and ARBs in patients who are volume depleted.	Avoid nondihydropyridine CCB (verapamil, diltiazem) in patients with left ventricular dysfunction or in combination with β-antagonists. Avoid carvedilol in patients with reactive airway disease owing to β₂ antagonism. Avoid nitroprusside and hydralazine (coronary steal). Avoid other diuretics.
Aortic dissection	Labetalol IV continuous infusion or esmolol IV, bolus, then continuous infusion Propranolol 1–10 mg IV bolus, then continuous infusion Verapamil, diltiazem IV Nicardipine IV continuous infusion (after β-blocker) Nitroprusside continuous infusion (after β-blocker)	Possible respiratory distress in patients with COPD and asthma given β-blockers; test dose of esmolol recommended; switch to diltiazem if esmolol intolerant. Always use β-blocker prior to vasodilators (nicardipine or nitroprusside). Avoid β-blockers, verapamil, and diltiazem in patients with aortic dissection complicated by aortic regurgitation: increased risk of reflex tachycardia.	Nitroprusside alone increases wall stress from reflex tachycardia; cyanide and thiocyanate toxicity in patients with reduced renal function or therapy >24–48 h. Avoid hydralazine: it increases wall shear stress and provides less accurate BP control.
Acute pulmonary edema	Nitroglycerin SL, topical, or IV continuous infusion Enalaprilat IV Nicardipine IV continuous infusion Nitroprusside IV continuous infusion Nesiritide IV	IV nitrates dilate capacitance vessels at low doses, higher doses dilate arterioles and lower BP. ACE inhibitors can worsen renal function, especially in patients who are volume-depleted. Use nicardipine with caution; some patients experience a negative inotropic effect. Nesiritide: Mixed outcomes; most recent ASCEND-HF trial showed no difference in dyspnea and mortality when compared with placebo.	Caution with nitroprusside: cyanide and thiocyanate toxicity in patients with reduced renal function or therapy >24–48 h.

(Continued)

TABLE 15.6 ■ Hypertensive Emergencies: Specific Therapeutic Agents—cont'd

Hypertensive Emergency	Agents to Use	Comments/Risks	Agents to Avoid
Neurologic Emergencies			
Hypertensive encephalopathy/ PRES	Clevidipine continuous IV infusion Nicardipine continuous IV infusion Labetalol continuous IV infusion Fenoldopam continuous IV infusion	Decrease MAP 10% to 15% in the first hour of presentation. Some recommend a target <160/100 mm Hg. Caution in the elderly and those with preexisting hypertension. Withdraw all immunosuppressive and cytotoxic drugs.	Cerebral perfusion autoregulation may be significantly impaired; avoid rapid reductions in BP. Avoid nitroglycerin; it may worsen cerebral dysautoregulation.
Subarachnoid haemorrhage	Nicardipine IV continuous infusion Labetalol IV bolus 10–20 mg or continuous infusion Esmolol IV bolus 500 µg/kg, then continuous infusion Clevidipine IV continuous infusion	All patients should receive nimodipine 60 mg PO q4h for vasospasm prophylaxis. The magnitude of BP control to reduce the risk of rebleeding has not been established, but current guidelines recommend that a decrease in SBP to <160 mm Hg is reasonable.	Avoid nitroprusside, as it requires more frequent titrations and increases the risk of iatrogenic hypotension and cerebral hypoperfusion.
Intracerebral hemorrhage	Nicardipine IV continuous infusion Labetalol IV bolus or continuous infusion	For patients with ICH presenting with SBP >220 mm Hg and without contraindication to acute BP treatment, acute lowering of SBP to 140 mm Hg is safe and can be effective for improving functional outcome.	Treatment with candesartan in the first week following intracerebral hemorrhage has been associated with worse functional outcomes.
Acute ischemic stroke	Labetalol 10 mg IV bolus, followed by IV continuous infusion or PO Nicardipine IV continuous infusion Lisinopril PO or SL	Antihypertensive treatment not recommended unless BP elevations are extremely high (SBP >220 mm Hg or DBP >120 mm Hg) or if the patient is eligible for thrombolysis. It is likely that the fate of the vulnerable ischemic penumbra has been determined by 10 h post-stroke onset. Once this period of vulnerability has lapsed, a benefit may be gained from BP reduction.	Caution with BP control efforts in patients taking oral β-blockers or clonidine; antihypertensive withdrawal syndrome may occur. Avoid ACE inhibitors and ARBs in patients who are volume depleted, as hypoperfusion may occur.

Condition	Drugs	Considerations
Renal insufficiency	Fenoldopam IV continuous infusion Nicardipine IV continuous infusion Clevidipine IV continuous infusion	Fenoldopam considered first line, as it improves natriuresis and creatinine clearance in these patients. Caution with ACE inhibitors and ARBs; they may cause hypotension and worsen renal function. Avoid β-antagonists, which reduce blood flow and GFR. Avoid nitroprusside owing to increased risk of cyanide and thiocyanate toxicity and no improvement in renal perfusion.
Preeclampsia/eclampsia	Labetalol 20mg IV bolus followed by 40mg, then 80mg Hydralazine 5–10mg IV bolus Nifedipine 10–20mg PO	Maximum 1 h IV labetalol dose of 220mg. Hydralazine lowers MAP more than labetalol; however, labetalol has a more rapid onset of action. Labetalol may cause fetal bradycardia. Women who receive oral nifedipine have faster BP reduction than those receiving intravenous labetalol or hydralazine. Avoid labetalol in patients with greater than first-degree heart block, bradycardia, or asthma. Avoid ACE inhibitors and ARBs; these are contraindicated in pregnancy. Avoid nitroprusside; it may cause maternal hypotension and is associated with fetal cyanide toxicity.
Perioperative hypertension	Clevidipine IV continuous infusion Nicardipine IV continuous infusion Labetalol IV bolus Esmolol IV infusion	Caution with IV β-antagonists in setting of myocardial ischemia or left ventricular dysfunction. Caution with nitrates in cardiac and vascular patients; a tachycardia may develop. Avoid ACE inhibitors and ARBs; their mechanism of action may be unpredictable and prolonged in a perioperative patient.
Hyperadrenergic state owing to sympathomimetic drugs	Benzodiazepine IV bolus Nitroglycerin SL, topical, or IV continuous infusion Phentolamine IV bolus or IM Dexmedetomidine IV infusion	Benzodiazepines are first-line agents; observe for respiratory depression. Dexmedetomidine adverse effects include hypotension, bradycardia, and sinus blockade. Use of mixed α-antagonists, β-antagonists (labetalol and carvedilol) is controversial; if given, administer along with a nitrate. Avoid all other β-adrenergic receptor antagonists owing to the potential of unopposed α-adrenergic stimulation, causing coronary vasoconstriction and BP increase.

(Continued)

TABLE 15.6 ■ Hypertensive Emergencies: Specific Therapeutic Agents—cont'd

Hypertensive Emergency	Agents to Use	Comments/Risks	Agents to Avoid
Hyperadrenergic state owing to abrupt cessation of anti-hypertensive agents	Restart original agent Labetalol IV bolus	Calcium channel blockers, phentolamine, nitrates may also be used.	
Hyperadrenergic state owing to pheochromocytoma and paraganglioma	Phentolamine IV bolus or IM	α-Receptor blockade is the cornerstone of BP control. There is a risk of reflex tachycardia with phentolamine, which can be treated with esmolol.	Avoid labetalol; paradoxic episodes of hypertension thought to be second-ary to incomplete α blockade may occur.
Hyperadrenergic state owing to autonomic dysreflexia	Nitroglycerin SL, topical, or IV continu-ous infusion Labetalol IV bolus Nicardipine IV infusion	Sit patient upright. First, address the underlying problem: pain, abdominal distension. Dexmedetomidine has been used with some success in refractory cases.	

ACE, Angiotensin-converting enzyme; *ARB*, angiotensin receptor blocker; *AV*, atrioventricular; *BP*, blood pressure; *CCB*, calcium channel blocker; *COPD*, chronic obstructive pulmonary disease; *GFR*, glomerular filtration rate; *HF*, heart failure; *ICH*, intracranial hemorrhage; *IM*, intramuscular; *IV*, intravenous; *MAP*, mean arterial pressure; *RAD*, reactive airway disease; *PRES*, posterior reversible encephalopathy syndrome; *SBP*, systolic blood pressure; *SL*, sublingual.

TABLE 15.7 ■ Therapeutic Agents for Hypertensive Emergency

Drug	Dosing (Intravenous)	Mechanism of Action	Adverse Effects/Risks
ACE Inhibitors			
Enalaprilat Onset: 15 min Duration: 6 h	0.625–1.25 mg q4–6 h Titrate at increments of 1.25 mg q12–24 h. Maximum of 5 mg q6h	Active metabolite of oral enalapril It blocks the formation of angiotensin II and causes a reduction in systemic vascular resistance and arterial BP.	Contraindicated in pregnancy. Patient's response may be unpredictable. First-dose hypotension is common, especially in high renin or volume-depleted patients. If first dose yields unsatisfactory results, use a second agent. Common side effects: angioedema, rash.
β-Receptor Antagonists			
Esmolol Onset: 1–2 min Duration: 10–20 min	Loading dose: 250–500 µg/kg over 1 min, then 50 µg/kg for 4 min, then increase dose by 50 µg/kg every 5 min up to 300 µg/kg/min.	β_1 receptor antagonist metabolized by bloodborne esterases Used primarily for short-term BP control (perioperative setting).	Avoid in patients with bradycardia, heart block, cardiogenic shock, decompensated heart failure, reactive airway disease. Avoid concomitant use of verapamil or diltiazem. Anemic patients will have prolonged half-life.
Labetalol Onset: 2–5 min Duration: 3–6 h Peak effect: 15 min	Bolus 10–20 mg (0.25 mg/kg for an 80-kg patient) over 2 min. May administer 20–80 mg as IV bolus every 10 min. Up to 300 mg total dose or 2 mg/min continuous infusion.	Nonselective β-antagonist with modest α_1-antagonist effects Has an α- to β-blocking ratio of 1:7.	Avoid in patients with bradycardia, heart block, cardiogenic shock, decompensated heart failure, reactive airway disease. Avoid concomitant use of verapamil or diltiazem. Prolonged effect in patients with liver impairment. Elderly may have a less predictable response, and increased risk of hypotension and adverse effects.
Calcium Channel Antagonists			
Clevidipine Onset: 2–4 min Duration: 5–15 min	Continuous infusion: start at 1–2 mg/h. Dose titration: double dose at short (90-sec) intervals initially. As BP approaches goal, increase dose by less than doubling and lengthen time between dose adjustments to every 5–10 min. Maximum dose: 16 mg/h.	Dihydropyridine L-type calcium channel antagonist Highly selective for vascular smooth muscle, reducing mean arterial BP by decreasing systemic vascular resistance. Has little or no effect on myocardial contractility or cardiac conduction. Metabolized by esterases in the blood and extravascular tissues; safe in patients with renal and liver dysfunction. Ideal for patients with labile BP.	Contraindicated in patients with egg or soy hypersensitivity Avoid in patients with advanced aortic stenosis. Avoid in patients receiving IV β-antagonists and in patients with decompensated heart failure. Lipid intake restrictions may be needed for patients with lipid metabolism disorders. Common side effects: headache, hypotension, vomiting, and tachycardia. Very limited data on doses at 32 mg/h

(Continued)

TABLE 15.7 ■ Therapeutic Agents for Hypertensive Emergency—cont'd

Drug	Dosing (Intravenous)	Mechanism of Action	Adverse Effects/Risks
Nicardipine Onset: 5–10 min Duration: 1–4 h	Continuous infusion: start at 5 mg/h, increase by 1–2.5 mg/h every 15 min. Maximum dose: 15 mg/h.	Dihydropyridine calcium channel antagonist Relaxes cardiac and smooth muscle cells and causes decrease in systemic vascular resistance, afterload, and arterial BP. Minimal negative inotropic effect.	Avoid in patients with advanced aortic stenosis. Avoid in patients receiving IV β-antagonists and in patients with decompensated heart failure. Dosing adjustment may be needed in patients with hepatic insufficiency. May cause worsening of GFR in patients with renal insufficiency. Common side effects: headache, hypotension, vomiting, and tachycardia.
Vasodilators			
Hydralazine Onset: 10–20 min Duration: 2–8 h	Bolus: 10–20 mg IV or 10–40 IM; repeat q4–6 h In pregnancy: bolus 5–10 mg IM or IV, then 5–10 mg every 20–40 min PRN or 0.5–10 mg/h infusion. Maximum total dose of 20–25 mg in pregnancy.	Preferentially relaxes arterial smooth muscle cells with little effect on veins, which reduces peripheral vascular resistance, afterload, and arterial BP with little or no change in preload or venous capacitance. Increases cardiac output, myocardial work, and myocardial oxygen demand.	Contraindicated in patients with acute aortic dissection. Avoid in patients with mitral valve disease (increases pulmonary artery pressure), renal impairment, volume depletion, CAD/ACS (reflex tachycardia), SLE and neurologic emergencies (increases ICP). Common side effects: reflex tachycardia, angina, fluid retention, headache, nausea, flushing, rash, dizziness.
Nitroglycerin Onset: 2–5 min Duration: 5–10 min	Continuous infusion: start at 5 µg/min. Increase by 5 µg/min every 3–5 min to 20 µg/min. If no response at 20 µg/min, increase by 10 µg/min every 3–5 min, up to 200 µg/min (many clinicians initiate with a higher infusion rate).	Nitroglycerin is converted by mitochondrial aldehyde dehydrogenase to nitric oxide, a potent venodilator. It causes venous capacitance vessel dilatation at low doses (5 µg/min) and arterial dilatation only at very high doses.	Avoid in cases of compromised cerebral and renal perfusion. Avoid concurrent use (within past 24–48 h) with phosphodiesterase 5 inhibitors (sildenafil, tadalafil, or vardenafil). Methemoglobinemia may occur. Common side effects: hypotension (especially in volume-depleted patients), reflex tachycardia, headache, nausea, vomiting.

Drug	Mechanism	Dosage	Considerations
Nitroprusside Onset: within seconds Duration: 1–3 min	Nitric oxide donor, which reduces both preload and afterload, can cause dose-related decreases in coronary, cerebral, and renal perfusion.	Continuous infusion: start at 0.5 µg/kg/min. Increase in increments of 0.5 µg/kg/min every 5–10 min; titrate to desired effect. Maximum dosage is 10 µg/kg/min IV for 10 min. For infusions 4–10 µg/kg/min, institute a thiosulfate infusion.	Avoid in patients with kidney or hepatic failure, atriovenous shunts, hereditary optic nerve atrophy (increases nerve ischemia), elevated ICP, or patients who are pregnant. Risk of cyanide and thiocyanate toxicity in patients with reduced renal function or therapy >24–48 h or at rates >2 µg/kg/min. Greater variability in BP response; needs more titrations than patients receiving nicardipine. Greater cardiac surgery mortality rates than with clevidipine. Nitroprusside is recommended only when other agents fail. Common side effects: hypotension, nausea, vomiting, cyanide, and thiocyanate toxicity.
Other Agents			
Dexmedetomidine Onset: 4–6 min Duration: 2–4 h	Centrally acting α₂-adrenergic agonist that is 8–10 times more selective to α₂-adrenergic receptors than clonidine. It decreases BP via a decrease in peripheral vascular resistance.	Loading dose: 1 µg/kg over 10 min, then 0.2–0.7 µg/kg/h (≤4 h).	Primarily used for light to moderate sedation in ICU settings; second agent for sympathomimetic hypertensive emergencies. Slight increase in blood pressure at the onset of infusion, lasting approximately 5–10 min. Common side effects: hypotension, bradycardia.
Fenoldopam Onset: 5–10 min Duration: 10–15 min	Peripheral dopaminergic-1 receptor agonist, which raises intracellular cyclic AMP and leads to vasodilation of most arterial beds, including renal, mesenteric, and coronary arteries.	Continuous infusion: 0.03–0.1 µg/kg/min Titrate no more than every 15 min by 0.05–0.1 µg/kg/min. Fenoldopam is approved for short-term use in adults (≤48 h) and children (≤4 h).	Avoid in patients with concomitant β-antagonist use and with elevated intraocular pressure or ICP. Avoid in patients with CAD (reflex tachycardia). May cause hypotension in patients receiving concomitant β-antagonist therapy. May cause hypokalemia or anaphylactic reactions in patients sensitive to sodium metabisulfite. Associated with hypokalemia (<3 mEq/L). Common side effects: headache, dizziness, reflex tachycardia, excessive hypotension, flushing

(Continued)

TABLE 15.7 ▪ Therapeutic Agents for Hypertensive Emergency—cont'd

Drug	Dosing (Intravenous)	Mechanism of Action	Adverse Effects/Risks
Phentolamine Onset: 1–2 min Duration: 10–30 min. Peak effect: 10–20 min.	Bolus 2–5 mg every 5–10 min (normally given IV, but also can be given IM).	Competitive α-adrenergic receptor antagonist $\alpha_1 > \alpha_2$ effects α_1 leads to relaxation of systemic vasculature, which leads to activation of the baroreceptor reflex, norepinephrine release, which is attenuated by phentolamine's effects on α_2-receptors, and a decrease in BP, which is accompanied by a rise, sometimes dramatic, in heart rate.	Contraindicated in patients with MI or CAD. Avoid in patients with neurologic hypertensive emergencies—has been associated with CVA owing to cerebral artery occlusion. Common side effects: hypotension, tachycardia, arrhythmias, angina, headache, nausea, vomiting.

ACS, Acute coronary syndrome; BP, blood pressure; CAD, coronary artery disease; CVA, cerebrovascular accident; GFR, glomerular filtration rate; ICP, intracranial pressure; ICU, intensive care unit; IM, intramuscular; IV, intravenous; MI, myocardial infarction; SLE, systemic lupus erythematosus.

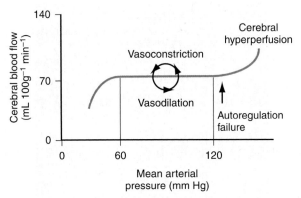

Fig. 15.2 Autoregulation of cerebral blood flow. Reprinted with permission from Elsevier, Vaughan CJ, Delanty N. Hypertensive emergencies. *Lancet.* 2000;356:411–417.

- A large percentage of patients have an autoimmune disorder, supporting theories of endothelial disruption.
- The diagnosis is made with T2-weighted fluid-attenuated inversion recovery (FLAIR) MRI (Fig. 15.3).
- Where neurologic deficits remain, the majority are believed to be caused by an intracerebral hemorrhage.
- The treatment goal is to reduce the SBP by 10% to 15% within the first hour and by 25% within the first few hours.
- Clevidipine, a dihydropyridine calcium channel blocker, has gained favor owing to its rapid action and ease of titration (see Table 15.6).

Subarachnoid Hemorrhage

- Subarachnoid hemorrhage (SAH) is a significant cause of morbidity and carries a mortality rate as high as 67%.
- Roughly half of survivors experience persistent neurologic deficits.
- The classic presentation is described as the "worst headache of my life" reaching maximal intensity within the first hour (thunderclap headache).
- Noncontrast head CT remains the cornerstone for diagnosis of SAH, with a negative predictive value of 99.9% if performed within 6 hours.
- The sensitivity of CT falls as time progresses, and to ensure a diagnosis, a lumbar puncture is required.
- Acute hypertension should be controlled after aneurysmal SAH and prior to aneurysm obliteration, but parameters for this have not yet been defined.
- The feared complication, cerebral vasospasm, occurs most frequently after 7 to 10 days.
- The cascade of events is initiated when oxyhemoglobin comes in contact with the abluminal side of the vessel.
- To prevent cerebral artery vasospasm, all patients should receive oral nimodipine.
  - Clinical trials have demonstrated a reduction in mortality by 74% and neurologic disability with nimodipine prophylaxis.
- If seizure prophylaxis is initiated, use caution with intravenous phenytoin and benzodiazepines, as these can further lower BP (see Table 15.6).

Intracerebral Hemorrhage

- Intracerebral hemorrhage (ICH) affects more than 1 million people worldwide annually.

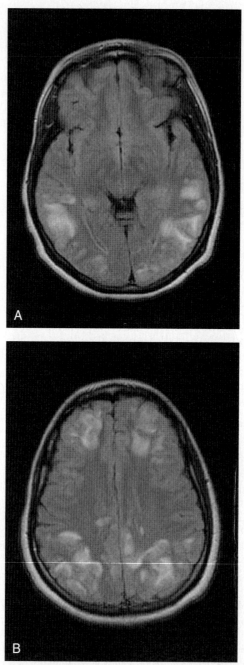

Fig. 15.3 Magnetic resonance (MRI) brain axial fluid-attenuated inversion recovery images showing radiographic features of posterior reversible encephalopathy syndrome. There is vasogenic edema resulting in a symmetric high signal within subcortical white matter of predominately parietal (A) lobes and occipital (B) lobes. These MRIs were obtained on a 16-year-old, postpartum female who presented with intractable headache and depressed sensorium.

- Elevated BP is extremely common, owing to stress, pain, increased intracranial pressure, and premorbid hypertension.
- The largest trial to date, the second Intensive Blood Pressure Reduction in Acute Cerebral Hemorrhage Trial (INTERACT II), demonstrated no statistically significant difference in the primary outcome of death or disability among patients randomized to an SBP target of less than 140 mm Hg compared with standard treatment (SBP <180 mm Hg).
- For patients with ICH presenting with SBP greater than 140 mm Hg, the American Heart Association (AHA) recommends consideration of antihypertensive therapy for improving functional outcome (Fig. 15.4).
- Nicardipine and labetalol are safe and effective in this population (see Table 15.6).

Ischemic Cerebrovascular Accident

- The acute hypertensive response is poorly understood, but because it occurs in transient ischemic attack as well as stroke, the Cushing reflex is likely not responsible.
- Up to 80% of patients with acute ischemic stroke are hypertensive on presentation.

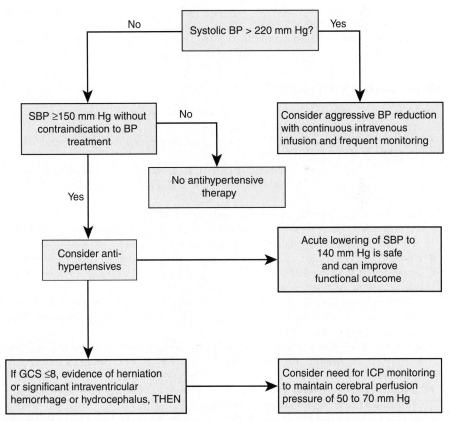

Fig. 15.4 Blood pressure management algorithm for patients with intracerebral hemorrhage. *GCS*, Glasgow Coma Scale; *ICP*, intracranial pressure; *SBP*, systolic blood pressure. Modified from Hemphill JC 3rd, Greenberg SM, Anderson CS, et al. Guidelines for the management of spontaneous intracerebral hemorrhage: a guideline for healthcare professionals from the American Heart Association/American Stroke Association. Stroke. 2015;46[7]:2032–2060.

- The elevated BP usually spontaneously resolves and, 10 days after the event, approximately two-thirds of patients are normotensive.
- In some, the response reflects poorly treated or long-standing hypertension.
- In others, it appears to be owing to other transient mechanisms, including anxiety surrounding the event or an abnormal autonomic response induced by the ischemic insult and direct injury to areas of the brain.
- Hypertension during acute ischemic stroke is an independent indicator of poor neurologic prognosis.
- Optimal management of BP remains unclear.
- Aggressive lowering of BP may reduce cerebral perfusion, aggravating brain ischemia and threaten the vulnerable ischemic penumbra.
- Conversely, very high BP may worsen cerebral edema and increase hemorrhagic transformation.
- Furthermore, evidence indicates that controlling hypertension immediately post stroke confers no benefit on short-term mortality or morbidity.
- Current guidelines recommend against lowering the BP unless BP elevations are extremely high (SBP >220 mm Hg or DBP >120 mm Hg) or if the patient is eligible for thrombolysis.
- Both US and European guidelines recommend BP reduction if thrombolysis is planned (goal <185/110 mm Hg).
- For the treatment of ischemic stroke, labetalol and nicardipine are the recommended agents. (see Table 15.6).

ACUTE RENAL INSUFFICIENCY

- Patients with acute renal insufficiency may present with peripheral edema, oliguria, loss of appetite, nausea and vomiting, orthostatic changes, or confusion.
- A patient with severely elevated BP with either new hematuria or a decline in renal function is a hypertensive emergency.
- Physicians should inquire about renovascular disease, renal parenchymal disease, autoimmune diseases (for possible vasculitis), renal artery stenosis, anatomic abnormalities, and renal transplantation.
- Patients should be asked about diuretics, and nephrotoxic and sympathomimetic agents.
- In patients with renal transplant, stenosis of the graft site, cyclosporine, steroids, and other immunosuppressants can predispose to a hypertensive emergency.
- Excessive renin secretion by the native kidney may also precipitate a hypertensive crisis.
- Evaluation of these patients includes a basic chemistry panel to reveal electrolyte abnormalities, creatinine elevation, and bicarbonate level.
- A bedside, postvoid residual sonogram may identify bladder outlet obstruction, in which case a bladder catheter should be placed followed by a renal sonogram to evaluate kidney size and higher urinary tract obstructions.
- BP management in renal hypertensive emergency cases includes fenoldopam, nicardipine, and clevidipine, because they reduce systemic vascular resistance while preserving renal blood flow.
- In patients presenting with severe hypertension owing to renal vasculitis, such as scleroderma and Takayasu arteritis, enalaprilat works well.

PREECLAMPSIA OR ECLAMPSIA

- Hypertensive disorders complicate up to 10% of pregnancies and account for up to 80,000 maternal and 500,000 perinatal deaths annually worldwide.

- From 1987 to 2004, the incidence of preeclampsia in the US increased 25%.
- This may be owing to the increased prevalence of obesity, changes in the diagnostic criteria, or earlier identification.
- Preeclampsia is characterized by severe hypertension (typically ≥ 160/110 mm Hg) beyond the 20th week of gestation.
- Diagnostic criteria no longer require the presence of proteinuria and instead incorporate other target organ damage (Fig. 15.5).
- Risk factors include maternal age 30 years or greater, high body mass index, nulliparity, absence of antenatal care, chronic hypertension, gestational diabetes, cardiac or renal disease, pyelonephritis or urinary tract infection, and severe anemia.
- Patients often complain of headache, visual changes, and nausea or vomiting. Health care providers need to remain vigilant even when mild disease is diagnosed.
- When seizures occur in the setting of elevated BP, this indicates progression to eclampsia.
- Patients with eclampsia can present from 20 weeks of gestation to 8 weeks postpartum.
- Impaired placentation of the trophoblast and incomplete vascular remodeling result in ischemia-reperfusion injury, oxidative stress, and a systemic inflammatory response.
- Endothelial dysfunction causes more vasoconstriction, BP elevation, and eventually end-organ damage (Fig. 15.6).
- Definitive treatment is delivery, but for preeclamptic women fewer than 34 weeks gestation, expectant management confers perinatal benefit with a minimum of additional maternal risk.
- In women 34 to 37 weeks gestation with nonsevere hypertensive disorders, delivery resulted in only minimal improvement in maternal outcome, with significant increases in neonatal morbidity.

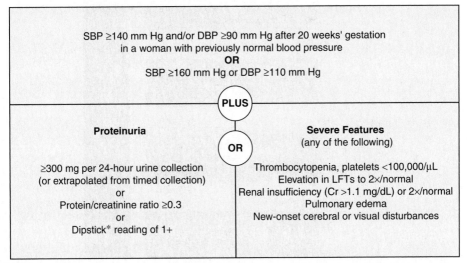

Fig. 15.5 Diagnostic criteria for preeclampsia. *Use only if other methods are not available. *Cr*, Creatinine; *DBP*, diastolic blood pressure; *LFTs*, liver function tests; *SBP*, systolic blood pressure. (Modified from Hypertension, Pregnancy-Induced—Practice Guideline. ACOG Task Force on Hypertension in Pregnancy. 2013;1–100. http://www.acog.org/Resources-And-Publications/Task-Force-and-Work-Group-Reports/Hypertension-in-Pregnancy.)

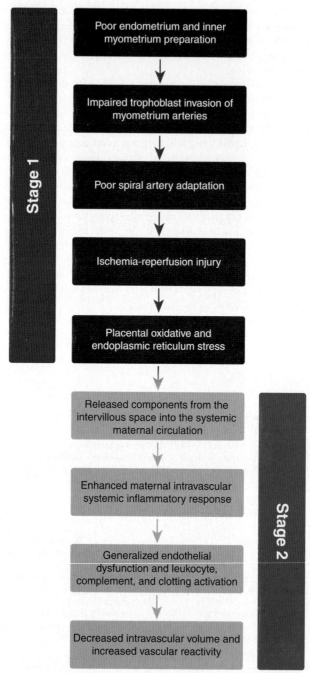

Fig. 15.6 Two-stage pathogenesis of preeclampsia. The first stage begins with poor preparatory remodeling and spiral artery adaptation, while the second stage is associated with exaggerated endothelial activation and a generalized inflammatory state. Reprinted with permission from Elsevier, Steegers EA, von Dadelszen P, Duvekot JJ, et al. Pre-eclampsia. *Lancet*. 2010;376[9741]:631–644.

- For preeclamptic cases of women with severe hypertension ($\geq$ 160/110 mm Hg) or elevated BP with target-organ damage, antihypertensive therapy is recommended with labetalol, hydralazine or nifedipine (see Table 15.6).
- Patients with severe preeclampsia or eclampsia should be given intravenous magnesium for seizure prophylaxis and treatment.

Perioperative Hypertension

- Perioperative hypertension generally occurs in patients with preexisting hypertension who are either untreated or inadequately treated preoperatively.
- The mechanism is multifactorial, including cessation of antihypertensive medications, sympathetic activation during induction and intubation, loss of vasodilation as anesthetic agents are weaned, and pain.
- Treatment of these patients can be difficult owing to hemodynamic instability: sudden changes in BP may be owing to release of catecholamines, fluid volume shifts, blunted baroreceptor response, renin-angiotensin activation, and reperfusion injury.
- The proinflammatory and hypercoagulable state of operative patients further contributes to vascular injury, platelet activation, and endothelial dysfunction.
- Complications include bleeding, cardiovascular events, and stroke and can occur in 5% to 35% of perioperative patients and carry a four-fold higher mortality risk.
- Postoperative hypertension may also lead to adverse events, including increased mortality, length of stay, and incidence of renal dysfunction.
- BP control in perioperative patients depends on the condition being managed operatively and what target organs are being affected or are at risk.
- The greatest experience in BP control has been in cases involving cardiac and vascular surgery.
- Perioperative BP control is associated with increased mortality in cases involving cardiac surgery.
- The composite safety endpoint of 30-day death, MI, stroke, or renal dysfunction did not differ among treatment groups (clevidipine, nitroglycerin, sodium nitroprusside, and nicardipine) in a recent study of cases involving cardiac surgery.
- In a meta-analysis, clevidipine was more effective in maintaining BP within prespecified ranges and demonstrated a reduction in failure rates compared with other agents.
- Other agents that have been used with success in patients undergoing cardiovascular surgery include nicardipine and labetalol (see Table 15.6).
- Following carotid procedures, patients frequently suffer from labile BPs that can last for days, owing to disruption of the baroreceptor reflex, carotid sinus, or vagus nerve during surgery.
- Hypertension can lead to hyperperfusion syndrome, in which resolution of the stenosis leads to hyperperfusion distal to the site, causing headache, seizure, intracranial hemorrhage, altered mental status, and focal neurologic changes.
- Intensive management of BP, with intravenous β-blockers or nitrates, decreases the incidence from 29% to 4%.
- Management of other perioperative hypertensive emergencies—such as myocardial ischemia, AD, left ventricular failure, and stroke—can be found in Table 15.6.

HYPERADRENERGIC STATES

Sympathomimetic Agents

- Sympathomimetic drugs—such as cocaine, amphetamines, phencyclidine hydrochloride (PCP), and lysergic acid diethylamide (LSD)—can precipitate a hypertensive emergency.
- Patients present with agitation, tachycardia, hypertension, mydriasis, and hyperthermia.
- Other agents include dietary supplements, such as *Ephedra sinica*, also known as *ma-huang*, which contains ephedrine generating an acute rise in BP and is associated with stroke, MI, and death.
- Although banned by the US Food and Drug Association in 2006, it can still be obtained via internet sources.
- Patients receiving monoamine oxidase inhibitor (MAOI) therapy who consume tyramine-containing foods may develop a hyperadrenergic state and resultant hypertensive crisis.
- Patients present with tachycardia, elevated BP, diaphoresis, chest pain, and—depending on the agent—mental status changes.
- Licorice can also cause acute elevations in BP, and complications may include PRES, as the active agent, glycyrrhizic acid, inhibits 11β-hydroxysteroid dehydrogenase, causing mineralocorticoid excess.
- Patients with MAOI toxicity often benefit from intravenous benzodiazepine.
- Phentolamine, nitroglycerin, and calcium channel blockers may also be used.
- Therapeutic options for these patients are presented in Table 15.6.

Abrupt Cessation of Antihypertensive Drugs

- An acute catecholaminergic syndrome may occur with the abrupt discontinuation of clonidine.
- This "rebound hypertension" often yields higher BP than pretreatment levels and is exacerbated by concomitant β-blocker therapy owing to unopposed α-mediated vasoconstriction.
- Elevations in BP have also been noted with acute cessation of β-antagonists, owing to adrenergic receptor up-regulation during the period of sympathetic blockade.
- Reinstitution of the original agent is preferred and will have the greatest effect on BP.
- Clonidine may be given orally at the patient's normal dose or, if unknown, 0.1 to 0.2 mg initially.
- A reduction in BP will occur within 30 to 60 minutes and peak at 2 to 4 hours.
- If additional BP control is needed, labetalol may be added.

Pheochromocytoma and Paraganglioma

- Tumors arising from chromaffin cells of the adrenal medulla and the sympathetic ganglia are referred to as pheochromocytomas and paragangliomas (extra-adrenal pheochromocytomas), respectively.
- Both have similar presentations and are managed in a comparable fashion.
- Patients may experience life-threatening hypertension, particularly in times of stress, that is, acute trauma, surgery, infection, or pregnancy.
- Patients with pheochromocytoma may present with ACS, prompting the term "the great imitator"; the diagnosis should be considered, especially in patients with normal coronary arteries.
- Features of pheochromocytoma include episodic headache, elevated BP, tachycardia, and flushed skin.
- Patient evaluation includes measurement of 24-hour urinary fractionated catecholamines and metanephrines in patients with a low suspicion of pheochromocytoma.

- In patients for whom there is a higher suspicion, free plasma metanephrines (drawn supine with an indwelling cannula for 30 minutes) is the best screening test owing to its high sensitivity (99%).
- This is also considered the best test for children at high risk, given its relative ease of collection compared with a 24-hour urine collection.
- Elevated metanephrines should prompt a search for the catecholamine-secreting mass, with CT as the initial diagnostic test.
- In patients for whom metastatic disease is suspected, MRI is preferred.
- Iodine metaiodobenzylguanidine (MIBG) scintigraphy can be done if suspicion is high, but no tumor is found with CT or MRI.
  - MIBG is a compound that resembles norepinephrine and is taken up by adrenergic tissue.
  - An MIBG scan is also helpful in identifying multiple tumors when the CT or MRI is positive.
- In patients with pheochromocytoma and a hypertensive emergency, intravenous phentolamine, a nonselective α-receptor blocker, is recommended.
- A short-acting β-antagonist, such as esmolol, may be needed to control reflex tachycardia.
- Definitive treatment is open surgical resection for large or invasive pheochromocytomas and for most paragangliomas and laparoscopic resection of isolated adrenal gland masses or small, noninvasive paragangliomas.
- In the preoperative setting, patients who are hypertensive but not in crisis may be treated and prepared for resection with oral phenoxybenzamine, a long-acting (irreversible), nonselective, α-receptor blocker for 7 to 14 days to allow adequate time to normalize heart rate and BP.
  - Phenoxybenzamine forms a permanent bond with α-receptors, preventing the binding of adrenaline and noradrenaline.
  - The α_1-receptor blockade in the walls of blood vessels leads to vasodilatation and a decrease in BP.

Autonomic Dysfunction

- Autonomic dysfunction caused by spinal cord or head trauma, intracerebral hemorrhage, or abnormalities, such as spina bifida, may present as a hypertensive emergency.
- Autonomic dysreflexia is well documented in patients with chronic spinal cord disease, but it can also occur <1 month after spinal cord injury.
- Typically, this occurs with injuries above T6, where exaggerated sympathetic responses to noxious stimuli below the level of the injury lead to diffuse vasoconstriction and hypertension.
- The parasympathetic response results in bradycardia and vasodilation above the level of the lesion and patients may complain of headache, flushing, and diaphoresis.
- This response, however, is insufficient to reduce elevated BP and may cascade into a hypertensive emergency and even cardiac arrest.
- Spinal cord injuries below T6 do not produce this complication, because intact splanchnic innervation allows for compensatory dilatation of the splanchnic vascular bed.
- Immediate interventions include sitting the patient upright and addressing causative factors—such as pain, fecal impaction, and abdominal distension (often owing to incomplete bladder emptying)—before pharmaceutical therapy.
- Agents for BP control include nitroglycerin, labetalol, and nicardipine.
- Several cases of paroxysmal autonomic instability with dystonia with BP control refractory to the aforementioned agents were successfully managed with dexmedetomidine, a central acting α_2 agonist.
- For additional guidance with pharmaceutical management of hypertensive emergencies, see Table 15.7.

CHAPTER 16

Acute Aortic Syndromes

Common Misconceptions

- A negative transthoracic echocardiogram excludes acute aortic dissection.
- All patients, irrespective of risk, presenting with symptoms suggestive of aortic dissection, need urgent CT to rule out acute aortic dissection.
- Coronary angiography must be performed on all patients prior to emergent surgical repair of aortic dissection.

Acute Aortic Dissection

- Acute dissection (AD) of the thoracic aorta is one of the most common catastrophic aortic conditions.
- The incidence is approximately 2.9 per 100, 000 per year.
- The variable clinical presentation in combination with a mortality rate of 1% per hour underscore the importance of a high index of suspicion and prompt diagnosis and therapy.
- There are two anatomic classification systems—the DeBakey and Daily (Stanford) systems—used to classify AD.
    - The DeBakey system is based on the site of origin of the dissection and recognizes three types (Fig. 16.1).
    - Because types I and II have a similar prognosis, the more widely used Stanford system classifies dissections that involve the ascending aorta as type A, and others as type B.
- Dissections are categorized as acute if the diagnosis is made within 2 weeks of symptom onset and chronic if more than 2 weeks, an important distinction as approximately 70% of patients with untreated AD die in the first 2 weeks after onset.

CLINICAL FEATURES

- AD most frequently affects patients in the fifth to seventh decades of life and is more common in men.
- In patients younger than 40 years, the incidence between genders is equal due to the occurrence of AD during pregnancy, with 50% occurring during the third trimester.
- Hypertension is present in 70% of type B dissections but only in 30% of type A dissections.
- Other major risk factors include bicuspid aortic valves and connective tissue disorders such as Marfan syndrome, Loeys Dietz syndrome, and Ehlers-Danlos syndrome.
- Additional predisposing factors for acute AD include pre existing aortic aneurysm (AA) and family history.
- Iatrogenic AD is an uncommon complication of invasive angiography and cardiac surgery and can usually be treated medically with serial examinations and noninvasive testing used to identify those in need of surgical therapy.
- Cardiac surgical procedures complicated by AD include those that cross-clamp or cannulate the ascending aorta, such as aortic valve replacement or coronary artery bypass grafting.

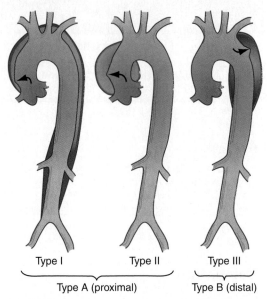

Type I   Type II   Type III

Type A (proximal)   Type B (distal)

Fig. 16.1 Classification of aortic dissection. Type I refers to a primary tear in the ascending aorta and dissection involving the aortic arch and descending thoracic aorta for a variable distance. Type II refers to dissection involving only the ascending aorta. Type III refers to a primary tear distal to the subclavian artery origin, extending distally for a variable distance. (Modified from DeBakey ME, Henly WS, Cooley DA, et al. Surgical management of dissecting aneurysms of the aorta. J Thorac Cardiovasc Surg. 1965;49:130–149.)

- Dissection usually occurs intraoperatively and is promptly diagnosed and treated, but chronic post operative AD has been reported.
- AD has also been reported in association with giant cell aortitis, Takayasu aortitis, rheumatoid arthritis, syphilitic aortitis, systemic lupus erythematosus, Noonan syndrome, Turner syndrome, fibromuscular dysplasia, annuloaortic ectasia, aortic coarctation, cocaine use, methamphetamine use, polycystic kidney disease, polyarteritis nodosa, trauma, and high intensity weightlifting.
- The patient with acute AD may have clinical manifestations of ischemia of various organ systems and symptoms and signs of cardiac disease which makes diagnosis difficult.
- Up to 55% of patients die without a correct diagnosis.
- The classic presentation of acute AD, present in over 70% of patients, is sudden severe anterior chest pain radiating to the back and moving distally.
  - Chest pain is more common with type A dissection (79%) vs. type B (63%), whereas back and abdominal pain are more common with type B dissection (64% and 43%) vs type A (47% and 22%).
  - Painless dissection is relatively uncommon but more likely in older patients or those with diabetes, AA, or recent cardiac surgery.
- A diastolic murmur of aortic regurgitation (AR) is heard in one-half to two-thirds of patients with type A AD.
- Heart failure, with proximal AD, is most often due to severe AR, but rupture into the atria or right ventricle have been reported.
- Myocardial infarction (MI), most commonly inferior, occurs in 5% of patients due to compromise of either coronary ostium by a hematoma or intimal flap.
- Peripheral pulse deficits are noted in 19% to 30% of patients, more commonly with type A AD, and are associated with a higher rate of in-hospital mortality.

- Acute lower extremity ischemia, as a result of dissection extending into the iliac arteries, occurs in 6% to 12% of patients.
- Syncope occurs in 5% to 10% of patients and is associated with a worse prognosis from either rupture into the pericardial space, producing cardiac tamponade, or involvement of the brachiocephalic arteries.
- Neurologic deficits—including cerebrovascular accident, disturbances of consciousness, ischemic paraparesis, and ischemic peripheral neuropathy—may also occur.
- Other, less frequent findings in association with acute AD include Horner syndrome, a pulsatile sternoclavicular joint, vocal cord paralysis, hemoptysis, superior vena cava syndrome, upper airway obstruction, hematemesis, pleural effusion, unilateral pulmonary edema, signs of mesenteric or renal infarction, fever, and deep venous thrombosis.

PATHOPHYSIOLOGY

- AD originates at an intimal tear in more than 95% of patients, exposing the media to pulsatile flow, creating a second or "false" lumen that dissects the outer layer of media, propagating distally and, occasionally, proximally.
- Ascending AD (50–65%) is twice as common as descending AD (20–30%).
- As the dissection encounters branches, it may pass around their origins, extend into them, or occlude them.
- Reentry of the dissection through a second distal tear may occur.
- Rupture of the AD into the pericardium is the most common cause of death, and acute heart failure is the second most common.
- Intimal tear without hematoma is an uncommon variant of AD without progression or separation of the medial layers.

INVESTIGATIONS

- The correct clinical diagnosis is made in less than 50% of patients, which can be improved by utilizing the AD risk score as follows.
  - Any high-risk condition (1 point) Marfan's syndrome, aortic valve disease, thoracic aortic aneurysm, recent aortic manipulation.
  - Any high-risk pain condition (1 point) Abrupt onset of chest, back or abdominal pain of severe intensity, ripping or tearing.
  - Any high-risk exam feature (1 point) Evidence of perfusion deficit (pulse deficit, systolic BP differential, or focal neuro deficit plus pain), new aortic insufficiency murmur (with pain), hypotension/shock.
- An AD risk score less than or equal to 1 and D-dimer less than 500 ng/mL rules out acute AD with sensitivity of 98.7%.
- The most common electrocardiographic (ECG) abnormality is left ventricular hypertrophy from hypertension.
- Acute changes occur in up to 55% of patients and include ST segment depression, T-wave changes, ST segment elevation and heart block.
- Chest radiography may be helpful in the diagnosis of AD, with abnormalities of the aortic silhouette being most common. (Fig. 16.2).
- Transthoracic echocardiography (TTE) demonstrating a dilated aortic root, widening of the aortic walls and a linear undulating echo representing the intimal flap has a positive predictive value of 100%, but a negative TTE does not exclude AD.
- Multiplane transesophageal echocardiography (TEE) has a sensitivity of 99% and a specificity of 98% in the diagnosis of aortic dissection.

- ■ CT with intravenous contrast is an accurate noninvasive screening test in patients with suspected AD.
  - ■ Advantages include ready availability at most hospitals and improved accuracy with spiral or multidetector CT. (Fig. 16.3).
  - ■ Disadvantages of CT include the need for iodinated contrast and nonportability.
- ■ MRI is a highly accurate noninvasive technique in the evaluation of patients with suspected AD.
  - ■ Advantages include being superior to TEE and CT in detecting arch vessel involvement and in identifying the anastomosis in patients managed with surgical therapy and may facilitate comparison of serial studies (Fig. 16.4).

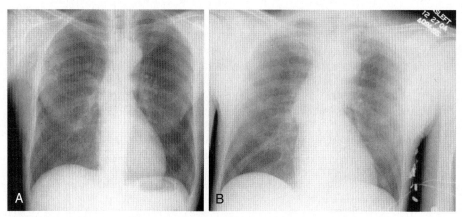

Fig. 16.2   Chest radiographs in a patient with aortic dissection. (A) Baseline anteroposterior chest radiograph before presentation with aortic dissection. (B) Chest radiograph 1 year later when the patient presented with acute aortic dissection. Note the increased diameter of the ascending aorta and aortic arch and new widening of the superior mediastinum.

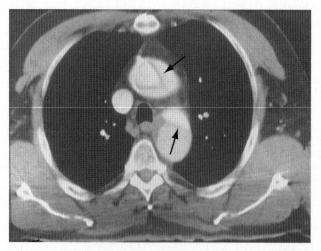

Fig. 16.3   Computed tomographic scan in a patient with type A aortic dissection. Note the complex intimal flap seen within the distal ascending aorta and descending thoracic aorta (arrows), and differential opacification of the true and false lumens.

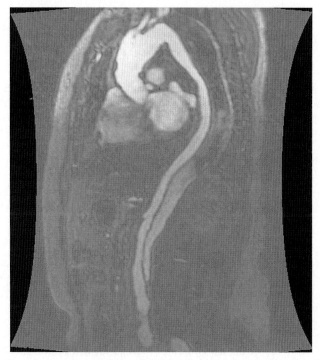

Fig. 16.4   Magnetic resonance imaging in the sagittal plane shows type A aortic dissection with an intimal flap extending into the distal abdominal aorta.

- Disadvantages of MRI include cost, time, reduced availability, and nonportability.
- Of the definitive noninvasive imaging techniques (TEE, CT, MRI), there is a pooled sensitivity (98% to 100%) and specificity (95% to 98%) between the three.
- The choice of test depends upon which is readily available and the patient's hemodynamic stability.

MANAGEMENT

- The initial treatment objectives are to reduce pain, blood pressure, and aortic shear stress to limit propagation of the dissection plane.
- In hypertensive patients, treatment consists of an intravenous (IV) β-adrenergic blocking agent, before, but often in combination with, IV sodium nitroprusside.
  - Intravenous labetalol in place of a β-blocker and sodium nitroprusside is an alternative, but it has the potential for hepatotoxicity with long-term therapy.
- In normotensive patients, an IV β-blocker may be used alone.
- Patients with acute AD type A should undergo emergent surgical repair unless significant comorbidities that limit survival to 1 year or less are present.
- **Coronary angiography before surgery does not improve survival and results in a delay in surgical intervention**.
- Resection of the ascending aorta and replacement with Dacron is the usual procedure in type A AD.

- With associated AR, resuspension of the valve is preferred, guided by intraoperative TEE.
- If there is associated annuloaortic ectasia or destruction of the aortic wall, a valved conduit may be used.
- The coronary arteries are reimplanted or bypassed.
- Aortic fenestration may be indicated in patients with organ or limb ischemia, which can effectively relieve the ischemia and can be performed safely in chronic AD.
- Operative mortality for AD type A at experienced centers varies from 7% to 36%, which is well below the 50% mortality without surgery.
- In-hospital mortality is approximately 14% to 27%, patients with cardiogenic shock and those requiring coronary artery bypass grafting being the highest-risk subgroup.
- Preliminary studies suggest that endovascular repair can be performed with minimal adverse effects on aortic valve function and sustained survival, but larger studies are needed to confirm the durability and to more accurately identify those patients most likely to benefit.
- With acute type B (type III) AD, urgent surgical intervention is reserved for patients who have a rupture, acute expansion or vascular occlusion.
  - Independent predictors of surgical mortality include age 70 years and older and hypotension or stroke on admission.
  - The optimal treatment for uncomplicated type III AD is less well defined, but the majority of patients are treated with medical therapy.
  - In-hospital mortality for these patients is approximately 10%.
  - Long-term medical therapy emphasizes control of blood pressure and periodic evaluation for progression of dissection, patency of the false lumen, aortic diameter greater than 5 cm, or saccular aneurysm.
  - The long-term survival rate with medical therapy is approximately 60% to 80% at 4 to 5 years and approximately 40% to 45% at 10 years.
  - The proximal descending thoracic aorta is the major site of aneurysm development; an enlarged false lumen in this region predicts poor outcome and subsequent aneurysm development.
  - Furthermore, partial false lumen thrombosis (34% of patients) predicts a significantly worse 3-year mortality rate.
  - An alternate approach is 2 to 3 weeks of pharmacologic therapy followed by surgical repair if the dissection becomes stable and the patient's general condition does not contraindicate surgery.
  - Endovascular intervention in AD type B may provide an alternative in highly selected patients.
  - Randomized trials comparing endovascular intervention and medical management have not demonstrated a significant difference in survival.
  - Postoperatively, continuation of β-blockade is essential, as hypertension and left ventricular ejection velocity play an important role in the recurrence of AD.
  - Following hospital discharge, noninvasive testing at periodic intervals (3, 6, and 12 months) to detect the development an aneurysm, dissection extension, false lumen patency, or progressive aortic dilation and then every 1 to 2 years if there is no evidence of progression.

Penetrating Aortic Ulcer

- Penetrating aortic ulcer (PAU) refers to an atherosclerotic lesion that undergoes ulceration, which penetrates the internal elastic lamina, resulting in formation of an IMH, a true saccular aneurysm, a pseudoaneurysm, or transmural aortic rupture.

- PAU shares several clinical features with AD, especially type B, but the absence of certain clinical signs suggests PAU.
- Results of noninvasive imaging studies are usually diagnostic.
- Differentiation between the PAU and AD is important as the natural history of PAU is less well defined; therefore, treatment may differ.

CLINICAL PRESENTATION

- The clinical presentations of PAU and acute AD are similar:
  - The most common presentation is an elderly patient with hypertension and the sudden onset of severe pain in the chest, back, and—less commonly—epigastrium.
  - Unlike AD, the pain is rarely migratory.
  - Since the most common site of PAU is in the descending thoracic aorta, a new murmur of AR, pericardial friction rub, and peripheral pulse deficits are not seen.
  - In addition, visceral vessel involvement has not been reported.
  - Neurologic deficits are very rare, but acute lower extremity paraplegia may occur.
  - In a patient with a history compatible with AD, the *absence* of physical findings suggests the diagnosis of PAU.
  - Asymptomatic PAU is usually incidentally discovered as enlargement of the descending thoracic aorta or a hilar mass on chest radiography or on CT.
  - The most common risk factors are advanced age, hypertension, and advanced atherosclerotic disease.
  - In contrast to AD, men and women are equally affected.
  - More than one-half of the patients have coronary, peripheral, or cerebrovascular disease.
  - An association of PAU and abdominal AA, and aneurysms in other locations, has also been reported.

INVESTIGATIONS

- Chest radiography may demonstrate mediastinal widening, focal or diffuse enlargement of the descending thoracic aorta, a hilar mass, left apical mass, bilateral or left pleural effusion.
  - Normal chest radiographic findings do not exclude PAU.
- The most common ECG abnormality is left ventricular hypertrophy from hypertension.
- The findings on CT, MRI, TEE, and aortography in patients with penetrating aortic ulcer are characteristic, differentiating PAU from AD.
  - In contrast to AD, an intimal flap or false lumen is not present; in addition, significant, often advanced atherosclerotic disease of the aorta, most commonly the descending thoracic aorta, is evident.
  - An echolucent intramural hematoma (IMH) with overlying advanced atherosclerotic disease is the most common TEE finding in patients with acute PAU.
  - When the IMH undergoes thrombosis, it becomes echogenic, creating the appearance of an increase in aortic wall thickness.
  - The IMH may extend proximally or distally for a variable distance from the entry site. Using CT, PAU manifests as focal involvement with adjacent subintimal hematoma and is often associated with aortic wall thickening or enhancement.
  - Magnetic resonance imaging is superior to conventional CT in differentiating acute IMH from atherosclerotic plaque and chronic intraluminal thrombus (Fig. 16.5).
- It should be noted that PAU is strongly associated with abdominal AA in 42% of patients, therefore imaging should be included in the initial evaluation.

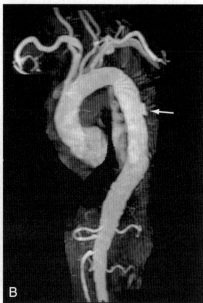

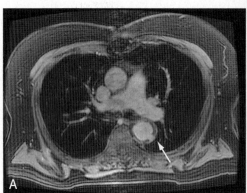

Fig. 16.5 Magnetic resonance (MR) imaging in a patient with multiple penetrating aortic ulcers. (A) Transverse imaging plane shows a penetrating aortic ulcer in the proximal descending thoracic aorta (arrow). (B) MR angiogram with gadolinium enhancement shows severe atherosclerotic changes of the descending thoracic aorta and a penetrating aortic ulcer in the proximal descending thoracic aorta (arrow).

MANAGEMENT

- The natural history of an IMH has been shown to follow a course of resorption of the hematoma and compensatory aortic dilation in the region in 85% of patients over 1 year.
- Patients with an IMH should be treated medically initially, preferably with a β-adrenergic blocking agent.
- Ascending aortic involvement, progressive aortic dilation, persistent symptoms, or hypertension that is difficult to control are indications for surgery.
- Thoracic endograft technology is being applied to patients with PAU involving the descending thoracic aorta with high procedural success and a low perioperative morbidity and mortality.

Aortic Intramural Hematoma

- Aortic intramural hematoma (IMH) is an acute, potentially lethal disorder pathologically distinct from acute AD.
- The prevalence of IMH among patients with acute aortic syndromes is 5% to 20%.
- The presentation and diagnosis of IMH are similar to AD, as are the classification scheme and general principles of management.

CLINICAL PRESENTATION

- Clinically, patients with acute IMH have a similar presentation to those with acute AD.
    - Sudden, severe chest and/or back pain are common in IMH.

- Anterior chest pain is more common with ascending (type A) lesions, whereas interscapular is more common with descending (type B) lesions.
- In contrast to AD, manifestations associated with aortic branch vessel disease (e.g., MI, stroke, AR, visceral vessel compromise, and paraplegia) are relatively uncommon.
- Patients with IMH are more likely to have type B lesions than those with classic AD (e.g., 60% vs. 35%).

PATHOPHYSIOLOGY

- Although hemorrhage into the aortic media occurs in both acute AD and IMH, an intimal tear with resultant false lumen is not present in IMH.
- Two mechanisms have been described: hemorrhage within the aortic wall owing to rupture of the vasa vasorum or rupture owing to an atherosclerotic PAU.
- IMH evolves very dynamically in the short term to regression, dissection, or aortic rupture.
- The most frequent long-term outcome of IMH is the development of aortic aneurysm (AA) or pseudoaneurysm.
- Lesions of the ascending aorta appear to represent the early stage of a classic dissection in some patients.
- Complete regression without changes in aortic diameter is observed in one-third of cases, and progression to classical dissection is less common (between 8% and 16%).
- A normal aortic diameter in the acute phase is the best predictor of IMH regression without complications, and absence of echolucent areas and atherosclerotic ulcerated plaque are associated with evolution to AA.
- IMH is most often associated with long-standing hypertension (50% to 84% of patients) but has also been reported in association with trauma in 6%.

INVESTIGATIONS

- The noninvasive imaging methods used to diagnose IMH are the same as those used in acute AD (TEE, CT, MRI).
- Exclusion of a dissecting intimal flap is a prerequisite for the diagnosis of IMH.
- Specific findings on TEE for IMH include crescentic or circumferential regional thickening of the aortic wall exceeding 7 mm, echolucent areas within the involved aortic wall, displaced intimal Ca^{2+}.
- CT and MRI will typically demonstrate a crescentic or circular high attenuation area along the aortic wall that does not enhance with contrast (Fig. 16.6).

MANAGEMENT

- The acute management of IMH and acute AD are similar.
- β-Blockade is indicated in all patients without absolute contraindications to their use.
- Surgical intervention is usually recommended in patients with type A IMH with a reduction in early mortality with surgical intervention as compared with medical management (14% vs. 36%), whereas aggressive medical therapy is the most common course for patients with type B IMH having a similar mortality with medical or surgical management (14% vs. 20%).
- Progression of disease in patients who are managed medically and survive the acute phase of the illness often occurs, although the rate of progression can be reduced in patients treated with β-blocker therapy acutely.
- Interestingly, in patients with ascending aortic IMH managed medically, the mortality rate is much lower as compared with patients with AD type A who do not undergo surgery.

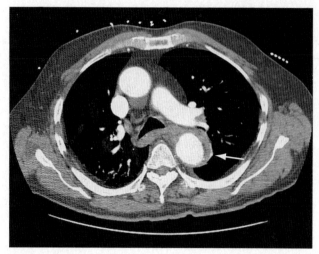

Fig. 16.6 Computed tomographic scan with contrast enhancement in a patient with sudden and severe chest pain shows a circumferential intramural hematoma involving the mid-descending thoracic aorta (arrow).

CHAPTER 17

Inotropic and Vasoactive Agents

Common Misconceptions

- Pulmonary artery catheterization plays no role in the evaluation and treatment of patients in the Cardiac Intensive Care Unit (CICU).
- Dobutamine is an appropriate treatment of hypotension, regardless of etiology.
- Milrinone is not used in combination with dobutamine.

Sympathomimetic Agents

DOPAMINE

- Inotropic and vasoactive agents are used to correct or stabilize hemodynamic function in the CICU setting (Table 17.1).
- Dopamine is the immediate precursor of epinephrine and norepinephrine.
- It has both cardiac and vascular sites of action, depending, in part, on the dose used.
- At low doses (1 to 3 µg/kg/min), dopamine directly activates dopaminergic receptors in the kidney and splanchnic arteries, thereby causing vasodilation of these beds.
- The resultant increase in renal blood flow leads to increased urine output and sodium excretion.
- At moderate doses (3 to 8 µg/kg/min), dopamine is a weak partial agonist of myocardial β_1-receptors and causes the release of norepinephrine from sympathetic nerve terminals in the myocardium and vasculature.
- The direct stimulation of myocardial β-adrenergic receptors exerts positive chronotropic and inotropic effects.

TABLE 17.1 ■ **Comparative Hemodynamic Effects of Commonly Used Positive Inotropic Agents**

	+ dP/dt	PCWP	SVR	CO
Dobutamine	↑↑	↓	↓	↑
Dopamine (low dose)	↔	↔	↓	↔↑
Dopamine (high dose)	↑↑	↑	↑↑	↑↔↓
Milrinone	↑	↓↓	↓↓	↑↑
Levosimendan	↑	↓↓	↓↓	↑

CO, Cardiac output; *dP/dt*, maximal rate of rise of LV pressure; *PCWP*, pulmonary capillary wedge pressure; *SVR*, systemic vascular resistance.

- The increased release of norepinephrine from nerve terminals (a tyramine-like effect) also contributes to myocardial stimulation but in addition may exert a mild vasoconstrictor effect due to stimulation of vascular α-adrenergic receptors.
- At high doses of dopamine (5 to 20 μg/kg/min), the effect of peripheral α-adrenergic stimulation predominates, resulting in vasoconstriction in all vascular beds and leading to increases in mean arterial pressure and systemic vascular resistance.
- At high doses, the vasoconstrictor effect overshadows the dopaminergic vasodilator effects so that renal blood flow decreases, and urine output may decline.
- However, in patients with acute decompensated heart failure, the dose required for improving systemic and renal hemodynamics may be higher (on the order of 4 to 6 μg/kg/min) than the usual low-dose range, leading to the suggestion that severe heart failure may impair the renal effects of dopamine.
- Low-dose dopamine is frequently combined with one or more other inotropic (e.g., dobutamine) or vasodilator (e.g., nitroprusside) agents.
- In patients with severe hypotension or frank cardiogenic shock, higher doses of dopamine are used to increase systemic vascular resistance.
- At these higher doses, the increased left ventricular afterload is partially offset by the positive inotropic action.
- In addition, when it is necessary to use vasoconstrictor doses of dopamine to manage systemic hypotension in the setting of myocardial failure, it is often useful to add dobutamine to augment the level of positive inotropic support beyond that provided by dopamine alone.
- When used alone at vasoconstrictor doses in patients with left ventricular failure, dopamine may increase both left and right heart filling pressures (Fig. 17.1).
- This effect reflects increased left and right ventricular afterload and increased peripheral venoconstriction, the latter causing increased return of venous blood to the heart.
- To counteract these actions, high-dose dopamine is sometimes combined with vasodilators (e.g., nitroglycerin).
- The inotropic responses to dopamine may be attenuated owing to desensitization of the β-adrenergic pathway and depletion of myocardial catecholamine stores, both of which are common in patients with chronic severe myocardial failure.
- Although generally well tolerated at low doses, higher infusion rates of dopamine may result in unwanted sinus tachycardia and/or arrhythmias (supraventricular and ventricular).
- Other adverse effects of dopamine include digital gangrene in patients with underlying peripheral vascular disease, tissue necrosis at sites of infiltration, and nausea at high doses.
- Local infiltration may be counteracted by the local injection of the α-adrenergic antagonist phentolamine.

DOBUTAMINE

- Dobutamine is a direct-acting synthetic sympathomimetic amine that stimulates β_1-, β_2-, and α-adrenergic receptors (Table 17.2).
- Clinically, dobutamine is available as a racemic mixture in which the (+) enantiomer is both a β_1- and β_2-adrenergic receptor agonist and an α-adrenergic receptor competitive antagonist, and the (−) enantiomer is a potent β_1-adrenergic receptor agonist and an α-adrenergic receptor partial agonist.
- The net effect of this pharmacologic profile is that dobutamine causes a relatively selective stimulation of β_1-adrenergic receptors.

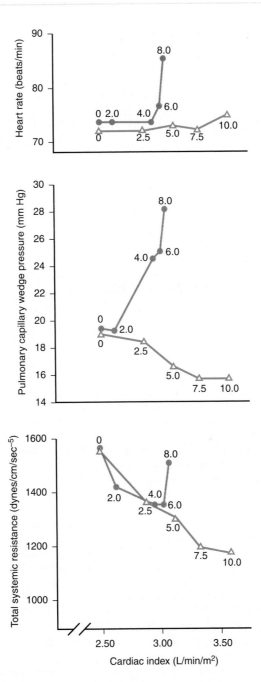

Fig. 17.1 Comparative effects of dopamine (*pink*) and dobutamine (*blue*) on heart rate, pulmonary capillary wedge pressure, and total systemic resistance in patients with moderate to severe heart failure. Each agent was titrated over the doses shown. These data illustrate that dopamine, when given alone at vasoconstrictor doses to patients with severe heart failure, increases left heart filling pressures. (Modified from Leier CV. Regional blood flow responses to vasodilators and inotropes in congestive heart failure. *Am J Cardiol*. 1988;62:86E.)

TABLE 17.2 ▨ **Receptor Activities of Several Sympathomimetic Agents**

	Myocardial	**Vascular**		
	β_1/β_2	α_1	β_2	**Dopaminergic**
Dobutamine	+++	++	++	0
Dopamine (low dose)	0	0	0	+++
Dopamine (high dose)	+++	+++	0	+++
Isoproterenol	+++	0	+++	0
Norepinephrine	+++	+++	+	0

0, No activity; +, low activity; ++, moderate activity; +++, high activity.

TABLE 17.3 ▨ **Intravenous Drug Selection in Patients With Elevated Left Heart Filling Pressures and a Reduced Cardiac Output**

Systemic Vascular Resistance	High	Normal	Low
Initial agents	Nitroprusside	Nitroprusside	Dobutamine
	Nitroglycerin	Milrinone	
		Dobutamine/nitroprusside	

- Dobutamine's primary cardiovascular effect is to increase cardiac output by increasing myocardial contractility with relatively little increase in heart rate.
- The drug causes modest decreases in left ventricular filling pressure and systemic vascular resistance owing to a combination of direct vascular effects and the withdrawal of sympathetic tone (Table 17.3).
- Dobutamine also directly improves left ventricular relaxation (positive lusitropic effect) via stimulation of myocardial β-adrenergic receptors.
- Although dobutamine has no effect on dopaminergic receptors and therefore no direct renal vasodilator effect, renal blood flow often increases with dobutamine in proportion to the increase in cardiac output.
- Dobutamine is a valuable agent for the initial treatment of patients with acute or chronic systolic heart failure characterized by a low cardiac output.
- It is often initiated at an infusion rate of 2.5 μg/kg/min (without a loading dose) and titrated upward by 2.5 μg/kg/min every 15 to 30 minutes until the hemodynamic goal is reached or a dose-limiting event occurs, such as unacceptable tachycardia or arrhythmias.
- Maximum effects are usually achieved at a dose of 15 μg/kg/min, although higher infusion rates may be used occasionally.
- If the maximally tolerated infusion rate of dobutamine does not result in a sufficient increase in cardiac index, a second drug (e.g., milrinone) may be added.
- In patients with elevated systemic vascular resistance and/or left heart filling pressures, the coadministration of a vasodilator, such as nitroprusside or nitroglycerin, may be required.
- In patients who remain hypotensive on dobutamine, consideration should be given to the addition of a pressor dose of dopamine and/or the use of mechanical support.
- Although dobutamine may increase heart rate, in some patients with very depressed cardiac output, the improvement in hemodynamic function may cause a withdrawal of sympathetic tone such that heart rate falls.

- Hypotension is uncommon, but it can occur in patients who are hypovolemic or who have unrecognized vasodilatory states, such as sepsis.
- Arrhythmias, including supraventricular and ventricular tachycardia, may limit the dose.
- Likewise, myocardial ischemia secondary to increased myocardial oxygen consumption may occur.
- Some patients with chronic severe heart failure may be tolerant to dobutamine, or tolerance to dobutamine may develop after several days of a continuous infusion.
- In this situation, the addition or substitution of a phosphodiesterase inhibitor may be helpful.
- Hypersensitivity myocarditis has also been reported with chronic infusions of dobutamine and should be suspected if a patient develops worsening hemodynamics in association with fever or peripheral eosinophilia.

ISOPROTERENOL

- A synthetic sympathomimetic structurally related to epinephrine, isoproterenol, is a nonselective β-adrenergic receptor agonist with little or no effect on α-receptors (see Table 17.2).
- Its cardiovascular effects include increased myocardial contractility, heart rate, and atrioventricular conduction owing to stimulation of myocardial β_1- and β_2-adrenergic receptors, and vasodilation of skeletal muscle and pulmonary vasculature owing to stimulation of vascular β_2-adrenergic receptors.
- Isoproterenol increases cardiac output and lowers both systemic and pulmonary vascular resistance.
- Owing to its propensity to increase heart rate, isoproterenol has relatively limited applications in the CICU.
- However, isoproterenol may be useful in the management of torsades de pointes that is refractory to magnesium, inotropic, and chronotropic support immediately following cardiac transplant, and treatment of pulmonary hypertension secondary to acute pulmonary embolism.
- Isoproterenol is usually administered as a continuous infusion at 0.5 to 5 μg/min. The dose of isoproterenol may be limited by tachycardia, increased myocardial oxygen consumption leading to ischemia, and atrial or ventricular arrhythmias.

EPINEPHRINE

- Like isoproterenol, epinephrine stimulates β_1- and β_2-adrenergic receptors in the myocardium, thereby causing marked positive chronotropic and inotropic responses.
- Unlike isoproterenol, it also has potent agonist effects at vascular α-adrenergic receptors causing increased arterial and venous constriction.
- Because of this latter effect, epinephrine (like high-dose dopamine and norepinephrine) plays little role in the acute management of heart failure, except when complicated by severe hypotension.
- Epinephrine may be useful for the treatment of low cardiac output, with or without bradycardia, immediately following cardiopulmonary bypass or cardiac transplantation.
- Continuous infusions may be started at a low dose (0.5 to 1 μg/min), and titrated upward to 10 μg/min, as needed.
- The use of epinephrine may be limited by tachycardia, arrhythmias, increased myocardial oxygen consumption leading to ischemia, and oliguria from renal vasoconstriction.
- In the setting of cardiac arrest, standard-dose epinephrine may be used as per the Advanced Cardiac Life Support (ACLS) protocol (1 mg intravenous push or via endotracheal tube

every 3 to 5 minutes) to manage asystole, ventricular fibrillation, pulseless ventricular tachycardia, or electromechanical dissociation.

■ In this scenario, high-dose epinephrine (0.1 to 0.2 mg/kg) is not recommended for routine use, except for special circumstances, such as for β-blocker or calcium channel blocker overdose.

■ Epinephrine may also be infused at 2 to 10 μg/min to manage symptomatic bradycardia that is unresponsive to atropine while awaiting placement of an external or temporary transvenous pacemaker.

NOREPINEPHRINE

■ The myocardial and peripheral vascular effects of this endogenous catecholamine are similar to those of epinephrine except that norepinephrine causes little stimulation of vascular β_2-adrenergic receptors and therefore causes more intense vasoconstriction (see Table 17.2).

■ Norepinephrine may be used to provide temporary circulatory support in the setting of hypotension (e.g., following cardiac surgery or with cardiogenic shock complicating acute myocardial infarction (MI) or pulmonary embolism).

■ Norepinephrine is infused at doses of 2 to 10 μg/min. As with epinephrine, the use of norepinephrine in the CICU may be limited by arrhythmias, myocardial ischemia, renal impairment, or tissue necrosis at the site of local infiltration.

MILRINONE

■ The breakdown of adenosine $3'$, $5'$-cyclic monophosphate (cyclic AMP [cAMP]) is mediated by a membrane-bound enzyme, phosphodiesterase (PDE).

■ In myocardium and vascular smooth muscle, the predominant isoform of this enzyme, termed type III, is inhibited by the type-III selective PDE III inhibitor milrinone, leading to an increase in intracellular cAMP concentrations.

■ In the myocardium, intracellular cAMP increases both contractility and the rate of relaxation (positive lusitropic effect).

■ PDE III inhibitors are also potent vasodilators in the systemic and pulmonary vasculature.

■ In patients with decompensated heart failure, type III PDE inhibitors increase cardiac output by increasing stroke volume.

■ Balanced arterial and venous dilation causes decreases in right atrial, pulmonary artery, pulmonary capillary wedge, and mean arterial pressures.

■ Because PDE inhibitors exert both positive inotropic and vasodilator actions, their net hemodynamic effects differ from those of dobutamine and nitroprusside.

■ For a comparable increase in cardiac output, milrinone decreases systemic vascular resistance and left ventricular filling pressure to a greater extent than dobutamine (see Table 17.3) (Fig. 17.2).

■ Conversely, for a comparable decrease in arterial blood pressure, milrinone increases cardiac output to a greater extent than nitroprusside (Table 17.4).

■ Milrinone is used to treat heart failure characterized by low cardiac output, high filling pressures, and elevated or normal systemic vascular resistance.

■ Milrinone may also be useful in the management of low cardiac output following cardiopulmonary bypass and as a bridge to cardiac transplant, especially in patients tolerant of dobutamine.

■ The positive inotropic effects of milrinone may be synergistic with those of sympathomimetics, such as dobutamine (Fig. 17.3).

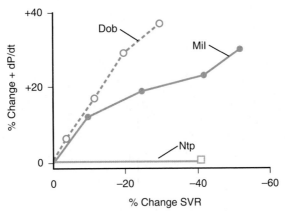

Fig. 17.2 The relative effects of dobutamine (Dob), milrinone (Mil), and nitroprusside (Ntp) on left ventricular contractility, as reflected by peak + dP/dt, and systemic vascular resistance (SVR) in patients with severe heart failure. Adapted from Colucci WS, Wright RF, et al. Positive inotropic and vasodilator actions of milrinone in patients with severe congestive heart failure. Dose-response relationships and comparison to nitroprusside. *J Clin Invest.* 1985;75:643.

TABLE 17.4 ■ Comparative Hemodynamic Effects of Intravenous Vasodilators

	PCWP	SVR	CO
Nitroprusside	↓↓	↓↓	↑
Nitroglycerin	↓↓	↔↓	↑↔↓
Milrinone	↓↓	↓↓	↑↑
Hydralazine	↓	↓↓	↔↑
ACE inhibitor	↓↓	↓↓	↑

ACE, Angiotensin-converting enzyme; *CO,* cardiac output; *PCWP,* pulmonary capillary wedge pressure; *SVR,* systemic vascular resistance.

- When excess β-blocking agents have been given, milrinone may be more effective than β-adrenergic stimulation for increasing cardiac output.
- In patients with heart failure, milrinone is administered as a 25 to 50 µg/kg intravenous bolus over 10 minutes followed by a constant infusion at 250 to 750 ng/kg/min.
- If a lower dose (i.e., 25 µg/kg) is used to initiate therapy and the response is not adequate, a second bolus of 25 µg/kg may be given before increasing the infusion rate.
- However, milrinone is frequently started without a bolus in order to avoid an excessive lowering of blood pressure.
- The dose is then titrated to the lowest dose at which the desired hemodynamic effect is obtained.
- With this approach, up-titration should occur at intervals of no less than 2 to 4 hours.
- The dose of milrinone tolerated may be limited by tachycardia or arrhythmias.
- In addition, patients who are relatively volume depleted may not tolerate its vasodilator effects and will experience hypotension that may necessitate stopping the drug.
- Thrombocytopenia is rarely seen with milrinone.

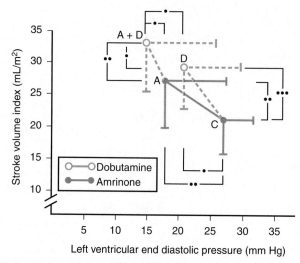

Fig. 17.3 Hemodynamic effects of dobutamine (D), amrinone (A) and the combination (A + D) in patients with moderate to severe heart failure. The additive effect of the two agents may exceed the effect of either agent alone. (Modified from Gage J, Rutman H, Lucido D, LeJemtel TH. Additive effects of dobutamine and amrinone on myocardial contractility and ventricular performance in patients with severe heart failure. *Circulation*. 1986;74:367.)

- Milrinone has a half-life of 30 to 60 minutes in patients with heart failure.
- It can be used alone or in combination with other agents (e.g., dobutamine or nitroprusside).

Calcium-Sensitizing Agents

- Positive inotropic agents, such as dobutamine and milrinone, act by increasing myocyte calcium influx; therefore, they may be associated with increased arrhythmias.
- An alternative approach that may avoid such complications is to enhance myocardial response to a given concentration of calcium with a class of molecules referred to as "calcium sensitizers," such as levosimendan.

LEVOSIMENDAN

- Levosimendan, the most widely studied calcium sensitizer, increases myocardial contractility by increasing myofilament sensitivity to calcium.
- Levosimendan is also a potent vasodilator owing to activation of adenosine triphosphate-dependent potassium channels in vascular smooth muscle cells leading to decreases in both preload and afterload.
- In patients with severe heart failure, levosimendan administration increases cardiac output and reduces pulmonary capillary wedge pressures and systemic vascular resistance (see Table 17.1).
- The hemodynamic effects are dose dependent at doses ranging from 0.05 to 0.6 µg/kg/min, with a higher incidence of side effects (headache, nausea, and hypotension) with doses above 0.2 µg/kg/min.
- Approximately 5% of a dose is converted to a highly active metabolite OR-1896 (that exhibits hemodynamic effects similar to those of levosimendan) with an elimination half-life of 75 to 80 hours (compared with 1 hour for levosimendan itself).

- Because of the long half-life of this active metabolite, these effects last for up to 7 to 9 days after discontinuation of a 24-hour infusion of levosimendan.
- Several clinical trials have evaluated the efficacy of levosimendan in patients with heart failure, compared with placebo or dobutamine.
- The data from these trials suggest symptomatic benefit with levosimendan in the short term in acutely decompensated patients, but with more frequent hypotension and arrhythmias.
- Levosimendan is approved for clinical use in several European and South American countries.

VASODILATORS

- For many patients with decompensated heart failure characterized by low cardiac output, high filling pressures, and elevated systemic vascular resistance, a parenteral vasodilator is the initial agent of choice, either alone or in combination with an inotropic agent (see Table 17.1).

NITROPRUSSIDE

- Nitroprusside is a sodium salt of ferricyanide and nitric acid, the reduction of which by intracellular glutathione leads to the local production of nitric oxide, which mediates the drug's potent vasodilator effect.
- The onset of action is rapid, in 1 to 2 minutes, making it an ideal agent for use in urgent situations that require rapid dose titration and a predictable hemodynamic effect.
- Nitroprusside is both an arterial and venous dilator; therefore, it reduces both filling pressures and vascular resistance (systemic and pulmonary).
- Stroke volume and cardiac output increase; pulmonary artery, pulmonary capillary wedge, and right atrial pressures decrease (Fig. 17.4).
- In patients with heart failure, heart rate is generally unchanged or may fall owing to reflex sympathetic withdrawal.
- The most common indication for nitroprusside is acute decompensated heart failure manifested by low cardiac output, elevated filling pressures, high systemic vascular resistance, and a systolic blood pressure adequate to maintain vital organ perfusion, usually 90 mm Hg or greater.
- This hemodynamic picture is often seen with acute MI, acute mitral or aortic regurgitation, and fulminant myocarditis.
- In acute MI, nitroprusside may be particularly useful if the infarction is complicated by significant hypertension, mitral regurgitation secondary to papillary muscle rupture, or rupture of the ventricular septum.
- Acute valvular regurgitation secondary to endocarditis, aortic dissection, or ruptured chordae is another situation in which nitroprusside may be used effectively, often as a bridge to more definitive therapy (e.g., valve replacement or repair).
- Nitroprusside is often used in patients with chronic heart failure owing to dilated cardiomyopathy, both to manage acute decompensation and to determine whether pulmonary hypertension is reversible during the evaluation for cardiac transplantation.
- Nitroprusside is often the parenteral agent of choice for treating hypertensive emergencies.
- A recent study showed increased cardiac output with nitroprusside administration in patients with severe aortic stenosis and left ventricular dysfunction presenting with severe heart failure, suggesting that it may be useful in this context as a bridge to aortic valve replacement or oral vasodilators.

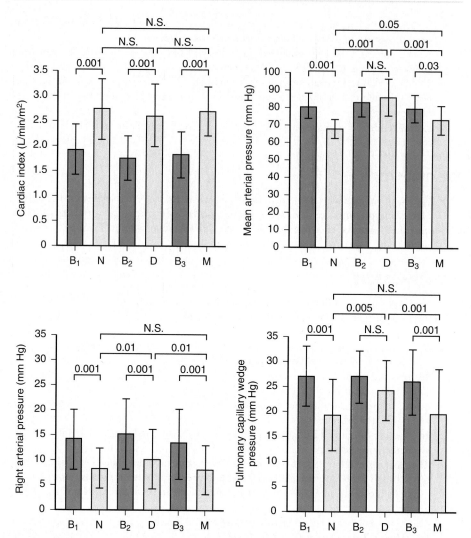

Fig. 17.4 Shown are the comparative effects of nitroprusside (N), dobutamine (D), and milrinone (M) on cardiac index, mean arterial pressure, right atrial pressure, and pulmonary capillary wedge pressure in patients with severe heart failure. The agents were administered in doses that caused comparable increases in cardiac index. Under these conditions, nitroprusside and milrinone significantly reduced mean arterial pressure, but dobutamine had no effect. All three agents reduced right atrial pressure, although the effect of dobutamine was less pronounced. Both nitroprusside and milrinone significantly reduced pulmonary capillary wedge pressure; this effect was significantly more pronounced than the effect of dobutamine. *N.S.*, non-significant. (Modified from Monrad ES, Baim DS, Smith HS, et al. Milrinone, dobutamine, and nitroprusside: comparative effects on hemodynamics and myocardial energetics in patients with severe congestive heart failure. *Circulation.* 1986;73:III168.)

- The infusion of nitroprusside should be guided by close hemodynamic monitoring, ideally with a pulmonary artery catheter and arterial line.
- Nitroprusside may be started at a rate of 10 to 20 µg/min and increased by 20 µg/min every 5 to 15 minutes until the hemodynamic goal is achieved (e.g., a systemic vascular resistance

of 1000 to 1200 dynes/sec/cm^5 and a pulmonary capillary wedge pressure of 16–18 mm Hg) while maintaining an adequate systolic blood pressure (generally ≥ 80 mm Hg).

- Doses of 300 μg/min or higher are seldom required and increase the risk of toxicity.
- Nitroprusside is a potent vasodilator and its use may be limited by hypotension.
- In patients with underlying coronary artery disease, drug-induced hypotension accompanied by reflex tachycardia may worsen myocardial ischemia.
- In patients with decompensated heart failure, hemodynamic deterioration may occur following the withdrawal of nitroprusside, apparently caused by a transient "rebound" increase in systemic vascular tone.
- Other adverse effects of nitroprusside are owing to the accumulation of its metabolites, cyanide and thiocyanate.
- The accumulation of cyanide results in lactic acidosis and methemoglobinemia and may manifest itself as nausea, restlessness, and dysphoria.
- Cyanide toxicity is most likely to occur in patients with liver dysfunction or following prolonged infusions, but may occur even in patients with normal hepatic function who have received the drug for only a few hours.
- If cyanide toxicity is suspected, serum levels should be drawn, and the infusion stopped.
- In severe cases, treatment with sodium nitrate, sodium thiosulfate, or vitamin B$_{12}$ may be necessary.
- Cyanide is converted in the liver to thiocyanate, which is cleared by the kidney.
- The half-life of elimination of thiocyanate is 3 to 7 days.
- Thiocyanate toxicity generally occurs gradually and is manifested by nausea, confusion, weakness, tremor, hyperreflexia, and, rarely, coma.
- Thiocyanate toxicity is more likely to occur in patients with renal insufficiency and with prolonged infusions or high rates of infusion.
- If mild, it can be managed by cessation of the drug; in severe cases, hemodialysis may be necessary.

NITROGLYCERIN

- When administered parenterally, nitroglycerin has an immediate onset of action and a plasma half-life of 1 to 4 minutes.
- It is cleared by vascular endothelium, hydrolyzed in the blood, and metabolized in the liver.
- At lower infusion rates, its main cardiovascular effect is venodilation, with a resultant fall in ventricular volumes and filling pressures.
- At higher infusion rates, nitroglycerin also causes arterial dilation, resulting in decreases in both pulmonary and systemic vascular resistances (see Table 17.4).
- In the setting of cardiogenic pulmonary edema, especially when caused by myocardial ischemia or MI, nitroglycerin provides immediate symptomatic relief and improves both hemodynamics and oxygen saturation.
- By causing direct coronary vasodilation, nitroglycerin also has the theoretic advantage of improving myocardial perfusion and limiting infarct size.
- Intravenous nitroglycerin is often useful in the treatment of patients with new-onset heart failure or acute decompensation of chronic heart failure, particularly in patients who are refractory to diuretic therapy and continue to manifest elevated right- and left-sided filling pressures, in patients with disproportionate right-sided failure, and in patients in whom nitroprusside is not tolerated.
- Intravenous nitroglycerin is usually started at a low infusion rate of 20 to 30 μg/min, and increased by 10 to 20 μg/min every 5 to 10 minutes until the desired response is observed or a dose of 400 μg/min is reached.

- In patients with decompensated heart failure, upward titration should be guided by filling pressures and systemic vascular resistance.
- While awaiting intravenous access, nitroglycerin can be administered by the sublingual, buccal, or transdermal route.
- Use of nitroglycerin may be limited by hypotension, which may require discontinuation of the drug and/or supportive care with intravenous fluids and leg elevation.
- Other common side effects related to vasodilation include headache, flushing, and diaphoresis.
- Some patients with significant right-sided failure and peripheral edema will not respond to the acute administration of nitroglycerin until they have been diuresed.
- In addition, patients may develop pharmacologic tolerance to nitroglycerin.
- Strategies to prevent the development of such tolerance include avoidance of excessive dosing, limiting fluid retention, and the use of intermittent dosing.

HYDRALAZINE

- Hydralazine is a potent direct-acting arteriolar smooth muscle dilator that causes both pulmonary and systemic vasodilation.
- Although nitroprusside and nitroglycerin are generally preferred as parenteral vasodilators in the acute management of heart failure, there are specific situations in which hydralazine given intravenously may be a useful or necessary alternative.
- In particular, hydralazine may be useful in patients who have become toxic with nitroprusside or continue to have an elevated systemic vascular resistance despite the use of a maximally tolerated dose of nitroprusside or nitroglycerin.
- In addition, hydralazine may be safely administered to pregnant patients with heart failure or severe hypertension.
- When used parenterally, hydralazine should be started at a low dose (5 mg given as an intravenous bolus every 4 to 6 hours), and increased gradually up to 25 to 30 mg, as tolerated.
- The onset of action is rapid, and the magnitude of the hemodynamic effects may be unpredictable.
- Blood pressure should therefore be monitored with an intraarterial line.
- Nausea may be a limiting side effect in the acute setting.

ENALAPRILAT

- Enalapril, a commonly used oral angiotensin-converting enzyme inhibitor, is cleaved by plasma and tissue esterases to form enalaprilat, the active form of the drug.
- When given parenterally, enalaprilat acts as a balanced vasodilator, resulting in decreased right- and left-side heart filling pressures.
- Enalaprilat is given as an intravenous bolus (0.625 to 1.25 mg every 6 hours).
- Although the onset of action is rapid (minutes), the duration of effect is prolonged (several hours).
- The major adverse effect is hypotension, which is more commonly seen in patients who are volume depleted.
- Enalaprilat may be of value in the treatment of acute decompensation in patients with chronic heart failure.
- However, owing to the somewhat unpredictable magnitude of the response and its prolonged duration of action, enalaprilat is not a first-line agent for the treatment of patients with heart failure.

Intensive Diuresis and Ultrafiltration

Diuretics

TYPES OF DIURETICS AND PHYSIOLOGIC EFFICACY

- Diuretics can be classified in terms of their site of action and behavior along the nephron (Table 18.1).
- With the exception of spironolactone and mannitol, diuretics are protein bound.
- Diuretics act from within the tubular lumen.
- Loop diuretics are transported from the plasma into the proximal tubular cells via organic anion transporters and from there are secreted into the luminal space.
- The quantity that enters the tubule depends on the intrinsic secretory capacity of the proximal tubule as well as the presence of other substances that also depend on cellular uptake via organic anion transporters, such as urea nitrogen and certain drugs.
- Loop diuretics selectively block the $Na^+/ K^+/Cl^{2-}$ cotransporter in the luminal membrane of the ascending loop of Henle and generate greater water loss than sodium loss, resulting in the production of hypotonic urine.
- Patients with an estimated glomerular filtration rate (GFR) of approximately 15 mL/min/1.73 m^2 secrete only 10% to 20% of the amount of loop diuretic secreted by patients with a normal GFR receiving the same dose.
- Patients with a reduced GFR require higher doses to elicit a diuretic response.
- In addition, in patients with a reduced GFR, the filtered load of extracellular fluid and sodium is lower, which limits the maximum achievable response to any further diuretic.
- Other factors that influence drug availability in the tubular lumen and diuretic response include the actual dose administered, absolute bioavailability (for orally administered drugs), renal blood flow, and the presence of competing drugs and metabolites.
- Diuretics have well-known side effects (see Table 18.1).

TABLE 18.1 ▓ Characteristics of Commonly Used Diuretics in Fluid Overload

Type of Diuretic	Site of Action	Physiologic Effect	Most Common Indications Related to Fluid Accumulation	Most Important Side Effects
Loop diuretics (furosemide, bumetanide)	Thick ascending limb of loop of Henle	Blockade of $Na^+/K^+/Cl^-$ cotransport system leads to inhibition of Na^+ reabsorption	AKI CKD CHF Chronic liver disease	Ototoxicity Hyperuricemia Electrolyte disorders Drug hypersensitivity
Thiazides (bendrofluazide, hydrochlorothiazide) Metolazone	Distal tubule; metolazone also acts on the loop of Henle	Blockade of Na^+/Cl^- transport system leads to inhibition of Na^+ reabsorption	CKD	Hyperglycemia Drug hypersensitivity Cholestatic jaundice Hepatitis Agranulocytosis
Aldosterone antagonists (spironolactone)	Aldosterone receptors in the distal tubule	Blockade of Na^+ retaining action of aldosterone	Chronic liver disease CHF	Gynecomastia Gastrointestinal side effects Drug hypersensitivity Agranulocytosis
Osmotic agents (mannitol)	Active in whole nephron following glomerular filtration	Reduced passive reabsorption of water	Cerebral edema	Skin necrosis (in case of extravasation) Renal failure Seizures
Potassium-sparing diuretics (amiloride, triamterene)	Late portion of the distal tubule and cortical collecting duct	Inhibition of K^+ secretion	To minimize K^+ loss during treatment with loop diuretics or thiazides	Hyperkalemia
ANP/BNP (nesiritide)	Afferent and efferent glomerular arterioles	Increase in GFR by dilation of afferent glomerular arteries and constriction of efferent arteries	Acute heart failure	Renal failure Skin necrosis (in case of extravasation)

AKI, Acute kidney injury; *ANP*, atrial natriuretic peptide; *BNP*, B-type natriuretic peptide; *CHF*, congestive heart failure; *CKD*, chronic kidney disease; *GFR*, glomerular filtration rate.

Indications for Intensive Diuresis

ACUTE DECOMPENSATED HEART FAILURE (ADHF)

- Volume overload and abnormal fluid distribution are defining features of ADHF and the main reason for hospital admissions and readmissions.
- Loop diuretics are administered in up to 90% of patients hospitalized for ADHF.
- The margin of safety of aggressive diuresis is determined by the amount of extravascular edema and the Starling curve of the individual patient.

- Patients with predominantly diastolic dysfunction are at greater risk of over diuresis than patients with severe systolic dysfunction.
- The management of fluid overload in ADHF is a clinical challenge owing to the lack of consistent data from randomized controlled trials and the resulting lack of formal evidence-based treatment guidelines.
- For decades, intravenous loop diuretics have formed the mainstay of therapy to reduce congestion and decrease ventricular filling pressures.
- However, many patients with ADHF with preserved ejection fraction are not substantially volume overloaded despite the presence of pulmonary or peripheral edema.
- In this case, removing too much volume may reduce the necessary preload and reduce stroke volume and cardiac output.
- Other potential risks from administering loop diuretics in this situation include the development of neurohormonal activation, hypovolemia and systemic vasoconstriction, electrolyte disturbances, and deterioration of renal function.
- For these reasons, aggressive diuresis should be avoided unless there is clear evidence of intravascular fluid overload.

CHRONIC KIDNEY DISEASE

- There are complex interactions between cardiac and renal function, and a large proportion of patients with CHF also suffer from CKD.
- In advanced CKD, urine output may be reduced, and patients often (but not always) develop progressive sodium and water retention.
- Loop diuretics are the preferred diuretics.
- Thiazides (with the exception of metolazone) cease to be effective when the estimated GFR falls to below 30 mL/min/1.73 m².
- Metolazone remains active in patients with a low GFR.
- As renal function deteriorates further and patients respond less well, renal replacement therapy (RRT) may be the only option to remove fluid.

CHRONIC LIVER DISEASE

- Chronic liver congestion and ascites are common features in patients with advanced heart failure.
- For large-volume ascites, there are two therapeutic strategies: paracentesis and administration of diuretics at increasing doses until an adequate amount of ascitic fluid has been removed.
- Randomized trials comparing both approaches support paracentesis as the method of choice.
- Although there is no difference with respect to long-term mortality, large-volume paracentesis is faster, more effective, and associated with fewer adverse events than diuretic therapy.
- Regardless of the strategy used, diuretics should be included in the maintenance therapy to prevent or delay recurrence of ascites.

Diuretic Resistance and Medical Management of Refractory Edema

- Diuretic resistance is a major problem as heart failure progresses and renal function deteriorates.

TABLE 18.2 ■ Mechanisms of Diuretic Resistance and Management Strategies

Mechanisms of Diuretic Resistance	Therapeutic Strategies
Variable enteral absorption owing to gut edema	Change from oral to intravenous administration
Worsening CKD	Increased doses of diuretics
Acute deterioration of renal function (owing to nephrotoxic exposure)	Discontinuation of nephrotoxins
Hypoalbuminemia	Correction of hypoalbuminemia
Severe proteinuria (binding of active diuretic within the tubular lumen)	Treatment of the underlying renal disease
Loop diuretic–induced compensatory distal tubular hypertrophy	Combination diuretic therapy
Co-administration of drugs that enhance fluid retention (fludrocortisone, minoxidil)	Discontinuation of competing drugs
Co-administration of drugs with high [Na⁺] (saline, piperacillin)	Discontinuation of competing drugs
Reduced cardiac output	Inotropic support
Intraabdominal hypertension	Measures to reduce intraabdominal pressure

CKD, Chronic kidney disease.

- Affected patients remain symptomatic and often need escalating doses of diuretics or combination therapies (Table 18.2).
- The significance of diuretic resistance is substantiated by data from large national registries showing that approximately 40% of hospitalized patients with heart failure are discharged with unresolved congestion.

COMBINATION OF DIURETICS

- The combination of alternative classes of diuretics creates a state of "sequential nephron blockade" in which multiple sites of sodium reabsorption are inhibited.
- Combinations of diuretics also reduce the risk of side effects from a single drug given at high dose.
- Thiazides and metolazone are often combined with loop diuretics.
- They inhibit sodium reabsorption in the distal convoluted tubule and thus can counteract compensatory distal tubular hypertrophy induced by loop diuretics.
- Although the combination can be effective in maintaining an acceptable fluid balance, few data suggest any mortality or morbidity benefit.

INTRAVENOUS BOLUS VERSUS CONTINUOUS INFUSION THERAPY

- Some evidence indicates that loop diuretics given as a continuous infusion are more effective than intermittent boluses, but the data are not consistent.
- In a randomized crossover study comparing bumetanide boluses with a continuous infusion in volunteers with CKD (mean estimated GFR 17 mL/min/1.73 m²), a greater net sodium excretion was observed during continuous infusion than with regular bolus administration despite comparable total 14-hour drug excretion.

- A randomized controlled trial comparing furosemide infusion versus bolus administration in 59 critically ill patients with fluid overload showed that patients in the bolus group needed a significantly higher total dose of furosemide to achieve target diuresis.
- Mean urine output per dose of furosemide was significantly higher in the infusion group, but there was no difference in hospital mortality, number of patients requiring ventilatory support, change in serum creatinine, or change in estimated GFR.
- The Diuretic Optimization Strategies Evaluation (DOSE) trial found no benefit of continuous-infusion furosemide compared with the same dose given intermittently in patient symptoms or change in renal function.
- However, the median furosemide infusion dose was only 6.7 mg/h.
- Based on these data, it appears that diuresis is easier to achieve with a continuous infusion of high-dose (20 to 40 mg/h) rather than low-dose furosemide, and the risk of toxicity appears to be reduced compared with high-dose intermittent bolus therapy.
- Superior diuresis has been found when a loading dose followed by higher infusion doses are used.

COMBINATION OF DIURETICS WITH ALBUMIN

- Severe hypoalbuminemia can contribute to diuretic resistance for several reasons.
    - First, albumin is necessary to deliver furosemide via renal blood flow to the proximal tubules, where it is secreted into the tubular lumen.
    - With hypoalbuminemia, the amount of diuretic delivered to the tubule is reduced.
    - Second, hypoalbuminemia reduces the intravascular volume available for removal.
    - Third, in patients with significant proteinuria, diuretics bind to albumin in the tubular fluid so that less active drug is available to interact with the tubular receptor.
- The role of albumin supplementation to overcome these problems remains unclear.
- In a study including patients with cirrhosis and ascites, the administration of premixed loop diuretic and albumin (40 mg of furosemide and 25 g of albumin premixed versus 40 mg of furosemide) did not enhance the natriuretic response.
- In contrast, a randomized controlled crossover study in 24 patients with CKD and hypoalbuminemia showed no significant differences in urine output between treatment with furosemide alone and furosemide and albumin at 24 hours.

Ultrafiltration

RATIONALE FOR MECHANICAL FLUID REMOVAL

- Ultrafiltration (UF) involves the removal of an iso-osmotic solution of plasma water and electrolytes from whole blood across a semipermeable membrane.
- During UF, the circulating blood volume is maintained by recruitment of interstitial fluid into the intravascular space (plasma refilling).
- The plasma refilling rate varies among patients and is dependent on the serum oncotic pressure and capillary permeability.
- Ideally, UF and plasma refilling should occur at a similar rate to prevent hemodynamic instability.
- When the rate of removal of plasma water exceeds the refilling capacity, hypotension develops.

OPTIONS FOR ULTRAFILTRATION

- Techniques to remove fluid mechanically include isolated UF and RRT with hemodialysis, hemofiltration, or peritoneal dialysis (Table 18.3).
- UF involves the removal of an iso-osmotic solution of plasma water and electrolytes, whereas RRT also provides clearance of metabolic and uremic solutes.
- Both techniques can be applied intermittently and continuously.
- Fluid removal is better tolerated when conducted with lower UF rates over longer periods of time.

TABLE 18.3 ▦ Options for Mechanical Fluid Removal

Modality	Blood Flow Rate (mL/min)	Fluid Removal Rate (mL/h)	Advantages	Disadvantages
SCUF	50–100	0–300	Slower and more sustained fluid removal	Immobilization
Intermittent UF	250–400	0–2000	Shorter procedure than continuous UF Anticoagulation not essential	Higher risk of hemodynamic instability
CRRT	50–100	0–300	Provision of UF and solute clearance Slower and more sustained fluid removal Less hemodynamic instability during fluid removal Adjustment of fluid removal to patient's needs at any time Requires some form of anticoagulation	Immobilization
IRRT	250–400	0–2000	Provision of UF and solute clearance Anticoagulation not essential	Higher risk of hemodynamic instability with fluid removal Fluctuating fluid balance Metabolic fluctuations
Peritoneal dialysis	Not applicable	0–500	UF and solute clearance No need for venous access Reduced risk of hemodynamic instability No need for anticoagulation	Need for peritoneal catheter Contraindicated in patients immediately after abdominal surgery Special expertise required

CRRT, Continuous renal replacement therapy; IRRT, intermittent renal replacement therapy; SCUF, slow continuous ultrafiltration; UF, ultrafiltration.
Modified from Rosner MH, Ostermann M, Murugan R, et al. Indications and management of mechanical fluid removal in critical illness. Br J Anaesth. 2014;113(5):764–771.

BENEFITS OF ULTRAFILTRATION

- Compared with diuretic therapy, fluid removal by extracorporeal techniques is fully controllable and adjustable.
- It is a strategy to reset fluid status to euvolemia (Fig. 18.1).
- The fluid removed with extracorporeal techniques is isotonic, whereas urine produced following diuretic administration is usually hypotonic.
- In patients with acute decompensated heart failure, the average urinary sodium concentration after furosemide administration is 60 mmol/L, leaving behind 80 mmol of excess sodium for every liter of urine output.
- This, combined with neurohormonal activation, may explain why the initial weight loss after diuretics is rapidly regained.
- By restoring euvolemia and removing sodium, UF may be successful at restoring diuretic responsiveness.

INDICATIONS FOR MECHANICAL FLUID REMOVAL

- The indications for mechanical fluid removal depend predominantly on the impact that fluid overload has on the patient, the expected clinical trajectory, the likelihood of successful fluid removal with pharmacologic measures, and the risk of serious side effects from diuretics (Fig. 18.2).
- The Acute Disease Quality Initiative (ADQI) expert group suggested the following indications for mechanical fluid removal:
  - Fluid overload after pharmacologic failure, that is, patients with fluid overload who have not responded adequately to diuretics.
  - Presence of serious adverse effects of diuretics, that is, patients with fluid overload who need to discontinue diuretics.

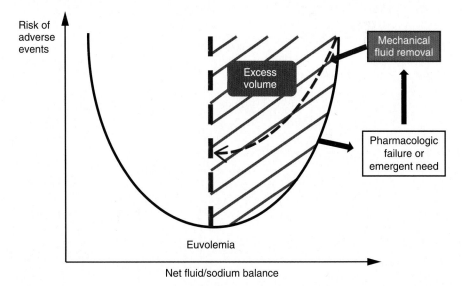

Fig. 18.1 Management of fluid overload during critical illness.

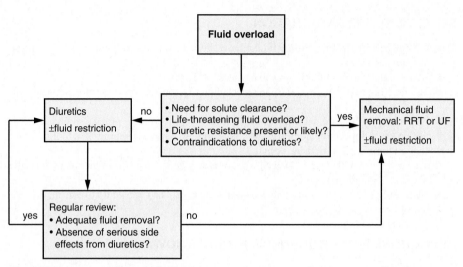

Fig. 18.2 Algorithm for management of cardiac cases involving patients with fluid overload. *RRT*, Renal replacement therapy; *UF*, ultrafiltration.

- High chance of diuretic failure, that is, patients with fluid overload and significantly impaired renal function in whom treatment with diuretics is unlikely to be effective in a timely manner and in whom the risk of prolonged and progressive fluid overload is high.
- Combined fluid overload and solute accumulation, that is, patients who need both fluid removal and solute clearance.
- In cases of localized fluid accumulation in a confined compartment, such as isolated pleural effusions or large-volume ascites, UF is less likely to be effective and fluid removal by direct drainage should be considered.

CHAPTER 19

Antidysrhythmic Electrophysiology and Pharmacotherapy

Common Misconceptions

- Lidocaine is used to prevent ventricular tachycardia following acute myocardial infarction.
- Only β-blockers with $β_2$ selectivity precipitate bronchospasm.
- Amiodarone should be avoided in patients with left ventricular dysfunction.

- Cardiac arrhythmias are common in critically ill patients.
- Patients with coronary artery disease (CAD), heart failure (HF), respiratory failure, or renal failure are at risk for different arrhythmias, and antidysrhythmic agents continue to be the mainstay for immediate arrhythmia management in the Cardiac Intensive Care Unit (CICU).

Classification of Antidysrhythmic Medications

- Two systems are used to classify antidysrhythmic medications.
- The oldest and most commonly used system remains the Vaughan-Williams system (Table 19.1), which classifies drugs based on mechanism of action.
- However, the Vaughan-Williams classification does not account for drugs having multiple effects, not working through ion channels, or those with different potencies.
- Because of this, the Sicilian Gambit system was introduced (Table 19.2), which links each medication to the relevant arrhythmia more directly (Table 19.3).

Antidysrhythmic Medications of Clinical Relevance in the CICU

- Table 19.4 lists the dosing and administration of the antidysrhythmic medications most commonly used in the CICU.

CLASS IA

- Procainamide is the only class IA agent that is commonly used in the CICU.
- It is metabolized via acetylation from a sodium channel blocker to N-acetylprocainamide (NAPA) that has potassium channel blocking properties, decreases conduction velocity, and prolongs the His-Purkinje action potential (AP) and the effective refractory period.
- It can also suppress automaticity in the sinoatrial node (SAN) and the atrioventricular node (AVN) and triggered activity in normal Purkinje fibers.
- Procainamide can prolong the QT interval.

TABLE 19.1 ▪ Modified Vaughan-Williams Classification of Antidysrhythmic Medications

	Drug Effects
Class I: Na⁺ Channel Blockers	
IA	Moderate slowing of conduction with prolonged refractoriness
Quinidine	
Procainamide	
Disopyramide	
IB	Slight slowing of conduction with minimal decrease in refractoriness
Lidocaine	
Mexiletene	
IC	Marked slowing of conduction with slight prolongation of refractoriness
Flecainide	
Propafenone	
Class II: β-Blockers	β-Adrenergic receptor antagonism
Metoprolol	
Atenolol	
Class III: K⁺ Channel Blockers	Prolongation of refractoriness
Amiodarone	
Dronedarone	
Sotalol	
Ibutilide	
Dofetilide	
Class IV: Ca²⁺ Channel Blockers	Block calcium entry
Verapamil	
Diltiazem	
Class V: Other	
Adenosine	
Digoxin	

Indications

- Historically, procainamide has been utilized as first-line therapy for management of stable ventricular tachycardia (VT).
- Procainamide also remains the treatment of choice for treating preexcited atrial fibrillation (AF) in the setting of Wolff-Parkinson-White syndrome.

Electrocardiographic Effects

- Patients demonstrate use-dependent widening of the QRS at faster heart rates or with high plasma concentrations.
- The PR interval and QT intervals can also lengthen.
- QRS widening by greater than 25% may suggest toxicity and be an indication to monitor therapy.

Side Effects

- In addition to QT prolongation, procainamide can be negatively inotropic and cause hypotension.
- Noncardiac effects, such as pancytopenia and agranulocytosis, can be life threatening.
- Headaches, gastrointestinal effects, and mental disturbances can also occur.

TABLE 19.2 ■ The Modified Sicilian Gambit

Mechanism	Arrhythmia	Desired Effect	Example Drugs
Automaticity			
Enhanced	Inappropriate sinus tachycardia	Decrease phase 4 depolarization	β-Blockers
	Idiopathic ventricular tachycardia (some)	Decrease phase 4 depolarization	Na^+ channel blockers
	Atrial tachycardia	Decrease phase 4 depolarization	Muscarinic receptor agonists
	Accelerated idioventricular rhythms	Decrease phase 4 depolarization	Ca^{2+} or Na^+ channel blockers
Triggered Activity			
EAD	Torsade de pointes	Shorten action potential	β-Blockers
		EAD suppression	Ca^{2+} channel blockers Mg^{2+} β-Blockers
DAD	Digoxin-induced arrhythmias	Block calcium entry	Ca^{2+} channel blockers
	Right ventricular outflow tract tachycardia	Block calcium entry DAD suppression	Ca^{2+} channel blockers β-Blockers
Na^+ Channel–Dependent Reentry			
Long excitable gap	Typical atrial flutter	Depress conduction and excitability	Class IA and class IC Na^+ channel blockers
	Atrioventricular reciprocating tachycardia	Depress conduction and excitability	Class IA and class IC Na^+ channel blockers
	Monomorphic ventricular tachycardia	Depress conduction and excitability	Na^+ channel blockers
Short excitable gap	Atypical atrial flutter	Prolong refractory period	K^+ channel blockers
	Atrial fibrillation	Prolong refractory period	K^+ channel blockers
	AV reciprocating tachycardia	Prolong refractory period	Amiodarone and sotalol
	Polymorphic and uniform ventricular tachycardia	Prolong refractory period	Class IA Na^+ channel blockers
	Bundle branch reentry	Prolong refractory period	Class IA Na^+ channel blockers and amiodarone
Na^+ Channel–Dependent Reentry			
	Atrioventricular nodal reentrant tachycardia	Depress conduction and excitability	Ca^{2+} channel blockers
	Atrioventricular reciprocating tachycardia	Depress conduction and excitability	Ca^{2+} channel blockers
	Verapamil-sensitive ventricular tachycardia	Depress conduction and excitability	Ca^{2+} channel blockers

DAD, Delayed afterdepolarization; *EAD*, early afterdepolarization.

TABLE 19.3 ▮ Actions of Antiarrhythmic Drugs Used in Critical Care

Drug	CHANNELS						RECEPTORS				PUMPS	CLINICAL EFFECTS			ECG INTERVAL EFFECT		
	Na+ Fast	Na+ Medium	Na+ Slow	Ca²⁺	Ca²⁺	γ	α	β	M2	A1	Na+/K+-ATPase	LV Function	Sinus Rate	Extracardiac	PR	QRS	QT
Lidocaine	Low											↑	↑	Med		↓	↓
Procainamide		ASB			Med							→	↑	High	↑	↑	↑
Verapamil	Low			High			Med					→	→	Low	↑		
Diltiazem				Med								→	→	Low	↑		
Sotalol					High			High				→	→	Low	↑		↑
Amiodarone	Low			Low			Med	Med				↑	→	High	↑	↑	↑
Propanolol	Low							High				→	→	Low	↑		
Adenosine										Agonist		?	→	Low	↑		
Digoxin									Agonist		High	↑	→	High	↑		↓

Potency of blockade: *Low*, low potency; *Med*, medium potency; *High*, high potency. *ASB*, Activated state blocker.

TABLE 19.4 ▮ Usual Dosing of Antidysrhythmic Drugs Used in Critical Care

Drug	INTRAVENOUS		ORAL (mg)		Peak Plasma Concentration (Oral Dosing in Hours)
	Loading	Maintenance	Loading	Maintenance	
Procainamide	6–15 mg/kg at 0.2–0.5 mg/kg/min	2–6 mg/min	500–1000	350–1000 q3–q6h	1
Lidocaine	1–3 mg/kg over 15–45 min	1 mg/kg/h			
Propanolol	1–3 mg at 1 mg/min			10–200 q6–8h	4
Ibutilide	1–2 mg				
Amiodarone	5 mg/kg over 10–30 min	720–1000 mg q24h	For VT: 1200–1600 qd for 1–2 wk then 600–800 qd for 2–4 wk. For SVT: 600–800 qd for 2 wk	For VT: 200–400 qd. For SVT: 200 qd	
Verapamil	10 mg over 1–2 min			80 mg q12h up to 320 mg/d	1–2
Adenosine	6–12 mg				
Digoxin	1 mg over 24 h in divided doses	0.125–0.25 mg q24h	1 mg over 24 h in divided doses	0.125–0.25 mg q24h	1–3

SVT, Supraventricular tachycardia; *VT*, ventricular tachycardia.

Administration

- Procainamide is used in the intravenous (IV) form in the CICU and is often initiated with a loading dose.
- One gram administered over 20 to 30 minutes is often used to convert preexcited AF.
- Procainamide can also be given as 6 to 15 mg/kg at 0.2 to 0.5 mg/kg/min.
- Care should be taken to reduce the dose in the setting of renal or cardiac impairment.
- Following the loading dose, maintenance should be administered at 1 mg/kg/h.
- The metabolism of this drug is widely variable, including the acetylation to NAPA; thus, levels of both procainamide and NAPA should be monitored with prolonged usage and should be less than 30 µg/mL combined.

CLASS IB

- Lidocaine is the only medication in this class useful in the CICU to treat ventricular arrhythmias.
- More recently, it has fallen out of favor compared with other agents, particularly amiodarone.
- Lidocaine exerts most of its actions on the Purkinje fibers and has little effect on the SAN or AVN.
- Lidocaine is a sodium channel blocker that decreases conduction velocity.
- Compared with other sodium channel blockers, it shortens the AP and decreases automaticity by decreasing the slow or phase 4 diastolic depolarization.
- It can be helpful in both reentrant and automatic arrhythmia suppression.

Indications

- Lidocaine is most commonly used for ventricular arrhythmias refractory to β-blockers and amiodarone.
- Prophylactic lidocaine was previously thought to be beneficial for patients with myocardial infarctions to prevent ventricular arrhythmias, but more recent studies demonstrated no benefit.

Electrocardiographic Effects

- Generally, no changes are seen on the ECG in patients receiving therapeutic doses of lidocaine.

Side Effects

- The most common toxicities of lidocaine are central nervous system (CNS) effects, particularly mental status changes.
  - In most cases, these are mild and resolve with cessation or dose reduction.
  - Elderly patients and those with HF are at higher risk of CNS toxicity.
  - In addition, because lidocaine is mostly cleared hepatically, liver failure predisposes to toxicity.
  - Tremors are the first CNS symptom observed with early toxicity; seizures occur at extremely high plasma concentrations.
- Bradyarrhythmia and hypotension only occur at very high plasma levels.

Administration

- The first-pass clearance of lidocaine is so high that it is administered only in IV form.
- It has a very short half-life of fewer than 3 hours.

- The metabolites have only weak antidysrhythmic properties.
- It is highly bound to α-acid glycoproteins, which are increased in patients with HF.
- Finally, the reduced volume of distribution in HF leads to higher concentrations of the drug.
- In general, a loading dose of 1 to 3 mg/kg is administered over several minutes followed by maintenance infusions of 1 to 4 mg/min.
- For acute arrhythmia treatment, patients can receive a bolus several times, if needed, until the steady state is reached by the maintenance infusion, which can take 3 to 4 hours.
- Therapeutic levels of lidocaine are between 1.5 to 5 μg/mL.

CLASS IC

- Flecainide and propafenone are the only two medications in this class left on the market, used in the outpatient setting, for atrial arrhythmias.
- They cannot be used in patients with structural heart disease or significant renal dysfunction and are available only in oral formulations.

CLASS II

- β-blockers have been shown to reduce mortality in a variety of situations, including HF, acute myocardial infarction, and CAD.
- They also decrease the rate of shocks for patients with implantable cardioverter-defibrillators and prevent degeneration of VT to ventricular fibrillation.
- β-Blockers may bind to β_1 receptors, β_2 receptors, or both.
- Some β-blockers also block α1 receptors.
- β_1 Receptors are found in the cardiovascular system.
- β_2 Receptors are noncardiac and lead to side effects, such as pulmonary bronchospasm.
- α_1 Receptor antagonism causes additional arteriolar vasodilation; drugs with α_1 receptor blockade tend to be used more commonly for hypertension or HF (Table 19.5).
- The myriad benefits of β-blocker therapy are mostly a result of blocking the effects of adrenergic stimulation, which can cause a variety of undesirable electrophysiologic changes, including increased automaticity, triggered activity, reentrant excitation, and delayed afterdepolarizations.
- Carvedilol, bisoprolol, and long-acting metoprolol, are indicated for long-term treatment of patients with HF in the setting of left ventricular (LV) dysfunction.

TABLE 19.5 ▪ **Dosing and Metabolism of Commonly Used β-Blockers**

Drug	β_1 Selective	IV Dosage	Half-Life	Elimination	Other Properties
Atenolol	Yes	5 mg q 10 min up to 10 mg	6–9 h	Renal	None
Esmolol	Yes	500 μg/kg loading; 50–300 μg/kg/min maintenance	9 min	Blood esterase	None
Labetalol	No	20 mg IV push; 2 mg/min infusion up to 300 mg	3–4 h	Hepatic	α-Blockade
Metoprolol	Yes	5 mg q 2–5 min up to 15 mg	3–4 h	Hepatic	None
Propanolol	No	1 mg/min up to 5 mg	3–4 h	Hepatic	Membrane stabilization

Indications

- β-Blockers can be used to suppress some forms of supraventricular tachycardia (SVT), including AVN reentrant tachycardia (AVNRT).
- They slow the ventricular response for AF and atrial flutter.
- They decrease ventricular arrhythmias in patients with acute myocardial infarction.
- Adrenergically mediated ventricular arrhythmias respond well to β-blockers, including right ventricular outflow tract tachycardia.
- β-Blockers reduce the risk of sudden cardiac death in patients with congenital long QT syndrome.

Electrocardiographic Effects

- β-blockers commonly slow the sinus rate and produce bradycardia.
- In high doses or in conduction system disease, PR prolongation can be seen.

Side Effects

- From a cardiovascular standpoint, all β-blockers can cause bradycardia and hypotension.
- The most common noncardiac side effect of β-blockers is bronchospasm in patients with asthma.
  - Bronchospasm is most commonly seen with β-blockers with β_2 selectivity, but also occurs from agents with predominantly β_1 selectivity in susceptible patients.
- Other uncommon noncardiac side effects include hypoglycemia, fatigue, and depression.

Administration

- Different β-blockers have different receptor selectivity, half-lives, and modes of elimination.
- For example, atenolol is not good for patients with severe renal impairment, because it is predominantly renally cleared.
- In addition, some β-blockers are available only in oral or IV forms.
- Table 19.5 outlines the IV β-blockers that are most commonly used in the CICU for arrhythmias.

CLASS III

- The weaknesses of the Vaughn-Williams classification system of antidysrhythmic drugs are apparent when reviewing the class III drugs.
- Nominally, these medications have potassium channel blocking properties.
- However, many of these drugs have other properties as well.
- In particular, amiodarone also has sodium channel blocking properties, calcium channel blocking (CCB) properties, and β-blocker properties.

Amiodarone

- Amiodarone is one of the most effective antidysrhythmic medications for both atrial and ventricular arrhythmias across a range of different mechanisms, including automatic and reentrant.
- It is available in both oral and IV forms; the oral form has high bioavailability.
- It has little proarrhythmic effects and does not cause significant QT prolongation.
- These features make it a very useful drug for treatment of arrhythmias, particularly in critically ill patients.
- Amiodarone has the potential for multiple side effects, some of which can be serious and life threatening.

- Amiodarone is classified as a class III medication owing to its ability to block IK_r and IK_s, leading to AP prolongation and increased refractory periods in atrial and ventricular tissues.
- It also decreases peripheral conversion of T4 to T3 and impairs T3 binding to myocytes, causing cellular hypothyroidism.
- The magnitude of the various effects is different in the oral versus IV forms, with the oral form demonstrating decreased automaticity, increased AP duration, and prolongation of the QT interval.

Indications

- Amiodarone is efficacious in converting and suppressing AF as well as in the acute treatment of ventricular arrhythmias, although it is approved by the US Food and Drug Administration only for the treatment of ventricular arrhythmias.
- Amiodarone is part of the advanced cardiac life support guidelines for management of ventricular fibrillation and pulseless VT.
- Nevertheless, amiodarone has been studied for multiple conditions over the last several decades and guideline statements for the treatment of AF and VT include amiodarone as a treatment option.
- It is important to note that amiodarone, unlike other antidysrhythmic drugs, is a vasodilator and not a negative inotrope, and thus it can be used safely in CAD or LV dysfunction.
- In the acute setting, IV amiodarone is the mainstay for treatment of lethal ventricular arrhythmias in most situations.
- Amiodarone is clearly superior to other antidysrhythmic medications for the treatment of AF.
- Restoration of sinus rhythm can improve hemodynamics in some patients with HF, renal failure, or sepsis.
- Amiodarone has been shown to decrease postoperative AF in patients having cardiac surgery.

Electrocardiographic Effects

- Sinus bradycardia and PR prolongation are common.
- Furthermore, mild QRS widening can be seen.
- QTc prolongation can also be seen, but it is usually mild and rarely proarrhythmic.
- Although administration of most class III medications requires inpatient monitoring of the QT interval, amiodarone can be started as an outpatient.

Side Effects

- The side effects of amiodarone occur mostly in the setting of long-term oral administration.
- In the inpatient setting, however, the most significant side effects are the development of hypotension, bradycardia, or proarrhythmia during intravenous administration.
- Table 19.6 lists the most common drug interactions with amiodarone.

Administration

- For acute management of arrhythmias, a 150-mg IV loading dose is given over 10 minutes.
- After this, an IV infusion of 1 mg/min is given for 6 hours followed by an infusion of 0.5 mg/min, which provides a total of just over 1 g of amiodarone in 24 hours.
- A maintenance infusion of 0.5 mg/min or intermittent IV loading doses can be continued for patients who cannot take oral medications.
- The oral form of amiodarone is very lipophilic and thus has a very large volume of distribution, and so it does not start to have an effect for several days and the half-life is extremely long.

TABLE 19.6 ▓ **Drug Interactions With Amiodarone**

Drug	Result	Risks	Mechanism of Interaction
Apixaban	Increases apixaban levels	Increased risk of bleeding	Inhibits CYP3A4 P-glycoprotein
Cyclosporine	Increases cyclosporine levels	Increased risk of CNS and GI side effects, hypertension	Inhibits CYP3A4 P-glycoprotein
Dabigatran	Increases dabigatran levels	Increased risk of bleeding	P-glycoprotein
Digoxin	Increases digoxin levels	Increased risk of arrhythmia, CNS, and GI side effects	P-glycoprotein
Rivaroxaban	Increases rivaroxaban levels	Increased risk of bleeding	Inhibits CYP3A4 P-glycoprotein
Simvastatin	Increases statin levels	Increased risk of liver toxicity and rhabdomyolysis	Inhibits CYP3A4
Warfarin	Increases INR	Increased risk of bleeding	Inhibits CYP2CP Inhibits CYP1A2

CNS, Central nervous system; *GI*, gastrointestinal; *INR*, international normalized ratio.

- To achieve steady state, a patient must have upward of 10 g to saturate the compartments.
- Amiodarone is entirely metabolized via the liver and the gut, which is another advantage in critically ill patients who may have acute renal failure.
- The liver metabolite desethylamiodarone is active and has a very long half-life.
- There should be adjustment of the dose for patients with liver dysfunction; liver function tests should be monitored closely.

Ibutilide

- Ibutilide blocks Ikr, leading to an increase in AP duration and atrial and ventricular refractoriness. It is available only in IV form.

Indications
- Ibutilide is indicated only for the acute conversion of AF and atrial flutter to sinus rhythm.
- It is more effective for atrial flutter than for AF and is more effective for episodes of shorter duration.
- Ibutilide can also be used to facilitate electrical cardioversion in patients who have AF refractory to prior electrical cardioversions.

Electrocardiographic Effects
Ibutilide can be a very potent QT-prolonging agent, with resultant risks of torsades de pointes.

Side Effects
- Ibutilide has few side effects beyond QT prolongation.
- The risk of torsades de pointes is not insignificant at 3.6% to 8.3%; very close monitoring is warranted with administration of this medication.

Administration

- Ibutilide should be administered in a controlled setting with patients on continuous monitoring.
- An external defibrillator must be immediately available.
- Potassium and magnesium levels should be optimized.
- The usual dosing is 1 mg infused over 10 minutes.
- The infusion should be stopped in the event of marked QT prolongation or cardioversion.
- A second dose can be given after 10 minutes if neither of the above occur.
- The drug is hepatically metabolized and renally excreted, with the half-life ranging from 2 to 12 hours.
- Continuous telemetry for at least 4 hours after the infusion with longer monitoring in patients with hepatic dysfunction.

CLASS IV

- The CCBs verapamil and diltiazem fall within this class.
- These medications slow phase 4 conduction and decrease conduction velocities in the SAN and AVN.

Indications

- The major use is for the treatment of atrial arrhythmias.
- Both IV diltiazem and verapamil decrease the ventricular response of AF and atrial flutter.
- They can also suppress forms of SVT, particularly AVNRT.
- As with other AVN blockers, they should not be used in Wolff-Parkinson-White syndrome.
- Right ventricular outflow tract VT and familial catecholaminergic polymorphic VT can be treated with CCB.

Electrocardiographic Effects

- For patients in sinus rhythm, CCB slow the sinus rate, leading to bradycardia and PR prolongation.

Side Effects

- Both diltiazem and verapamil can cause hypotension and flushing owing to the vasodilator effects.
- They should be used with caution in conjunction with other drugs that have similar electrophysiologic effects, particularly β-blockers and digoxin.
- Verapamil cannot be used with dofetilide, because verapamil affects the renal clearance of that drug and can lead to severe QT prolongation, and it also interacts with amiodarone, causing profound bradycardia.
- Thus, when rate control medications are needed, β-blockers are preferable to CCB in the CICU.

Administration

- Verapamil and diltiazem are often given in the IV form because they both undergo significant first-pass elimination.
- Verapamil can be loaded at 5 to 20 mg over several minutes.
- A maintenance infusion at 0.005 mg/kg/min is given when patients are unable to take oral medications.
- Diltiazem can be loaded with a 20-mg bolus. Repeated boluses can be given as well as maintenance infusions.

ATYPICAL ANTIDYSRHYTHMICS (CLASS V)

Digoxin

- Digoxin is a cardiac glycoside that has many electrophysiologic effects, the most important of which are autonomic, increasing parasympathetic nervous system activity and decreasing sympathetic nervous system activity.
- It also decreases automaticity in the SAN and increases refractoriness of the AVN.

Indications

- The only indication is as a second-line agent for rate control of AF or atrial flutter, when β-blockers and CCBs are not completely effective, but unlike those, digoxin does not cause hypotension.

Electrocardiographic Effects

- Patients often develop downsloping of the ST segment, known as the digoxin effect.
- At toxic doses, patients can have a variety of arrhythmias, including AV block, atrial tachycardias, junctional tachycardias, and bidirectional VT.

Side Effects

- Clearance is substantially affected by renal function, and patients can become toxic easily, with changes in renal function.
- Low potassium levels increase the risks of toxicity, as digoxin competes with potassium for the binding site on Na^+/K^+-adenosine triphosphatase (ATPase).
- At toxic levels, digoxin causes a wide variety of noncardiac side effects including nausea, vomiting, headaches, and visual disturbances.
- Digoxin has a variety of drug interactions.
    - One of the most important is the interaction with amiodarone. Digoxin is a substrate for the P-glycoprotein system, of which amiodarone is a potent inhibitor.
    - Administration of digoxin and amiodarone together can increase digoxin levels dramatically by increasing bioavailability and decreasing clearance.
- Treatment of digoxin toxicity is urgent.
    - The medication should be stopped and electrolyte levels corrected, though pseudohyperkalemia may develop owing to potassium displacement from the myocytes.
    - The only exception to this is the administration of calcium, which should be avoided as it can precipitate arrhythmias owing to the Na^+/K^+-ATPase blockade.
    - In urgent settings, the digoxin immune FAB antibody can be administered.
- Digoxin is not removed by dialysis.

Administration

- Digoxin is principally excreted via the kidney; thus, renal insufficiency places patients at an increased risk for toxicity through reductions in both volume of distribution and clearance, requiring doses to be lowered.
- Regular monitoring of digoxin levels is important for preventing toxicity.
- In general, serum digoxin concentrations should be less than 2.0 ng/mL.
- For patients with HF, they should be less than 1.0 ng/mL.
- If rapid effects are needed, digoxin can be loaded IV.
    - Up to 1 mg can be infused in divided doses over 24 hours.
    - Owing to the relatively long distribution time, the recommended dosing strategy is 50% of the total loading dose followed by 25% for the subsequent two doses, spaced 6 hours apart.
- Oral maintenance doses should be 0.125 mg or 0.25 mg daily, depending on the renal function.

Adenosine

- Adenosine is an endogenous nucleoside that affects potassium and calcium channels via α_1 and α_2 receptors, in addition to G proteins.
- The half-life is only seconds, and the primary activity is the outward potassium current (I_{KAdo}) found in atrial tissue.
- It inhibits the I_f channel, which decreases sodium influx in the SAN and AVN, resulting in a negative chronotropic effect.
- Adenosine slows automaticity and conduction in the SAN and AVN.

Indications

- The primary indication of adenosine is for the termination of SVTs that depend on the AVN for a reentrant circuit.
- This would include AVNRT and AV reentrant tachycardia.
- Adenosine should be used with caution in patients with AV reentrant tachycardia, because it can induce AF, which can be life threatening in rapid conduction down the accessory pathway.
- Adenosine can terminate some atrial tachycardias owing to its effects in atrial tissue.
- It is thought that about 10% of atrial tachycardias may be adenosine responsive.
- Right ventricular outflow tract tachycardia may be adenosine responsive as well.
- Adenosine can also be used for diagnostic purposes when the diagnosis of atrial flutter or AF is unclear.
- For these rhythms, the AVN blocks and the absence of QRS complexes allow for evaluation of the underlying atrial waveforms, particularly the flutter waves.
- Adenosine is sometimes used to differentiate VT from SVT with aberrancy, but this can be misleading and unsafe.

Electrocardiographic Effects

- Adenosine causes transient AV block.
- This leads to termination of AVN-dependent reentrant arrhythmias or slowing of the ventricular response in AF or atrial flutter.

Side Effects

- The extremely short half-life of adenosine makes side effects very limited.
- Facial flushing and chest pain can occur owing to vasodilator effects.
- It can also cause bronchospasm in patients with reactive airways.
- There is approximately a 10% chance of inducing AF with adenosine administration.

Administration

- Adenosine needs to be given as a rapid IV bolus in order to be effective.
- Preferably, it should be given via a central venous IV.
- Doses of 6 to 12 mg can be given as a rapid IV push followed by a saline flush.
- If no evidence of AVN blockade is seen, another larger bolus, up to 18 mg, can be given.
- The half-life is so short that repeat doses can be given within 30 seconds.

CHAPTER 20

Central Venous and Arterial Access Procedures

Central Venous Access: General Principles and Preparation

- Patients in the Cardiac Intensive Care Unit (CICU) require reliable intravenous access.
- Central venous access is indicated for vasopressor administration, hemodynamic monitoring, temporary transvenous pacing, and hemodialysis.
- Contraindications are relative, depending on alternative options and clinical urgency.
- Anatomic distortion, local infection, and existing hardware justify avoiding specific sites when possible.
- Coagulopathy is not an absolute contraindication, but the risk and benefits should be carefully weighed.
- Although consent should be obtained prior to attempting central venous access, it is often required emergently and obtaining consent may not be practical.
    - Infection, bleeding, arterial injury, venous thrombosis, and pneumothorax are all important to discuss.
- Most nonemergent central venous catheters in the CICU are placed in the internal jugular or subclavian vein.
- Ultrasound guidance is recommended, and the site should be investigated prior to skin preparation and draping.
- Abnormal vascular anatomy or visible clots may disqualify a preferred site.
- The Trendelenburg position is recommended for subclavian and jugular access if the patient can safely tolerate repositioning.
- Once the site is selected and the patient is positioned, the skin should be cleaned, ideally with chlorhexidine-based solutions.
- Full sterile precautions should be used for all central access procedures.
- The central line kit should be ergonomically positioned on a large table, but not on the sterile drape, because patients can unexpectedly move.
- The insertion site should be anesthetized with 1% lidocaine.

Technique

- The modified Seldinger technique is standard for central access procedures.
- Vessel puncture is obtained with a large-bore, 18-gauge introducer needle or catheter-over-needle assembly.
- Needle trajectory and depth should be monitored closely throughout.
- Continuous negative pressure is applied to the aspirating syringe during needle advancement and withdrawal.
- Venous puncture confirmation is important for central venous access procedures to avoid inadvertent arterial cannulation.
- Blood color, pulsatility, and ultrasound visualization may be misleading.
- A 30-cm length of pressure tubing can be connected to the access needle and used to transduce venous pressure prior to wire introduction.
- The guidewire is next advanced through the introducer needle to approximately 20 cm.
- The needle must remain stationary before wire insertion.
- The guidewire should pass easily with minimal resistance; if not, remove the wire, reconfirm blood aspiration, or reposition the needle trajectory or guidewire J-tip orientation prior to readvancing.
- With the wire stabilized at 20 cm, the needle is removed and a small stab incision at the guidewire exit site is performed with a No. 11 scalpel.
- While stabilizing the guidewire, the tissue tract dilator is advanced over the guidewire through the skin and connective tissue to the vessel.
- Care must be taken to avoid advancing the wire and dilator together because this can bend the wire and damage the vessel.
- The wire should always slide easily within the dilator.
- Next, the dilator is removed while keeping the wire stationary and maintaining hemostasis with firm pressure.
- The vascular catheter is then advanced into position over the guidewire.
- Finally, the guidewire is removed, the catheter lumens are flushed, and the catheter is secured to the skin at the appropriate depth (usually 15 to 20 cm, depending on access site and patient size).

Internal Jugular Venous Cannulation

RELEVANT ANATOMY

- The internal jugular vein originates at the jugular foramen and descends to join the subclavian vein.
- In the mid to lower neck, it lies lateral and then anterolateral to the carotid artery.
- At the level of the thyroid cartilage, the vein lies deep to the sternocleidomastoid muscle.
- The vessel emerges from behind the muscle into the triangle created by the sternal and clavicular insertions of the sternocleidomastoid muscle, just above the clavicle.
- Right-sided jugular cannulation is preferred owing to the direct path to the superior vena cava and to avoid risk to the left-sided thoracic duct.

ULTRASOUND-GUIDED TECHNIQUE

- Ultrasound-guided central line placement aids in identifying anatomic variations and is associated with improved success and reduced complications.

- Real-time dynamic ultrasound allows the provider to visualize the needle tip during insertion, which is important because the needle shaft and tip have a similar appearance.
- Vigilantly monitor needle insertion depth during the procedure.

COMPLICATIONS

- Carotid artery puncture with immediate needle withdrawal and application of firm pressure is usually uncomplicated.
- Major bleeding can lead to neck hematoma and airway compromise.
- Arterial cannulation however, can result in cerebrovascular insufficiency, thrombosis, or pseudoaneurysm.
  - If this occurs, leave the catheter in place and consult a vascular surgeon.

Subclavian Venous Cannulation

- Subclavian venous access is an often the preferred access site based on the low risk of complications.
  - Contraindications include clavicle distortion or local hardware (i.e., pacemakers) and severe coagulopathy at this noncompressible site.

TECHNIQUE

- Steps for subclavian central venous line placement are shown in Fig. 20.1.
- The left subclavian vein is preferred owing to the low incidence of catheter malposition and direct insertion trajectory for emergency transvenous pacemaker or pulmonary artery catheter placement.
- Set up for the central line as described above with proper position and full sterile equipment.
- Consider having an assistant apply gentle caudal traction to the ipsilateral arm.
- Ultrasound guidance for subclavian cannulation is not standard, but is described.
- Inject 1% lidocaine at the injection site for anesthesia.
- The introducer needle is inserted 2 cm lateral and inferior to the midclavicular point.
- Aim for the suprasternal notch and pass beneath the clavicle.
- Intentionally contacting the clavicle to "walk" the needle down the clavicle helps to maintain the needle in a plane parallel to the floor to reduce the risk of pneumothorax.
- Following vessel puncture, insert the catheter via the Seldinger technique as described above.

COMPLICATIONS

- Pneumothorax and subclavian arterial puncture are common concerns, but the rate of mechanical complication remains low.

Femoral Venous Cannulation

- Femoral venous catheters still have a role in certain scenarios, such as emergency situations and for hemodialysis access when the right internal jugular vein is not an option.
- The femoral site has historically been associated with an increased risk of infection and venous thrombosis.
- Steps for inserting a femoral central venous line are shown in Fig. 20.2.
- The ipsilateral leg should be slightly abducted and externally rotated for access site exposure.

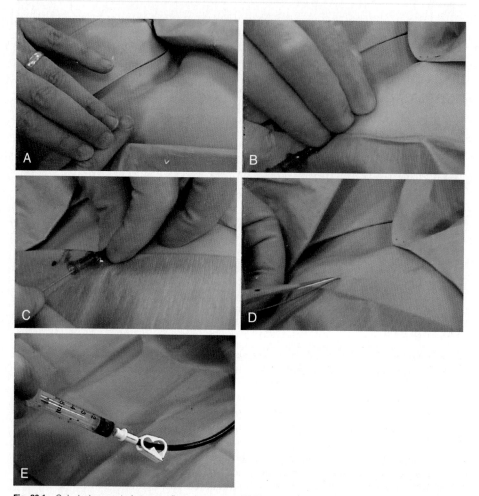

Fig. 20.1 Subclavian central venous line placement. (**A**) The needle should target the sternal notch, but always angle away from the lungs. If the needle needs to be depressed, press down on top with three fingers so that the whole needle goes down flat as a single unit rather than just pointing the tip down. (**B**) The needle is in the clavicle and the upper fingers are pressing the needle down as a unit so that it goes down but is still inclined away from the lung. (**C**) Once the needle is in, the subclavian area has a distinct advantage over the internal jugular vein area, as the needle is held between the clavicle and the first rib and is better secured. (**D**) Wire, nick, dilate, and flush. Do not go too medially to avoid getting stuck between the first rib and the clavicle. (**E**) Aspirate, flush, sew, and dress.

- The introducer needle is inserted 1 to 2 cm below the inguinal crease with the aim of puncturing the femoral vein as it emerges beneath the inguinal ligament.
- The needle is advanced at a 20- to 30-degree angle to the skin toward the arterial pulsation.

COMPLICATIONS

- Vessel puncture and instrumentation above the inguinal ligament risks retroperitoneal hemorrhage from posterior vessel injury without any evidence of superficial bleeding or hematoma formation and may go unrecognized.

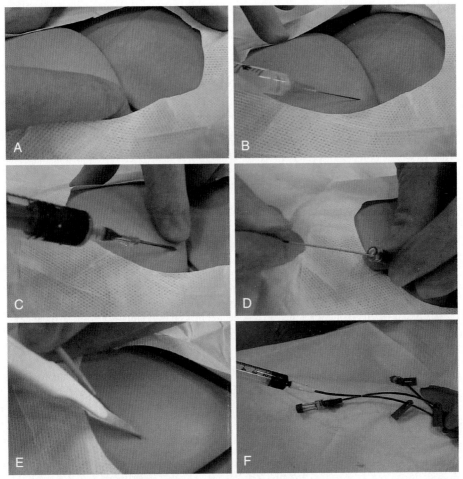

Fig. 20.2 Femoral central venous line placement. (**A**) The mnemonic NAVEL is very useful for reviewing the anatomic landmarks (*n*erve, *a*rtery, *v*ein, *e*mpty space, *l*ymphatics). (**B**) Apply local anesthesia generously. (**C**) Using the hollow needle, advance until dark venous blood is observed. (**D**) Hold the needle steady, wire it up, and proceed using the standard Seldinger technique. (**E**) Nick the skin, dilate, and pass the line. (**F**) Aspirate, flush, sew in place, and apply dressing.

Radial Arterial Cannulation

- Continuous invasive arterial access is indicated for blood pressure monitoring and serial blood gas sampling.
- The radial artery is the most commonly selected site.
- This site is contraindicated in cases of preexisting arterial insufficiency to the hand.

EQUIPMENT

- Equipment for radial arterial line placement includes the following:
  - Antiseptic skin preparation
  - A wrist board

- Tape
- 1% lidocaine in a small syringe with a 25-gauge needle
- 20-gauge vascular cannula—a prefabricated arterial catheter-over-needle assembly with attached guidewire and sheath
- Transducer and pressure tubing

TECHNIQUE

- Steps for inserting a radial arterial line are shown in Fig. 20.3.
- Set up all equipment prior to starting the procedure.
- Sitting in a comfortable position at the bedside is recommended over standing and bending over the target.
- Extend the target site wrist 20 degrees to flatten the thenar eminence and gain exposure to the site.
- Tape the hand to maintain this position.
- Apply chlorhexidine-based antiseptic skin preparation solution and allow it to dry followed by infiltration of local anesthetic at the intended puncture site.
- Target the distal vessel just proximal to the flexor crease.
- Puncture the skin and slowly advance the needle or catheter-over-needle assembly at a 15- to 30-degree angle along the long axis of the target vessel.
- The vessel lies less than 0.5 cm deep in most situations.
- Once inserted beyond the anticipated target depth, slowly withdraw the needle under close guidance while monitoring for blood flash.
- Once punctured, pressurized arterial blood should flow from the catheter or up the attached sheath.
- A flexible, straight guidewire is advanced over the wire to maintain access to the vessel.
- A 20-gauge catheter is then advanced in place over the guidewire and the needle and guidewire are removed.

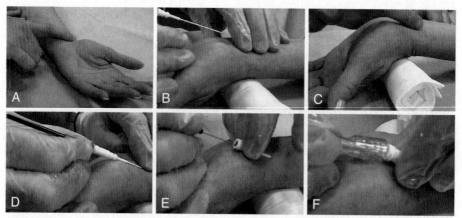

Fig. 20.3 Radial arterial line placement. (**A**) To approach the radial artery, one needs to go over the thenar eminence. (**B**) Extending the wrist allows a straight shot to the radial artery. (**C**) Approach at a shallow angle to get the needle in, then slide up a little more to get the catheter in as well. (**D**) Make sure that the blood keeps flowing as you advance. (**E**) Slide the catheter in, then hold down above the line so that the blood does not squirt out. (**F**) It is recommended to use a Luer-Lok to avoid disconnecting the line.

- Following confirmation of arterial blood withdrawal, connect the pressure tubing to the catheter.
- Check the arterial tracing to ensure an appropriate waveform.
- Secure the catheter and wrist position with an arm board.
- If the first attempt fails, apply pressure to maintain hemostasis and reinsert at the same site or just proximal.

COMPLICATIONS

- Distal arterial ischemia is the most feared complication, but it is uncommon.
- Despite tradition, the Allen test is not a good screening test for arterial collateralization of the hand.
- Other important complications include infection, dissection, vasospasm, arterial aneurysm, and vascular sclerosis.

Femoral Arterial Cannulation

INDICATIONS AND CONTRAINDICATIONS

- Femoral arterial access is indicated for close blood pressure monitoring and arterial access for frequent blood sampling.
- The femoral site is often selected for patients in shock or with absent or diminished radial pulses.
- This site is contraindicated in patients with recent femoral or iliac artery surgery, local infection, and severe aortoiliac disease.

EQUIPMENT

- The equipment for femoral arterial line placement includes the following:
  - Antiseptic skin preparation and sterile barrier equipment
  - 1% lidocaine in a small syringe with a 25-gauge needle
  - 18- or 16-gauge single-lumen cannula—often contained in prefabricated arterial or venous access kits
  - Transducer and pressure tubing

TECHNIQUE

- Steps for inserting a femoral arterial line are shown in Fig. 20.4.
- If the operator is right-handed, the right femoral artery is easier to approach.
- Prepare and drape in sterile fashion and have an assistant nearby.
- Apply local anesthetic.
- The ipsilateral leg should be slightly abducted and externally rotated for access site exposure.
- The needle is inserted 1 to 2 cm below the inguinal crease in anticipation of puncturing the femoral artery as it emerges beneath the inguinal ligament.
- Needle puncture above the inguinal ligament risks procedure-related hemorrhage that may be concealed in the retroperitoneum and is noncompressible.
- The needle is inserted at a 20- to 30-degree angle to the skin toward the arterial pulsation.
- Following arterial puncture, the arterial cannula is inserted via the Seldinger technique as described earlier.

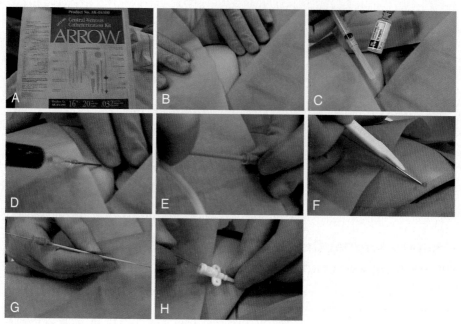

Fig. 20.4   Femoral arterial line placement. (**A**) Shown is a good kit for a femoral arterial line. The needle is soft-tipped so that it does not erode and cause retroperitoneal bleeding. (**B**) Palpate the femoral pulse and remember the mnemonic NAVEL for anatomic structures going lateral-to-medial (*n*erve, *a*rtery, *v*ein, *e*mpty space, *l*ymphatics). (**C**) Apply local anesthetic generously. (**D**) Using the big hollow needle, advance until bright blood is observed. (**E**) Once the needle is in, proceed with the Seldinger technique, making sure that the wire goes in easily. (**F**) A small nick is enough for the 16-gauge catheter to go in easily. (**G**) Dilate with caution to avoid a major bleed. (**H**) Slide the catheter up, check the location again, connect the tubing, sew in place, and apply dressing.

COMPLICATIONS

- Vascular complications—including hemorrhage, arterial thrombosis, pseudoaneurysm, dissection, and arteriovenous fistula—are rare, but well recognized.
- The absence of superficial hematoma formation does not exclude the presence of a retroperitoneal hemorrhage.

CHAPTER 21

Temporary Cardiac Pacing

Common Misconceptions

- The indication for a pacemaker is solely based on the patient's heart rate.
- Transcutaneous pacing may be performed on conscious patients without sedation.
- A temporary transvenous pacemaker may be placed from the femoral vein without fluoroscopic guidance.

Bradyarrhythmias

- Bradyarrhythmias can be classified into five groups:
  - Sinus bradycardia
  - Sinus pause
  - Junctional rhythm
  - Sinoatrial (SA) exit block
  - Idioventricular rhythm (Table 21.1).
- Atrioventricular (AV) conduction blocks may also result in bradycardia and require pacemaker implantation.
  - AV blocks are defined in three groups (Table 21.2).

SIGNS AND SYMPTOMS OF BRADYARRHYTHMIAS

- The decision for pacemaker implantation depends on the hemodynamic consequences of bradycardia, such as hypotension along with:
  - Dizziness
  - Dyspnea
  - Fatigue
  - Confusion
  - Syncope

Permanent Versus Temporary Cardiac Pacing

- All indications for permanent cardiac pacing are indications for temporary cardiac pacing (see Table 21.2), but when the cause is reversible or unknown, a temporary pacemaker is preferred.

Types/Forms of Temporary Pacing

- Transcutaneous and transvenous pacing are most commonly used (Table 21.3).
- Epicardial pacemakers are used following cardiothoracic surgery in which the pacemaker leads are attached to the epicardium of the atrium and/or ventricle.

TABLE 21.1 ■ **Different Types of Bradyarrhythmias**

Bradyarrhythmias	Definition	ECG Changes
Sinus bradycardia	• Rate: < 60 beats/min • Rhythm: regular • P waves: normal in morphology and duration • PR interval: between 0.12 and 0.20 sec	> 1 sec
Sinus pause	• Sinus node fails to generate an impulse • No P wave or its associated QRS and T wave • Lasting from 2.0 sec to several minutes	
Junctional rhythm	• AV node becomes the principal pacemaker • Rate: 40–60 beats/min	
Idioventricular rhythm	• Ventricle becomes the principal pacemaker • Wide QRS complexes (> 120 msec) • Rate: lower, between 20 to 40 beats/min	
Sinoatrial Exit Block[a]		
Second-degree type 1 SA block	• Shortening of the PP interval until a P-QRS-T complex is dropped • Takes progressively longer for each SA node impulse to exit the node until an impulse fails to exit the node	
Second-degree type 2 SA block	• Impulse generated in the SA node occasionally fails to propagate into the atria, which appears as a dropped P-QRS-T complex • PP interval surrounding the dropped complexes is two times (or a multiple) the baseline PP interval	
Third-degree SA exit block	• None of the generated impulses exits the SA node • Pause or junctional rhythm	> 1.5 sec

[a]First-degree SA block, which is a delay between generation of impulse in SA node and its exit from the node, is not detectable on surface ECG.
AV, Atrioventricular; *ECG,* electrocardiogram; *SA,* sinoatrial.

TRANSCUTANEOUS PACING

■ Transcutaneous pacing is the fastest method to initiate temporary cardiac pacing.
■ Because transcutaneous cardiac pacing may be associated with a burning sensation and/or skeletal muscle contractions, patients who are conscious should be sedated.

TABLE 21.2 ■ **Indications and Contraindications for Permanent and Temporary Cardiac Pacing Based on Causes**

	Indications	Contraindications
Permanent cardiac pacing	• Any symptomatic bradycardia • Sinus node dysfunction • Acquired Mobitz II or third-degree atrioventricular block in adults • Hypersensitive carotid sinus syndrome and severe neurocardiogenic syncope • After cardiac transplantation • Pacing to prevent ventricular tachycardia • Patients with congenital heart disease	• Local infection at implantation site • Active systemic infection with bacteremia • Severe bleeding tendencies (relative contraindication) • Active anticoagulation therapy (relative contraindication)
Temporary cardiac pacing	• Reversible injury to the sinus node or other parts of the conduction system after cardiac surgery (e.g., injuries, postcoronary bypass) • Chest and cardiac trauma associated with temporary sinus node or AV node dysfunction • Metabolic and/or electrolyte imbalance (e.g., hyperkalemia) • Drug-induced bradyarrhythmia (e.g., digitalis toxicity) • Infectious diseases (e.g., Lyme disease or bacterial endocarditis)	• Asymptomatic patient with stable rhythm (e.g., a first-degree AV block or a Mobitz 1 or stable escape rhythm)

AV, Atrioventricular.

TABLE 21.3 ■ **Advantages and Disadvantages of Different Types of Temporary Pacing**

	Advantages	Disadvantages
Transcutaneous pacing	• Method of choice in case of emergencies (asystole or cardiac symptoms)	• Least reliability • Least convenient • Skin tingling, burning • Musculoskeletal contractions
Transvenous pacing	• Enhanced patient comfort • Greater reliability • The ability to pace the atrium • Stability of pacing system	• Requires central venous access • Complications that result from obtaining venous access (venous thrombosis, inadvertent arterial puncture)
Temporary permanent transvenous pacing	• Higher stability • Provides data by interrogation	• Expensive

■ Transcutaneous cardiac pacing equipment consists of a pacing unit, pads (cardiac electrodes), and a cardiac monitor (Fig. 21.1).
  ■ First, wipe the patient's skin with alcohol and shave body hair carefully.
  ■ The anterior electrode has negative polarity and should be placed either over the cardiac apex or at the position of lead V_3.
  ■ The posterior electrode, which has positive polarity, should be placed inferior to the scapula or between the right or left scapula and the spine.
  ■ The pacemaker is then turned on and the pacing mode selected.

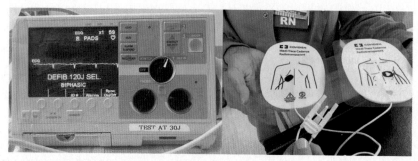

Fig. 21.1 External defibrillator and transcutaneous pacing system. Three knobs on the pacing system allow setting the device for pacing, choosing the rate, and then choosing the output to have appropriate cardiac capture. Two external pads are attached to the appropriate part of the chest and the back of the patient, as shown on the pads.

- If the patient is in cardiac arrest with bradycardia or asystole, pacing should be initiated at the maximum current output to ensure that capture is achieved as soon as possible.
- Then, the current can be gradually reduced to 5 to 10 mA above the threshold for capture.
- A wide QRS complex after each pacing stimulus suggests capture, but it is only confirmed by assessing the pulse, blood pressure, and clinical status of the patient
- The pacing threshold is usually less than 80 mA, but can be increased by obesity, myocardial ischemia, metabolic derangements, pneumothorax, and by poor electrode contact.

TRANSVENOUS PACING

- Transvenous pacing requires central venous access (see Chapter 20).
- This method has several advantages over the transcutaneous method, such as patient comfort and stability, but it cannot be initiated as rapidly as transcutaneous pacing.
- The requirements for transvenous pacing are a central venous access kit, a pacing lead, a temporary external transvenous pacing generator and external defibrillator, along with the following:
    - Sterile gown, gloves, cap, and face shield
    - Drapes or towels for skin preparation
    - Lidocaine, sterile gauze, syringes, scalpel, saline flush, catheter, dilator, needle, wire, suture, needle driver
    - Fluoroscopy is commonly used for intracardiac lead placement.
    - If fluoroscopy is not available, electrocardiographic (ECG) guidance or echocardiography may be used instead.
- The first step in transvenous pacing is obtaining venous access.
- The most common access site is the right femoral vein with fluoroscopic guidance or the internal jugular and subclavian veins without fluoroscopic guidance.
- The following steps are taken to insert a temporary pacer at the bedside using ECG guidance, with insertion of a temporary pacer under fluoroscopic guidance being more straightforward.
    - A balloon-tipped catheter is inserted through the sheath into the vein and is advanced 20 cm. It is then inflated to be advanced with blood flow.
    - The distal electrodes of the catheter are connected to the V_1 lead of the ECG device to record a unipolar ECG.
    - This allows sensing of atrial and ventricular ECGs as the lead enters these chambers.

- The catheter is advanced through the vein until it reaches the right atrium (RA).
- When the catheter enters the RA, atrial waves are recorded that confirm the catheter position or, if the lead is paced at maximum output, then the atrial position of the lead is confirmed by atrial capture on the ECG.
- Advancing further, when the catheter passes the tricuspid valve and enters the right ventricle (RV) and the catheter is in contact with the RV endocardium, the ventricular signal is very large (usually > 4 mV) and produces ST segment elevation as an indication of an injury current.
- From the morphology of the paced QRS on the surface ECG, one can determine the catheter position within the RV.
- In an emergency, the highest output should be tried first; output should then be gradually reduced until the capture is lost and the pacing threshold is determined.
- If the situation is not an emergency, the rate is set 10 to 20 beats/min above the intrinsic heart rate and the output is initially set low and then gradually increased until capture occurs.
- The output should be set to a value at least three times higher than the threshold to ensure a safe margin for any change that occurs in the capture threshold.
- The ideal capture threshold is less than 1 mA.
- The lead and sheath are secured to the skin with suture and a transparent dressing applied.
- The patient is reevaluated daily, checking for infection, threshold testing, and the ECG.

PERMANENT TEMPORARY PACEMAKER

- The permanent temporary pacemaker (PTPM) is a permanent pacing system with an active fixation lead that is used for temporary purposes with the lead externalized through the skin to a standard pacemaker pulse generator.
- PTPM is indicated when temporary pacing is required for a longer period of time.
- Patients with PTPM have a more stable and reliable pacing system and may, therefore, be monitored and treated outside of the Cardiac Intensive Care Unit.
- With this method, the lead usually is implanted via either the internal jugular or subclavian vein under fluoroscopic guidance (Fig. 21.2):
  - A peel-away sheath is used to obtain venous access.
  - Fluoroscopy is required for insertion of the active fixation lead and the lead is then inserted through the sheath and advanced to the RV.
  - The ideal position is usually in the mid to apical portion of the RV septum.
  - The tip-screw mechanism is then activated to fix the lead in the appropriate position.
  - After measuring sensing, impedance, and pacing threshold and finding a position with satisfactory measurements, the peel-away sheath is removed, the lead suture sleeve is advanced to the puncture site, and the lead is sutured over the sleeve to the skin.
  - The lead is then connected to a standard pacemaker pulse generator.
  - This pacemaker can be taped to the neck or upper chest, depending on the access site.
- Uses of the PTMP include following transcatheter aortic valve replacement in which patients may develop transient complete heart block after the procedure or patients who are pacer-dependent with pacemaker infections in whom the infected permanent system is removed and they require safe and stable temporary pacing.

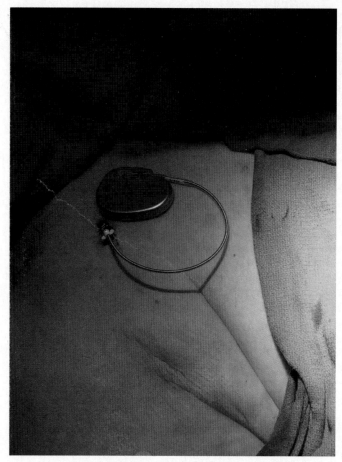

Fig. 21.2 A permanent temporary pacemaker is used for pacing for longer than the usual indications and when more stability is required. The active fixation lead is inserted into the right ventricle under fluoroscopic guidance. The sleeve is sutured to the skin, and the pulse generator is connected to the lead and then covered by a dressing.

Pericardial Tamponade

Clinical Presentation

- The clinical presentation is dependent on the acuity of presentation, the etiology, the patient's underlying comorbidities (e.g., ventricular dysfunction, volume status, valvular disease), and the ability to sustain a compensatory physiologic response.
- Patients with a hemodynamically significant pericardial effusion usually present with chest pain, breathlessness, and fullness along with signs and symptoms related to impaired cardiac function—such as fatigue, dyspnea, hypotension, pulsus paradoxus, elevated jugular venous pressure (JVP), and edema—all of which can also be present in cardiomyopathy or disease processes affecting the right heart.
- The classic triad of hypotension, elevated JVP, and diminished heart sounds (one of Beck's triads) is present in only a minority of patients.
- Less commonly, compression of adjacent intrathoracic structures results in hoarseness, hiccough, and nausea.
- It is important to be mindful of the ways in which pericardial disease may also simulate ischemic syndromes, listed in Table 22.1.
- On physical examination, patients with pericardial tamponade usually appear anxious and uncomfortable.
- Depending on the hemodynamic effects of the pericardial effusion, signs such as tachycardia, tachypnea, elevated JVP, pulsus paradoxus, and diminished pulse pressure may be present.
- A pericardial friction rub may be detected with a small effusion in the setting of pericarditis.
- If pericardial fluid compresses the adjacent lung, dullness to percussion, egophony, and bronchial breath sounds at the angle of the left scapula may be elicited (Ewart sign).

Pathophysiology

- The normal pericardium consists of a double-layered membranous sac that envelops the heart and proximal portions of the great vessels.
- The outer layer, or parietal (fibrous) pericardium, serves to anchor the heart within the thorax, and becomes contiguous with the adventitia of the great vessels.
- The inner layer, or visceral pericardium, is a serosal monolayer that adheres firmly to the epicardium, reflects over the origin of the great vessels creating the oblique and transverse sinuses and pericardial recesses (major contributors to the pericardial reserve volume), and fuses with the tough, fibrous parietal layer.

TABLE 22.1 ▨ **Major Ways in Which Pericardial Disease May Simulate Ischemic Syndromes**

Pericardial pain simulating ischemic pain
ST segment deviation suggesting myocardial ischemia
Dressler syndrome mistaken for reinfarction
Cardiac tamponade misinterpreted as heart failure
Severe tamponade mistaken for cardiogenic shock
Friction rub mistaken for murmur of acute mitral regurgitation
Friction rub mistaken for murmur of rupture of the ventricular septum

- Under normal physiologic conditions, there is typically less than 50 mL of pericardial fluid (largely an ultrafiltrate of plasma) between the pericardial layers.
- The pericardium limits distention of the cardiac chambers, facilitates ventricular interaction and coupling of the atria and ventricles, equalizes physical forces across the entire myocardial surface, minimizes friction with surrounding structures, and provides an anatomic barrier to the spread of infection.
- The accumulation of pericardial fluid is usually owing to inflammation or infection of the pericardium and adjacent structures.
- *Hemopericardium* can result spontaneously from coagulation abnormalities or as a result of surgical complications, trauma, dissection of an aortic aneurysm, or myocardial rupture.
- *Chylopericardium* is a pericardial effusion composed of chyle—a milky white and opaque fluid, with a triglyceride level greater than 500 mg/dL and a cholesterol/triglyceride ratio less than 1.
- Although the cholesterol content is high, chylopericardium should not be confused with cholesterol pericarditis, in which the fluid is clear and contains cholesterol crystals, foam cells, macrophages, and giant cells.
  - Primary chylopericardium is rare.
  - Secondary chylopericardium may be owing to radiation, subclavian vein thrombosis, infections (e.g., tuberculosis), mediastinal tumors, following cardiac and aortopulmonary surgeries, or from any process that damages the thoracic duct.
- *Pneumopericardium* is rare, occurring in the setting of chest trauma, following medical interventions (e.g., catheter ablation of arrhythmias), fistula formation, and a variety of gas-forming infections.
- Table 22.2 summarizes the most important causes of pericardial effusion.
- The rate of fluid accumulation is the critical factor in determining the hemodynamic effects and associated clinical signs and symptoms.
- A slow accumulation of a large amount of pericardial fluid may have no significant hemodynamic effect, whereas with an acute pericardial effusion, even a small volume can result in tamponade physiology.
- Cardiac tamponade is a hemodynamic condition generally characterized by an equal elevation of atrial (pulmonary capillary wedge and right atrial) and pericardial pressures, an exaggerated (> 10 mm Hg) inspiratory decrease in aortic systolic pressure (pulsus paradoxus) and hypotension or tachycardia (Fig. 22.1).
- Although the pericardium has some degree of elasticity (part of the pericardial reserve volume), once the elastic limit is reached, the heart must compete with the intrapericardial fluid for a fixed intrapericardial volume.
- As the total pericardial volume reaches the stiff portion of its pressure–volume relation, tamponade rapidly ensues.

TABLE 22.2 ▨ **Causes of Pericardial Effusion**

Categories	Examples
Idiopathic	
Infections	• Bacteria (e.g., staphylococci, streptococci, pneumococci, *Haemophilus influenzae, Mycoplasma* species, *Neisseria* species, *Borrelia burgdorferi, Chlamydia* species, *Legionella* species, *Salmonella* species, *Mycobacterium tuberculosis*, *Mycobacterium avium*).
	• Viral (e.g., coxsackievirus, adenovirus, Epstein-Barr virus, echovirus, cytomegalovirus, infectious mononucleosis, parvovirus B19, influenza, mumps, varicella, hepatitis B, HIV)
	• Fungal (e.g., histoplasmosis, aspergillosis, blastomycosis, coccidioidomycosis, *Candida* species, *Nocardia* species)
	• Rickettsial organisms
	• Parasitic (toxoplasmosis, amebiasis)
Neoplasm	• Metastatic (e.g., lung or breast carcinoma, lymphoma, leukemia, melanoma)
	• Primary (e.g., rhabdomyosarcoma, lipoma, teratoma, fibroma, fibrosarcoma, angioma, angiosarcoma, mesothelioma)
Myocardial infarction	• Rupture of ventricular aneurysm
Drugs	• Procainamide
	• Hydralazine
	• Warfarin
	• Heparin
	• Thrombolytics
	• Methysergide
	• Isoniazid
	• Cyclosporine
Autoimmune diseases	• Systemic lupus erythematosus
	• Rheumatoid arthritis
	• Scleroderma
	• Polyarteritis nodosa
	• Temporal arteritis
	• Mixed connective tissue disorder
	• Inflammatory bowel diseases
	• Sarcoidosis
	• Behçet disease
	• Myasthenia gravis
Trauma	• Blunt
	• Penetrating
	• Iatrogenic (e.g., perforation caused by catheter insertion or pacemaker implantation, status postcardiopulmonary resuscitation)
Others	• Hypothyroidism
	• Amyloidosis and autoimmune diseases
	• Chylopericardium
	• Uremia
	• Radiation
	• Pneumopericardium
	• Postcardiothoracic surgery
	• Idiopathic thrombocytopenic purpura
	• Postpericardiotomy syndrome
	• Dissecting aortic aneurysm

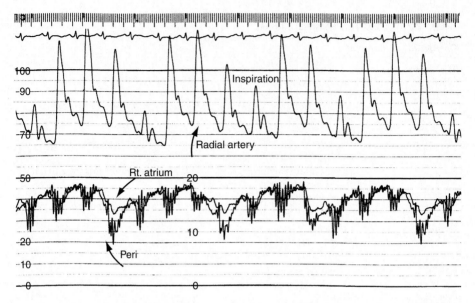

Fig. 22.1 Hyperacute cardiac tamponade caused by penetration of a saphenous vein graft during angioplasty of the graft. The radial arterial tracing shows tachycardia and extreme pulsus paradoxus. The right atrial and pericardial pressures are equilibrated at a very high level. The volume of blood in the pericardium was small.

- As cardiac tamponade progresses, the cardiac chambers become smaller, transmural chamber pressures (i.e., preload) decrease, and diastolic chamber compliance and ventricular filling decrease owing to enhanced ventricular interdependence, which lead to the characteristic elevation and equalization of diastolic filling pressures and decreases in stroke volume and blood pressure.

Investigations

- The chest radiograph may show an enlarged cardiac silhouette (often flask-shaped), typically seen when at least 250 mL of fluid has accumulated.
  - Lungs are usually clear unless the patient is in left-sided heart failure or has additional lung disease.
- Electrocardiographic (ECG) signs of acute pericarditis in the form of diffuse ST segment elevation and PR segment depression may be seen.
  - The ECG hallmark of pericardial effusion is low-voltage QRS complexes (QRS amplitude < 0.5 mV in the limb leads and < 1 mV in the precordial leads), reflecting the electrical insulation of the pericardial fluid, but it is neither a sensitive nor specific sign for pericardial effusion; therefore, it should not be used to confirm or refute a working diagnosis of pericardial effusion.
  - Electrical alternans, the beat-to-beat variation of the amplitude of QRS voltage, is another ECG finding suggestive of a large pericardial effusion or cardiac tamponade.
- Routine laboratory studies prior to pericardiocentesis should include complete blood count, prothrombin time/international normalized ratio, activated partial thromboplastin time, and a basic metabolic panel.
- Routine tests on pericardial fluid often include cell count with differential, lactate dehydrogenase, protein, glucose, Gram stain, and routine bacterial cultures.

- Smears for acid-fast bacilli; adenosine deaminase; mycobacterial, fungal, and viral cultures; and cytology are indicated, depending on the degree of suspicion for specific infectious or malignant etiologies.
- Most pericardial effusions are exudates, but no biochemical or cell-count parameter is useful for differentiating among the individual causes of pericardial disorders.
- Echocardiography is the best method for making the diagnosis of pericardial effusion and pericardial fluid appears as an echolucent space between the pericardium and the epicardium (Fig. 22.2).
  - Echocardiography can detect a pericardial effusion as small as 30 mL. Pericardial effusions are classified according to their onset, size, distribution, hemodynamic impact, and composition.
  - The detection of a pericardial effusion often has important implications for diagnosis (e.g., acute pericarditis after myocardial infarction), prognosis (e.g., patients with cancer), or both (e.g., acute aortic dissection).
  - Small nonloculated pericardial effusions usually present in the posterior pericardial space with the patient in the supine position. As the amount of fluid increases, it starts to accumulate anteriorly and laterally.
  - Large effusions are usually circumferential, allowing free motion of the heart within the fluid (swinging of the heart).
  - Important echocardiographic findings may include right atrial (RA) collapse, right ventricular (RV) collapse, reciprocal changes in right and left ventricular volume, and transvalvular flow velocities and inferior vena cava dilation with reduced respiratory change in dimension.
    - Cardiac chamber collapse occurs when the intrapericardial pressure exceeds the intracardiac pressure in a given chamber; the RV free wall buckles or invaginates in early diastole when RV pressure is at a minimum.
    - This is often best visualized in the subcostal view with an M-mode cursor through the affected chamber wall to determine timing within the cardiac cycle.
    - Early diastolic RV collapse is highly specific for tamponade, although other conditions can reproduce this finding in the absence of a hemodynamically significant effusion.

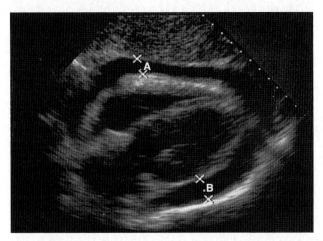

Fig. 22.2 Echocardiogram showing a large circumferential pericardial effusion. Anterior *(A)* and posterior *(B)* aspects of the effusions are shown. (From Shabetai R. Pericardial disease. In: Brown DL, ed. Cardiac Intensive Care. Philadelphia: Saunders; 1988:469–475.)

- At end-diastole when RA pressure is at its nadir, pericardial fluid pressure exceeds right atrial pressure, resulting in RA collapse, often best appreciated in the four-chamber view (Fig. 22.3).
- If persistent for longer than one third of diastole, the sensitivity, specificity, and positive predictive values approach 100% in patients with tamponade.
- The degree of invagination has no predictive value for the presence of tamponade.
- It is important to note that the absence of any chamber collapse has a nearly 90% negative predictive value for clinically significant tamponade.
- Collapse of the left atrium and the left ventricle are less common; the latter is usually in the presence of right ventricular pressure and volume overload or when tamponade is regional (e.g., after cardiac surgery).
- In normal individuals, there is minimal variation in flow velocity during normal respiration.
- In tamponade, exaggerated respiratory variation in transvalvular velocities results from enhanced ventricular interdependence and suggests the presence of pulsus paradoxus.
  - With inspiration, tricuspid flow velocity increases markedly, with a concomitant decrease in mitral flow velocity. By recent consensus, the percentage of respiratory variation for mitral and tricuspid inflow is calculated as: 100 × (expiration − inspiration)/expiration.
  - In tamponade, tricuspid flow variance usually exceeds 60%, whereas mitral flow exceeds 30%.
  - It is important to note that transvalvular flow velocity should not be the sole criterion used for the diagnosis of tamponade.
  - Inferior vena cava plethora is present in many patients with tamponade; although this finding is highly sensitive, it lacks specificity, because many other conditions are associated with increased RA pressure and have the same echocardiographic finding.

Management
- The choice between pericardiocentesis and open surgical drainage is based on local preference and experience, etiology, hemodynamic status of the patient, and characteristics of the pericardial fluid/contents.

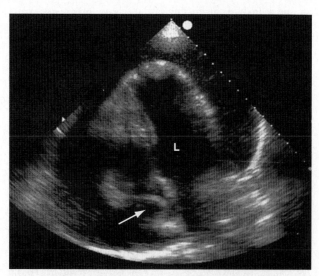

Fig. 22.3 Echocardiogram showing severe right atrial compression *(arrow)* in a patient whose pericardial effusion had caused cardiac tamponade. *L*, Left ventricle. (From Shabetai R. Pericardial disease. In: Brown DL, ed. Cardiac Intensive Care. Philadelphia: Saunders; 1988:469–475.)

- Generally, for a majority of free-flowing or uncomplicated effusions, echo-guided percutaneous drainage is preferred in the hands of a skilled operator.
- Conversely, the presence of loculated or organized fluid, hemopericardium, a traumatic etiology of the effusion, or concern for aortic dissection may be best served with surgical evacuation of the pericardium.
- Pericardiocentesis can be performed under fluoroscopic or echocardiographic guidance.
- The latter allows the operator to select the shortest route to the effusion and the puncture site with the largest collection of fluid.
- In the largest published series, the paraapical location was utilized in 66%, whereas the subxiphoid location was ideal in only 15%.
- Surgical pericardiectomy with drainage, although less commonly performed than pericardiocentesis, is recommended by the 2015 European Society of Cardiology (ESC) guidelines only in patients with symptomatic effusions in whom medical therapy and repeated pericardiocenteses were not successful.
- Patients who are diagnosed with a large pericardial effusion with minimal or no evidence of hemodynamic compromise may be treated conservatively with careful hemodynamic monitoring, serial echocardiographic studies, avoidance of diuretics and vasodilators (a IIIC recommendation), and therapy aimed at the underlying cause of the pericardial effusion.
- Effusions that progressively enlarge, lead to worsening symptoms suggesting cardiac tamponade, or that are otherwise refractory to a conservative approach should be treated with pericardial fluid drainage.
- There is no role for medical therapy of cardiac tamponade, but fluid resuscitation may be helpful while preparing for pericardial drainage.
- Mechanical ventilation should be avoided whenever possible.
- In asymptomatic patients, pericardiocentesis is rarely indicated.
- In addition, if the amount of pericardial fluid is small, it may be very difficult to access and drain.
- Occasionally, pericardial fluid drainage is required for diagnostic purposes even if the patient is asymptomatic from the effusion.
- The indications for pericardiocentesis are as follows:
  - Pericardial tamponade or large pericardial effusions
  - Symptomatic pericardial effusions
  - Suspicion of purulent pericarditis
  - Effusions of unclear etiology
  - Pericardial effusions that compress other organs (e.g., trachea, lung)

The Pericardiocentesis Procedure

- Elective or urgent pericardiocentesis should be performed by experienced individuals; otherwise, the surgical approach should be pursued.
- An echocardiogram should be obtained prior to the pericardiocentesis procedure to confirm that the effusion is at least of moderate size and is not loculated.
- Echocardiographically guided pericardiocentesis can be performed at the bedside with no exposure to radiation from fluoroscopy.
- If the clinical situation permits, any clotting abnormality should be corrected.
- The pericardiocentesis tray and associated equipment should include:
  - An 18- to 20-gauge cardiac needle or long central venous catheter with needle introducer
  - A three-way stopcock
  - Syringes (10, 20, and 60 mL)
  - Antiseptic chlorhexidine and alcohol or povidone-iodine solution

- ECG monitor
- Specimen collection tubes for fluid analysis and cultures; fluid receptacle (1 L vacuum bottle)
- Small-gauge needle for local anesthesia and 1% to 2% lidocaine
- Sterile gloves, mask, gown, dressing materials (sterile transparent plastic drape), and gauze
- Surgical blade (No. 11)
- Sterile isotonic sodium chloride solution (for flushing catheter)
- Emergency medications (e.g., atropine, lidocaine, epinephrine)
- Defibrillator with monitor
- 4-0 silk sutures and needle holder
- Position the patient at a 30- to 45-degree, head-up angle to permit pericardial fluid to pool on the inferior surface of the heart.
- Palpate the subxyphoid process, about a finger-width below the edge of the rib. This location avoids difficulty in advancing the catheter through fibrous tissue closer to the lower part of the sternum itself.
- Using the echo probe, first find the maximal effusion, which will determine the position and angle of your needle, and then measure the distance from the probe to skin and then probe to the myocardium (in diastole), which will determine the depth you are aiming for and the buffer zone.
- Prepare the site in a sterile manner and drape, covering everything but a small area around the subxyphoid process.
- After infiltration of the skin and subcutaneous tissues with lidocaine, make a small incision (~ 5 mm) to decrease the resistance during needle insertion.
- Advance the pericardial needle through the skin, first perpendicularly to the chest and then angled lower to a plane nearly parallel with the floor, moving under the subxyphoid process toward the left shoulder.
- More lidocaine can be given gently through the pericardial needle as it is advanced.
- If the patient is obese, a longer needle and some force may be required to tip the syringe under the subxyphoid process toward the heart.
- Advance the needle into the pericardial space.
- Passage of the needle through the skin causes the needle to become occluded by subcutaneous tissue.
- Flush any tissue that may have accumulated during passage before entering the pericardium, a tough fibrous membrane.
- Use caution when advancing the needle through the diaphragm; excessive forward pressure may result in a sudden jump through the pericardium into a cardiac chamber.
- Confirm the intrapericardial position with echo contrast imaging. As the needle advances, colored fluid or blood in the syringe signals likely entry into the pericardium (note that chronic effusions are often clear yellow, occasionally serosanguineous, or, less commonly, dark brown).
- Acute effusions resulting from trauma, cancer, myocardial rupture, or aortic dissection are frankly bloody.
- After entering the pericardial space, an injection of 5 to 10 mL of agitated saline through the needle appears as microbubble contrast and confirms the intrapericardial needle position.
- If the needle tip is in the RV, the bubbles will be seen in the RV cavity and will be dispersed rapidly by RV systole.
- When the needle tip is inside the pericardial space, a soft floppy-tip guidewire is passed through the needle.
- This guidewire should be advanced posteriorly around the heart.

- This wire position is important to ensure that the needle has not punctured the heart and the wire is not inserted into the RV, in which case the wire will go up the RV outflow tract and will induce frequent premature ventricular contractions or ventricular tachycardia.
- The needle is exchanged over a guidewire for a multiple side-hole pericardial drainage catheter.
- If the catheter will not drain or the exact position of the catheter is uncertain, a further amount of echo contrast medium may be injected to assess the problem.
- Contrast medium pools in the dependent portion of the pericardial space, but rapidly washes out of a vascular space.
- Bloody pericardial fluid may be owing to chronic disease or to acute trauma during the procedure and has a lower hematocrit value than blood and will not clot as rapidly.
- Secure the catheter in place with anchor sutures using 4.0 silk.
- Obtain serial echocardiograms before and after removal of the pericardial drainage catheter to confirm the absence of fluid reaccumulation.
- In the absence of significant fluid reaccumulation, the pericardial drain can usually be removed after 24 to 48 hours.
- Should there be a large or hemodynamically significant effusion, consider a surgical pericardial window.

Complications

- Potential complications of pericardiocentesis include:
  - Ventricular puncture
  - Cardiac arrest
  - Pneumothorax
  - Liver laceration
  - Laceration of a coronary artery or vein
  - Hemorrhage
  - Ventricular and atrial arrhythmias
- Contraindications to pericardiocentesis include:
  - Myocardial rupture
  - Aortic dissection
  - Skin infection at the access site
  - Severe bleeding disorders

CHAPTER 23

Invasive Hemodynamic Monitoring

Common Misconceptions

- Invasive hemodynamic monitoring should be used in all patients in the Cardiac Intensive Care Unit (CICU).
- The pulmonary capillary wedge pressure is always a surrogate for left ventricular end-diastolic pressure.
- Mixed venous oxygen saturation can be sampled from any right heart chamber.

- Hemodynamics is derived hydrodynamics, the physics of the motion and action of water.
- The dimensions of hemodynamics include flow, pressure, static resistance, dynamic imped- ance, reflectance and compliance, branching effects, viscosity, fluid friction, turbulence, and other physical characteristics.
- The goals of hemodynamic assessment and manipulation in the critically ill patient are to ensure adequate organ blood flow, oxygen supply, and, ultimately, to improve survival.
- Noninvasive parameters to measure organ perfusion include systolic and diastolic blood pressure, body temperature, heart rate, urine output, and respiratory frequency.
- The development of bedside intravascular catheterization procedures allowed, for the first time, meaningful application of hemodynamic monitoring in the care of selected critically ill patients.

Systemic Arterial Blood Pressure

- The continuous measurement of arterial pressure is essential in hemodynamic monitoring of critically ill patients.
- Arterial pressure is the input pressure for organ perfusion.
- In the CICU, insertion of an indwelling arterial catheter into either the arm (brachial or radial sites) or groin (femoral arterial site) is often used to provide more precise monitoring.
- The advantages of arterial catheterization over noninvasive techniques are continuous monitoring of arterial pressure and its waveform and providing a site for repetitive blood sampling.
- Arterial pressure is a function of both vasomotor tone and cardiac output (CO).
- Local metabolic demands determine local vasomotor tone that, in turn, determines blood flow distribution.
- Perfusion pressure and local vascular resistance determine organ perfusion of all capillary beds.
- Flow is proportional to local metabolic demand if there is no hemodynamic instability to cause increased sympathetic tone.
- CO primarily determines arterial pressure in the setting of varying degrees of local blood flow and, because it is proportional to local metabolic demand, there is no normal value in an unstable, metabolically active patient.

TABLE 23.1 ■ **Arterial Catheterization**

Probable Indications for Arterial Catheterization

- Guide to management of potent vasodilator drug infusions to prevent systemic hypotension
- Guide to management of potent vasopressor drug infusions to maintain a target mean arterial pressure
- As a port for the rapid and repetitive sampling of arterial blood in patients in whom multiple arterial blood samples are indicated
- As a monitor of cardiovascular deterioration in patients at risk for cardiovascular instability

Useful Applications of Arterial Pressure Monitoring in the Diagnosis of Cardiovascular Insufficiency

- Differentiating cardiac tamponade (pulsus paradoxus) from respiration-induced swings in systolic arterial pressure; tamponade reduces the pulse pressure but keeps diastolic pressure constant. Respiration reduces systolic and diastolic pressure equally, such that pulse pressure is constant.
- Differentiating hypovolemia from cardiac dysfunction as the cause of hemodynamic instability. Systolic arterial pressure decreases more following a positive pressure breath as compared with an apneic baseline during hypovolemia. Systolic arterial pressure increases more during positive pressure inspiration when left ventricular (LV) contractility is reduced.

Modified from Polanco PM, Pinsky MR. Practical issues of hemodynamic monitoring at the bedside. *Surg Clin North Am*. 2006;86(6):1431–1456.

- The literature currently suggests maintaining patients who were previously nonhypertensive at a mean arterial blood pressure (MAP) of 65 mm Hg, consistent with the initial MAP target recommended by the Surviving Sepsis Guidelines.
- In a clinical trial that examined the effects of resuscitative efforts with fluid and vasopressors in patients with circulatory shock to varying MAP targets, ranging from 60 to 90 mm Hg, no increased organ blood flow could be determined above a MAP of 65 mm Hg.
- However, evidence in the septic shock literature indicates that a MAP of 75 to 85 mm Hg may reduce the development of acute kidney injury in patients with chronic arterial hypertension.
- As a result, it has been suggested to consider more individualized targets for older patients with hypertension or atherosclerosis and in patients with septic shock.
- The indications for arterial catheterization (Table 23.1).
- In most cases, the choice of location for insertion of the catheter is the radial artery because femoral artery cannulation is more often associated with displacement during patient movement and hemorrhage that is more difficult to control.
- Although arterial catheterization is an invasive procedure with inherent risks (temporary vascular occlusion 20% and hematoma 14%), most complications are not severe, with permanent ischemic damage, sepsis, and pseudoaneurysm occurring in less than 1% of cases.

Pulmonary Artery Catheterization

- Pulmonary artery (PA) catheterization permits additional measurements of CO, right heart, and pulmonary pressures that make it possible to calculate other derived hemodynamic parameters, such as cardiac work indices and systemic and pulmonary vascular resistance.
- These fundamental hemodynamic variables help further describe the disordered physiologic state with sufficient precision to enhance management decisions and aid in the care of critically ill patients.

- The PA catheter allows for determination of various fundamental hemodynamic parameters, including measurement of CO by thermodilution (TD), right atrial (RA), right ventricular (RV), PA, and pulmonary capillary wedge pressures (PCWP), and sampling of blood from the PA, RV, and RA.
- Pulmonary vascular and systemic resistance, as well as RV and left ventricular (LV) stroke work, can then be derived.

Pulmonary Artery Catheter

- The most commonly used PA catheter is a 7.5 Fr thermodilution, triple-lumen, radiopaque catheter, 110 cm long made of polyvinylchloride.
- Most catheters are heparin coated to reduce thrombogenicity.
- The outside is marked with black rings every 10 cm from the tip that allow determination without fluoroscopy of the appropriate catheter length at which to inflate the distal balloon.
- The distal lumen terminates at the tip of the catheter, whereas the RA lumen terminates 30 cm proximal to the tip. There is a venous infusion lumen 1 cm proximal to the RA lumen.
- A thermistor bead located 3 to 5 cm from the tip is connected to an external thermistor connector by a wire.
- The external thermistor is, in turn, linked to a computer that allows for determination of CO by the TD method.
- A soft latex balloon with a maximum inflating capacity of 1.0 to 1.5 mL is affixed to the distal tip of the PA catheter.
- Upon inflation, the balloon engulfs the catheter tip, cushioning the transmitted force, limiting injury of endocardial surfaces, and reducing the frequency of arrhythmias.
- The inflated balloon facilitates flow-directed advancement of the catheter through the right heart into the PA.
- Once inflated in a distal branch of the PA, the balloon occludes the vessel and allows for measurement of PCWP through the catheter tip.
- The catheter can serve multiple functions, including measurement of CO by TD, PA temperature, and intracardiac pressures (RA, RV, PA, PCW).
- Blood sampling can be done through the active lumens of the catheter.

EQUIPMENT AND SIGNAL CALIBRATION

- The fluid-filled PA catheter is connected via semirigid pressure tubing to pressure transducers.
- These transducers consist of a fluid-filled dome, a diaphragm, and a strain gauge Wheatstone bridge arrangement.
- An electric current directly proportional to the fluid motion is amplified and transmitted to the oscilloscope equipment for display.
- The system must have a frequency response of flat to 15 to 20 Hz to be adequate for human studies.
- Pressure waveforms are not reliable in patients with excessively rapid heart rates of greater than 180 beats/min.
- The length of the pressure tubing determines the natural frequency of fluid-filled systems.
- Excessively long tubing will drop the natural frequency to below physiologic range, causing an overamplification of signal, resulting in falsely elevated pressure readings.
- The recommended length of pressure tubing is 3 to 4 feet.
- Damping is the opposite effect, with a loss of physiologic signal that most commonly results from air trapped in the circuit.
- Damping of the PA pressure signal may make it difficult to discern from the PCWP tracing.

TABLE 23.2 ▪ Equipment Required for Pulmonary Artery Catheter Insertion

Appropriate PA catheter
Dilator-sheath-side arm assembly
Three-way stopcocks
Pressure tubing
Transducers
18-gauge, thin-walled Cook needle
Sterile gowns, drapes, gloves
1% lidocaine
Heparinized saline
J-tipped guidewire
Towel clips, syringes, suture material
Electrocardiography and pressure-monitoring equipment
Intravenous line
Atropine
Defibrillator unit
21-gauge Micropuncture Access Set (Cook Medical)
Ultrasound

- Catheter whip artifact from motion imparted to the catheter with each cardiac contraction can be eliminated by high-frequency filters.
- Accurately measuring pressure signals requires proper calibration of the monitoring system.
  - With a patient supine, the pressure transducer is aligned with the fourth intercostal space midway between the front and back of the chest.
  - This site serves as the standard zero reference point.
  - The calibration of the monitor involves the introduction of a known pressure signal. This can be done either internally or externally.
  - Zero reference and calibration should be checked each day of hemodynamic monitoring.
- Required equipment for PA catheter insertion (Table 23.2).

CATHETER INSERTION

- Catheter equipment should be inspected and calibrated.
- All lumens should be flushed with normal saline and should be free of air.
- Potential insertion sites include the internal jugular, subclavian, and femoral veins (Table 23.3).
- The right internal jugular vein is the preferable access route because of the straight course to the superior vena cava.
- Ultrasound-guided insertion of the needle and a micropuncture system are commonly used to further reduce complications.
- Meticulous preparation of the chosen site with aseptic technique is crucial.
- The operator and any assistants should be in sterile gown, gloves, face masks, and caps.
- The patient should be properly prepared, draped, and placed in the Trendelenburg position.
- The site is then accessed percutaneously through a modified Seldinger technique.

TABLE 23.3 ■ **Comparison of Venous Access Routes**

Vein	Advantages	Disadvantages
Internal jugular	Rapidly accessible Does not interfere with CPR Provides a straight route to the heart Less restrictive to patient movement	Air embolism, carotid artery puncture, and tracheal injury may occur. Pneumothorax (more common in the left than the right internal jugular vein). Thoracic duct injury (left internal jugular vein only).
Subclavian	Rapidly accessible Allows free neck and arm movement Easier to keep sterile	Air embolism, more frequent pneumothorax and hemothorax; subclavian artery puncture; injury to nerve bundle may occur.
Femoral	Rapidly accessible Does not interfere with CPR	Sepsis, *in situ* thrombosis, and pulmonary embolism may occur. Usually requires fluoroscopy.

CPR, Cardiopulmonary resuscitation.

- After local anesthesia, an 18-gauge, 7.6-cm Cook needle with attached syringe is inserted bevel up at approximately 45 degrees between the heads of the sternocleidomastoid muscles toward the ipsilateral nipple while palpating the ipsilateral carotid artery.
- After free-flowing venous blood is obtained, the syringe is disconnected from the needle and a 40-cm long J-tipped guidewire is inserted into the needle and passed gently into the vein.
- The guidewire should pass without any resistance and should never be advanced if any resistance is encountered.
- The needle is then removed, and the skin puncture is enlarged with a scalpel blade.
- The dilator sheath system is then advanced over the guidewire into the vein with a gentle rotating movement.
- Once the sheath is properly positioned, the wire and dilator should be removed, and the sheath sutured in place.
- Prior to insertion, the PA catheter should be inspected for bends and kinks and the balloon tested with air inflation underwater to evaluate for leaks.
- The catheter then should be connected with pressure tubing to calibrated pressure transducers.
- Finally, a plastic sleeve is placed over the catheter to preserve the sterile length of the catheter outside of the body for future manipulation.
- The catheter is then inserted and advanced approximately 10 cm before the balloon is inflated with 1 to 1.5 mL of air.
- In most patients, the catheter will reach the RA 10 to 15 cm from the internal jugular or subclavian vein.
- Once in the RA, the catheter should be advanced quickly under continuous pressure and electrocardiographic monitoring across the tricuspid valve, through the RV, PA, and into the PCWP position.
- The catheter should reach the PA approximately 50 to 55 cm from the internal jugular vein.
- Typical pressure waveforms (Fig. 23.1).
- After achieving the wedge position, deflation of the balloon should allow the deflated catheter to recoil into the proximal PA.
- The balloon should be slowly inflated while PA pressure is continuously monitored.

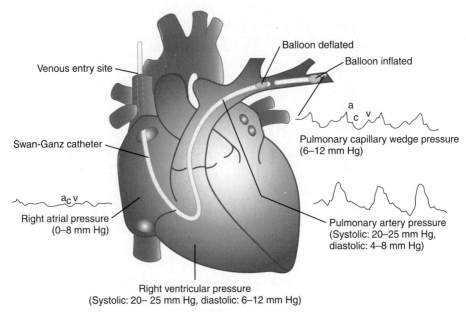

Fig. 23.1 Normal hemodynamic pressures. (Modified from Swan HC. The pulmonary artery catheter. Dis Mon. 1991;37:518.)

- With inflation, the catheter should then float to a wedge position.
- The goal is occlusion of a distal pulmonary artery branch impeding blood flow to that area.
- PCWP tracings without inflation of the distal balloon indicates distal migration of the catheter.
  - If distal migration occurs, the catheter should be repositioned by slow withdrawal of the catheter 1 to 2 cm at a time with the balloon deflated.
- Inability to secure a proper PCWP tracing can be caused by patient movement, mechanical ventilation, positive end-expiratory pressure (PEEP) and eccentric balloon inflation.
- Catheter position should be checked routinely by chest radiographs.
- To minimize the risk of endothelial damage to the PA, PA rupture, or pulmonary infarction, time in the wedge position should be kept to a maximum of about 10 seconds.
- End-expiration diastolic PA pressures should approximate mean PCWP in the absence of increased pulmonary arteriolar resistance, such as with pulmonary hypertension or pulmonary embolus.
- Assuming no anatomic or functional interruptions, the pressure recorded through a wedged end-hole catheter is that of the next active vascular system which, in most circumstances, is the left atrium (LA) or LV at end-diastole.
- The ideal placement of the catheter is the lower lung zone.
  - In zone 3, the most dependent portion, both PA and venous pressures exceed alveolar pressure, thereby maintaining an open vascular system from the catheter tip to the LA.
  - In the upper lung, or zone 1, alveolar pressure exceeds PA and venous pressures, keeping the capillaries closed, disrupting the system, and preventing accurate measurement of LA pressures.

- The arterial pressures in the central lung, or zone 2, should exceed alveolar pressure, but low pulmonary venous pressure may prevent retrograde transmission of pressures from the LA.
- Fortunately, most of the lung in the supine position is in zone 3 and flow-guided catheters will usually enter this zone. A lateral chest radiograph can confirm position of the catheter tip below the LA.

Pulmonary Capillary Wedge Pressure

- PCWP is a phase-delayed, amplitude-damped version of LA pressure.
- During diastole with a nonstenotic mitral valve, the pulmonary venous system, LA, and LV is a continuous circuit and the PCWP is then reflective of the LV diastolic pressure.
  - The PCWP provides the measure of hydrostatic pressure that is responsible for forcing fluid out of the pulmonary vascular space.
  - In addition, the capillary pressure is directly related to diastolic fiber stretch according to Starling's principle, which states that the strength of contraction is proportional to myocardial fiber length/LV volume.
  - When applied to construct a cardiac function curve, it is often called LV filling pressure or preload.
- The natural oscillation in intrathoracic pressure associated with respiration directly affects intraluminal pulmonary vascular pressure.
  - During spontaneous breathing, the highest pulmonary pressures occur at end-expiration.
  - This is the opposite of mechanical positive pressure ventilation, in which the lowest pulmonary pressures occur at end-expiration.
  - To minimize this artifact, recorded pressures should be made at end-expiration.
  - Even at end-expiration, PCWP measures still can be overestimated if pleural pressures are elevated at end-expiration.
  - Factors, such as hyperinflation, air trapping, and PEEP in relation to lung and chest wall compliance, increase pleural pressure to varying degrees.

Cardiac Output and Mixed Venous Oxygen Consumption

- Although CO can be measured by several techniques, the two most commonly used are the indicator thermodilution technique and the Fick oxygen technique.
- Both are based on the theoretic principle devised by Adolf Fick in 1870, which states that the total uptake or release of any substance by an organ is the product of blood flow to the organ and the arteriovenous (AV) concentration difference of the substance.

INDICATOR DILUTION METHOD

- The most commonly used indicator today is the "cold" indicator in the TD method.
- This technique measures the change in the temperature of blood caused by the introduction of a known quantity of cold liquid upstream from a point of temperature measurement.
- Typically, cold saline injected into the RA results in cooling of the blood that is measured downstream by a thermistor to produce a TD curve.
- The area under the curve represents the integral of the instantaneous mixing temperature at the sensing point (Fig. 23.2).
- CO is automatically computed from these measurements using a small microprocessor.
- The validity of results depends on the precision of the technique.
- The injection technique should be smooth and rapid to avoid dispersion of the injectate.
- Multiple measures should be taken and averaged to avoid ventilatory cycle-specific patterns.

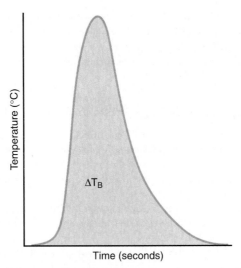

Fig. 23.2　Sample thermodilution curve shows the change in instantaneous mixed temperature at the sensing point (thermistor) versus time. (Modified from Ehlers KC, Mylrea KC, Waterston CK, et al. Cardiac output measurements: a review of current techniques and research. Ann Biomed Eng. 1986;14:219–239.)

FICK METHOD

- With the Fick method of CO measurement, pulmonary blood flow is determined by measuring the AV difference of oxygen across the lungs and the rate of uptake by blood across the lungs.
- If there are no intracardiac shunts, pulmonary and systemic blood flow should be equal, and the CO equals oxygen consumption divided by AV oxygen difference.

$$CO\ (vol\ /\ time) = \frac{O_2\ consumption\ (mass\ /\ time)}{[arterial - venous\ O_2\ content]\ (mass\ /\ vol)}$$

- The oxygen consumption can be either directly measured or calculated.
  - Direct measurement is performed with exhaled breath analysis using a spirometer, such as the metabolic rate meter or the Deltatrac II (Datax-Ohmeda).
  - In a steady state, oxygen consumption can be determined by having the patient breathe pure oxygen from the spirometer with a carbon dioxide absorber and measuring oxygen uptake directly by the net gas flux.
  - Normal oxygen consumption in a resting individual is approximately 250 mL O_2/min.
- Calculation of the $\dot{V}/O_2$ can be done by rearranging the Fick equation: $\dot{V}/O_2$ (mL O_2/min) = CO × (Cao_2 − Cvo_2), where Cao_2 is the arterial oxygen content and CVo_2 is the mixed venous blood content.
  - Normal Cao_2 and CVo_2 are 20 mL O_2/dL and 15 mL O_2/dL, respectively.
- Oxygen consumption can also be estimated using a nomogram based on age, sex, height, and weight.

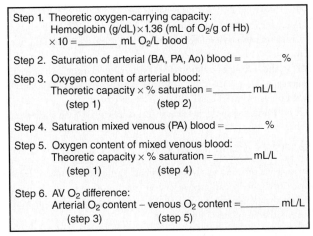

Step 1. Theoretic oxygen-carrying capacity:
Hemoglobin (g/dL) × 1.36 (mL of O_2/g of Hb)
× 10 = _____ mL O_2/L blood

Step 2. Saturation of arterial (BA, PA, Ao) blood = _____%

Step 3. Oxygen content of arterial blood:
Theoretic capacity × % saturation = _____ mL/L
(step 1)   (step 2)

Step 4. Saturation mixed venous (PA) blood = _____%

Step 5. Oxygen content of mixed venous blood:
Theoretic capacity × % saturation = _____ mL/L
(step 1)   (step 4)

Step 6. AV O_2 difference:
Arterial O_2 content − venous O_2 content = _____ mL/L
(step 3)   (step 5)

Fig. 23.3 Calculation of oxygen content and arteriovenous (AV) oxygen difference when using the reflectance oximetry method. *Ao,* Aorta; *BA,* brachial artery; *PA,* pulmonary artery. (Modified from Baim DS, ed. Grossman's Cardiac Catheterization, Angiography, and Intervention, ed 7. Philadelphia: Lippincott Williams & Wilkins; 2006:154.)

- The AV difference is calculated by obtaining blood from a peripheral artery and the pulmonary artery for a mixed venous sample.
- The oxygen saturation is then multiplied by theoretic oxygen-carrying capacity to yield the oxygen content of the sample (Fig. 23.3).
- Mixed venous oxygen saturation (Svo_2) reflects the relationship between oxygen consumption ($\dot{V}/O_2$) and oxygen delivery (DO_2).
- It should be measured from blood drawn from the distal tip of the PA catheter to allow for adequate mixing of superior vena cava, inferior vena cava, and coronary sinus samples.
- The normal range of Svo_2 is 60% to 80%.
  - If the Svo_2 is normal, one can assume that tissue perfusion is adequate, whereas high or low values reflect an imbalance between oxygen supply and demand.
  - A low Svo_2 reflects either decreased oxygen delivery (i.e., decreased haemoglobin (Hb), Sao_2, or cardiac output) or increased oxygen demand.
  - Conversely, high Svo_2 reflects increased oxygen delivery or decreased oxygen demand, such as in the case of sepsis or, more generally, the systemic inflammatory response syndrome.

Pulmonary and Systemic Vascular Resistance

- The pulmonary vascular resistance (PVR) and systemic vascular resistance (SVR) are computed values using measurements from the PA catheter.

$$PVR\ (dyne \times sec/cm^5) = 80 \times \frac{MeanPAP - PCWP}{CO}$$

$$SVR\ (dyne \times sec/cm^5) = 80 \times \frac{MAP - RA}{CO}$$

- Normal PVR is less than 250 dyne × sec/cm^5.
- If pulmonary hypertension is associated with increased PVR, causes are primarily within the lung, such as pulmonary embolism, pulmonary fibrosis, essential pulmonary hypertension, or pulmonary venoocclusive disease.
- Normal PVR in the setting of pulmonary hypertension is more indicative of elevation of LV filling pressures.
- Normal SVR ranges from 800 to 1200 dyne × sec/cm^5.
  - Low SVR indicates a vasoplegic state, whereas increased SVR indicates vasoconstriction.

Complications of Pulmonary Artery Catheterization

- As with any invasive procedure, complications are an inherent risk of PA catheterization.
- Complications occur with catheter insertion (pneumothorax, arrhythmia, atrioventricular block) and after the catheter is in place (pulmonary infarction, local thrombosis, pulmonary artery rupture, catheter-related infection).

Indications for Pulmonary Artery Catheterization

- Hemodynamic data derived from PA catheterization may aid in diagnosis as well as guide management.
- Despite the widespread use of PA catheters, the effect on patient outcome remains controversial.
- The accepted indications for PA catheterization have been based largely on expert opinion.
- The decision to place a PA catheter should be based on a clinical question regarding a patient's hemodynamic status that cannot be answered with noninvasive assessment (Table 23.4).
- Carefully obtained hemodynamic data can influence choice of therapy (Table 23.5).

CONTROVERSIES

- The PA catheter became a widely used monitoring device in critically ill patients after its introduction in 1971, but its initial use was based only on assumed benefit and the desire to understand the hemodynamic profiles of various disease states.
- Retrospective analyses from the 1980s studying PA catheter use in acute myocardial infarction found no difference in mortality after adjusting for illness severity.
- In 1996, a retrospective observational study of more than 5500 cardiac and noncardiac critically ill patients concluded that, after adjustment for treatment selection bias, use of a PA catheter was actually associated with increased mortality and length of stay.
- In 2005, two large multicenter randomized trials were published examining the effectiveness of PA catheterization in the management of critically ill patients.
- The first reported on more than 1000 critically ill patients enrolled between 2001 and 2004.
  - Patients were randomized to PA catheter insertion or no PA catheter.
  - There was no statistical difference in hospital mortality between the groups (68% vs. 66%; adjusted hazard ratio, 1.09; 95% confidence interval, 0.94–1.27; $P = .39$).
  - The less than 10% complication rate did not directly lead to an increase in mortality.
  In the second trial, patients admitted with severe symptomatic and recurrent heart failure from 2000 to 2003 were randomized to PA catheter insertion or no PA catheter.
  - The authors found that therapy in both groups led to a substantial reduction in symptoms, jugular venous pressure, and edema.

TABLE 23.4 ■ How Hemodynamic Profiles Differentiate Cardiopulmonary Disorders

Disorder	Hemodynamic Profile	Comments
Acute ischemic RV dysfunction	Increased RA, decreased SV, decreased CO, decreased AP, RA greater than or equal to PCWP	Steep y descent RV diastolic dip and plateau (square root sign) Volume loading may unmask hemodynamic changes
Acute mitral regurgitation	Increased PCWP, prominent v waves, sometimes reflecting onto the PA tracing as well	V waves may not always differentiate mitral regurgitation from ventricular septal rupture
Acute ventricular septal rupture	Oxygen step-up from RA to RV and PA	RV forward output exceeds LV forward output Early recirculation on the thermodilution curve
Shock		
Ventriculopenic	Increased RA, decreased SV, decreased CO, decreased AP, increased SVR	
Hypovolemic	Decreased or low-normal PCWP, decreased SV, decreased CO, decreased AP, increased SVR	Orthostatic tachycardia
Early septic	Increased PA, increased PVR, increased CO, decreased AP, decreased SVR	SVR is elevated and cardiac output is lowered in later stages
Noncardiac pulmonary edema	Normal PCWP	Normal heart size
Acute massive pulmonary embolism	Decreased SV, decreased CO, decreased AP, increased PA, increased PVR, normal PCWP	PCWP normal despite elevated pulmonary artery systolic and diastolic pressures
Chronic precapillary pulmonary hypertension	Increased RA, increased RV systolic pressure, increased PA, increased PVR, normal PCWP	Left-sided pressures often normal PA and RV systolic pressures may reach systemic levels
Acute cardiac tamponade	Increased RA, increased PCWP, RA equal to PCWP, decreased SV, decreased CO, decreased AP	Paradoxic pulse Blunted y descent Prominent x descent on RA tracing
Constrictive pericarditis	Increased RA, increased PCWP, dip and plateau in RV pressure, M- or W-shaped jugular venous pressure with preserved x and steep y descent	Paradoxic pulse rare Positive Kussmaul sign common May simulate ischemic RV dysfunction or restrictive cardiomyopathy
Restrictive cardiomyopathy	Findings are similar to those described for constrictive pericarditis, but PCWP may be higher than RA; difference between PCWP and RA may be exaggerated by exercise	Simulates constrictive pericarditis; however, PA systolic pressure is usually > 50 mm Hg and diastolic plateau is less than one-third peak RV systolic pressure. Thus, other tests are often needed for differentiation from constrictive pericarditis
Tricuspid regurgitation	Increased RA, increased RV end-diastolic pressure	Blunted x descent, prominent v wave, steep y descent Ventricularization of RA pressure

AP, Mean arterial pressure; CO, cardiac output; LV, left ventricular pressure; PA, mean pulmonary artery pressure; PCWP, pulmonary capillary wedge pressure; PVR, pulmonary vascular resistance; RA, mean right atrial pressure; RV, right ventricular pressure; SV, stroke volume; SVR, systemic vascular resistance.

TABLE 23.5 ■ **Using Hemodynamic Data to Choose Therapy**

Clinical Diagnosis	Hemodynamic Data	Suggested Therapy
Acute pulmonary edema	Increased PCWP, decreased CO	Diuretics, vasodilators Hemofiltration/dialysis if edema is associated with oliguria or anuria Intraaortic balloon counterpulsation support in special circumstances
Low-Output or Shock Syndromes		
Absolute or relative hypovolemia	Decreased PCWP	Volume expansion
Ischemic right ventricular dysfunction	Increased RA, normal PCWP, normal PA	Volume expansion with or without inotropic agents
Early sepsis	Increased CO, decreased SVR, decreased AP	Volume loading Vasopressors/inotropic drugs Specific treatment for causative organism
Ventriculopenia	Increased PCWP, increased PA, decreased CO, decreased AP	Reduce preload with diuretics and/or vasodilators Inotropic agents and intraaortic balloon counterpulsation in special circumstances
Pulmonary embolism	Increased RA, decreased CO, decreased AP, increased PA, normal PCWP	Thrombolytic or anticoagulant therapy after scintigraphic or angiographic confirmation
Cardiac tamponade	Increased RA, RA equals PCWP, paradoxic pulse	Echocardiographic confirmation, if time permits Pericardiocentesis

AP, Mean arterial pressure; *CO*, cardiac output; *PA*, mean pulmonary artery pressure; *PCWP*, pulmonary capillary wedge pressure; *RA*, mean right atrial pressure; *SVR*, systemic vascular resistance.

■ The use of a PA catheter did not significantly affect the primary endpoint of 6-month mortality, indicating that basing the decision to administer vasodilator and diuretic therapy on PAC data plus clinical judgment was not superior to decisions based on clinical judgment alone.

■ Ultimately, the data from both trials found PA catheter use to be safe and did not substantiate previous retrospective reports of excessive mortality associated with PA catheter use.

■ Safe and effective PA catheter use should be predicated on careful catheter placement, attention to measurement techniques, meticulous catheter care, and thoughtful interpretation of the data.

CHAPTER 24

Temporary Mechanical Circulatory Support Devices

- Clinicians practicing in the cardiac intensive care unit are challenged with increasingly complex patients who often require hemodynamic support to improve end-organ perfusion and reduce mortality.
- Numerous devices to augment left ventricular or right ventricular cardiac output (CO) have been developed that can be placed surgically or percutaneously (Fig. 24.1).
- Each approach has device-specific characteristics (Table 24.1).
- Each device has different effects on hemodynamics (Table 24.2).
- The different complication profiles of each device must be taken into consideration when selecting the optimal type of hemodynamic support for each patient (Table 24.3).

Intraaortic Balloon Pump

- The intraaortic balloon pump (IABP) is one of the most frequently placed mechanical circulatory support devices.
- The IABP is used in managing cardiogenic shock, intractable angina, myocardial ischemia, during high-risk percutaneous coronary intervention (PCI), in cardiac surgery, and for patients with refractory heart failure or arrhythmias awaiting definitive therapy.
- It relies on the concept of diastolic augmentation and afterload reduction to improve the function of ischemic and/or failing myocardium.

PHYSIOLOGIC PRINCIPLES

- The primary goal of IABP counterpulsation is to increase myocardial oxygen supply while decreasing oxygen demand.
- During diastole, the balloon inflates, resulting in a volume of blood being displaced toward the proximal aorta.
- During systole, the balloon rapidly deflates, creating a vacuum effect resulting in a decrease in left ventricular (LV) afterload and a reduction in myocardial workload.
- To optimize these two hemodynamic effects, the IABP must inflate and deflate in synchrony with the cardiac cycle.

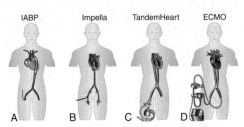

Fig. 24.1 A, intraaortic balloon pump (IABP); B, Impella; C, TandemHeart; D, venoarterial (VA) extracorporeal membrane oxygenation (ECMO). (From Werdan K, Gielen S, Ebelt H, et al. Mechanical circulatory support in cardiogenic shock. Eur Heart J 2013;35(3):156–67.)

TABLE 24.1 ▮ Characteristics of Temporary Mechanical Circulatory Support Devices

Device Characteristics	IABP	Impella	TandemHeart	VA ECMO
Pump mechanism	Pneumatic	Axial flow	Centrifugal	Centrifugal
Cannula size	8 Fr	13–23 Fr	21 Fr inflow, 15–17 Fr outflow	18–21 Fr inflow, 15–17 Fr outflow
Insertion	Percutaneous	Percutaneous or surgical cutdown	Percutaneous	Percutaneous and surgical
Maximum implant duration	7–10 days	7–21 days (model dependent)	14–21 days	21–28 days
Delivered flow	0.5–1 L/min	1.5–5 L/min (model dependent)	4 L/min	3–6 L/min

IABP, Intraaortic balloon pump; *VA ECMO,* venoarterial extracorporeal membrane oxygenation.
From Combes A, Brodie D, Chen Y, et al. The ICM research agenda on extracorporeal life support. *Intensive Care Med.* 2017;43:1306–1318.

■ The single most important determinant of effective counterpulsation is the timing of the IABP relative to the cardiac cycle.
■ Once proper timing has been established, IABP counterpulsation improves myocardial oxygen delivery via an increase in coronary perfusion pressure, reduces cardiac work by decreasing systolic blood pressure and afterload, and improves forward blood flow in patients with impaired cardiac contractile function.
■ The majority of patients exhibit a decrease in systolic pressure, an increase in diastolic pressure (which may subsequently enhance coronary blood flow to a territory perfused by an artery with a critical stenosis), a reduction in heart rate, a decrease in the mean pulmonary capillary wedge pressure (PCWP), and an increase in CO of 0.5 to 1.0 L/min.
■ Two indices measured during IABP counterpulsation are the tension-time index (TTI), which is the time integral of LV pressures during systole, and the diastolic pressure-time index (DPTI), which is the time integral of the proximal aortic pressures during diastole.
■ Proper balloon inflation augments diastolic pressure (i.e., increases DPTI), whereas rapid balloon deflation decreases LV afterload (i.e., decreases TTI).

TABLE 24.2 ■ **Effect of Temporary Mechanical Circulatory Support Devices on Hemodynamics**

Hemodynamic Parameter	IABP	Impella	TandemHeart	VA ECMO
MAP	Increase	Increase	Increase	Increase
Afterload	Reduced	Neutral	Increased	Increased
Coronary perfusion	Slightly Increased	Unknown	Unknown	Unknown
LV stroke volume	Slightly Increased	Reduced	Reduced	Reduced
LV preload	Slightly Reduced	Slightly Reduced	Reduced	Reduced
LVEDP	Slightly Reduced	Reduced	Reduced	Increased
Peripheral tissue perfusion	Neutral	Improved	Improved	Improved

IABP, Intraaortic balloon pump; *LV*, left ventricular; *LVEDP*, left ventricular end-diastolic pressure; *MAP*, mean arterial pressure; *VA ECMO*, venoarterial extracorporeal membrane oxygenation.
Modified from Werdan K, Gielen S, Ebelet H, et al. Mechanical circulatory support in cardiogenic shock. *Eur Heart J*. 2014;35:156–167; and Combes A, Brodie D, Chen Y, et al. The ICM research agenda on extracorporeal life support. *Intensive Care Med*. 2017;43:1306–1318.

TABLE 24.3 ■ **Complications of Temporary Mechanical Circulatory Support Devices**

Complication	IABP	Impella	TandemHeart	VA ECMO
Limb ischemia	+	++	+++	+++
Hemolysis	+	++	++	++
Hemorrhage	+	++	+++	+++

IABP, Intraaortic balloon pump; *VA ECMO*, venoarterial extracorporeal membrane oxygenation.
From Combes A, Brodie D, Chen Y, et al. The ICM research agenda on extracorporeal life support. *Intensive Care Med*. 2017;43:1306–1318.

■ The endocardial viability ratio (DPTI:TTI), which reflects the relationship between myocardial oxygen supply and demand, will increase with optimal IABP counterpulsation.

MONITORING OF IABP COUNTERPULSATION

■ The appropriate timing of balloon counterpulsation to the mechanical events of the cardiac cycle must be monitored to ensure that the patient is deriving maximal hemodynamic benefit (Fig. 24.2).
■ To maximize diastolic augmentation, the balloon should inflate at end systole, immediately after closure of the aortic valve.
■ Mean diastolic pressure correlates well with coronary perfusion and, hence, oxygen delivery.
■ Maximal coronary perfusion occurs when balloon inflation coincides with end systole.
■ The timing of balloon deflation, which decreases LV oxygen consumption, should occur at end diastole.
■ Loss of the optimal hemodynamic effect occurs when balloon IABP counterpulsation is not appropriately timed to the mechanical events of the cardiac cycle.

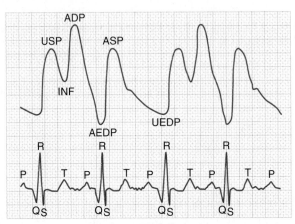

Fig. 24.2 Optimal timing of an intraaortic balloon pump (IABP). Arterial pressure tracing from a patient with an IABP. The balloon was set at 2:1 to evaluate timing. Inflation (INF) was timed to the dicrotic notch to follow aortic valve closure. There is augmentation of diastolic pressure (ADP) and reduction of the end-diastolic pressure with augmented beats (AEDP) compared with the unaugmented end-diastolic pressure (UEDP). The augmented systolic pressure (ASP) is often lower than the unaugmented systolic pressure (USP) as well. (Modified from Hollenberg S, Saltzberg M, Soble J, Parrillo J. Heart failure and cardiomyopathy. In: Crawford MH, Dimarco JP, Paulus WJ, eds. Cardiology. London: Mosby; 2001.)

- Four different scenarios involving faulty coupling of balloon IABP counterpulsation with the cardiac cycle have been described (Fig. 24.3).
  - During early inflation, the balloon inflates before closure of the aortic valve. Pressure augmentation is thus superimposed upon the systolic aortic pressure tracing, leading to a decrease in LV emptying (a decrease in stroke volume), a decrease in cardiac output, an increase in LV afterload, and an overall increase in myocardial oxygen consumption.
  - In this scenario, there is loss of the distinct systolic peak of the central aortic pressure waveform and loss of the dicrotic notch (see Fig. 24.3A).
  - To correct early inflation, the timing interval should be slowly increased until the onset of inflation occurs at the dicrotic notch.
  - During late inflation, the dicrotic notch on the aortic pressure waveform is clearly visualized.
  - The balloon inflates well beyond closure of the aortic valve. In this scenario, diastolic augmentation of the central aortic pressure is decreased, whereas LV afterload is minimally affected.
  - The classic morphologic finding on the central aortic pressure tracing is the presence of a distinct dicrotic notch, with the augmented diastolic pressure wave occurring well afterward (see Fig. 24.3B).
  - To correct late inflation of the IABP, the timing interval should be gradually decreased until the onset of inflation coincides with the dicrotic notch on the arterial pressure waveform.
  - During early deflation, the balloon deflates prematurely; consequently, the benefits of diastolic augmentation are lost.
  - Analysis of the arterial pressure tracing reveals the presence of a peaked diastolic augmentation wave along with a U-shaped wave preceding the onset of systole (see Fig. 24.3C).
  - To correct early deflation, the timing interval should be increased until the augmented diastolic wave becomes appropriate.

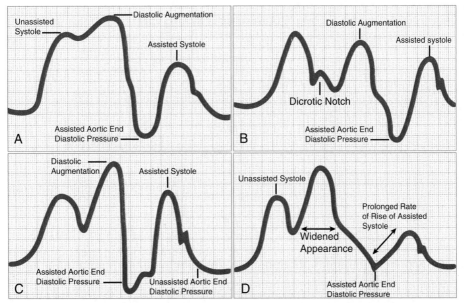

Fig. 24.3 Incorrect timing in intraaortic balloon counterpulsation. (**A**) Early inflation: loss of dicrotic notch and distinct systolic peak of the aortic pressure waveform. (**B**) Late inflation: dicrotic notch is clearly visualized with the augmented diastolic pressure curve occurring well afterward. (**C**) Early deflation: peaked augmented diastolic wave along with a U-shaped wave preceding the onset of systole. (**D**) Late deflation: loss of a distinct valley representing the end-diastolic pressure before the central aortic systolic waveform. (From Krishna M, Zacharowski K. Principles of intra-aortic balloon pump counterpulsation. Continuing education in anaesthesia. Crit Care Pain. 2009;9(1):24–28. Reproduced with permission from Datascope.)

- During late deflation, the balloon is deflated after the onset of systole and the opening of the aortic valve.
- The resultant hemodynamic profile is like the one observed with early inflation: afterload is increased, leading to increased LV work and myocardial oxygen consumption along with reduced stroke volume and CO.
- Analysis of the arterial pressure tracing usually reveals the loss of a distinct valley representing the end-diastolic pressure before the central aortic systolic wave (see Fig. 24.3D)
- To correct late deflation, the timing interval should be decreased gradually until the balloon deflates before the onset of systole.

CONTRAINDICATIONS TO IABP COUNTERPULSATION

- Absolute contraindications include significant aortic regurgitation, suspected aortic dissection, clinically significant abdominal or thoracic aortic aneurysm, distal aortic occlusion or severe stenosis, and chronic end-stage heart disease with no anticipation of recovery.
- Relative contraindications include severe peripheral arterial disease (PAD), contraindications to anticoagulation, uncontrolled sepsis, and sustained tachyarrhythmias (heart rate > 160 beats/min).

INSERTION, REMOVAL, AND COMPLICATIONS

- The most commonly used approach for percutaneous placement is cannulation of the femoral artery (Table 24.4).

TABLE 24.4 ■ **Insertion and Removal of the Intraaortic Balloon Pump**

The following steps are involved during insertion of an intraaortic balloon pump:

1. An initial physical examination focusing on peripheral vasculature should be conducted, including palpation and demarcation of the femoral, popliteal, dorsalis pedis, and posterior tibial pulses and auscultation for femoral and abdominal bruits.
2. The side with the better arterial pulsations should be selected for insertion.
3. The inguinal region should be inspected for landmarks and the femoral artery should be identified.
4. The inguinal region should be prepared and draped in a sterile fashion.
5. Following administration of a local anesthetic agent, a skin incision is made 2 to 3 cm below the inguinal ligament.
6. Using a modified Seldinger technique, the femoral artery is cannulated with a needle and a J-tipped guidewire is then advanced through the needle after brisk flow of arterial blood is confirmed.
7. The guidewire should be advanced to the level of the descending aorta under fluoroscopic guidance.
8. A dilator is inserted and removed until an arterial sheath can be safely placed.
9. The intraaortic balloon is passed over the guidewire to a position just distal to the origin of the left subclavian artery.
10. The guidewire is subsequently removed and the catheter lumen is aspirated to remove any residual air or thrombus.
11. The intraaortic balloon is connected to the drive system console and counterpulsation can subsequently begin.
12. The hemodynamic tracing should be inspected for proper timing.
13. A chest radiograph should be obtained to document correct positioning.
14. The intraaortic balloon catheter and femoral sheath should be secured with sutures.

- Once it is concluded that the patient no longer requires circulatory support, the removal of the IABP is also a straightforward process (Table 24.5).
- No conclusive data support the requirement for intravenous anticoagulation in the setting of IABP use.
- A trial of 153 patients found no difference in vascular complications in patients undergoing IABP therapy with and without continuous heparin anticoagulation.
- Industry guidelines do not require continuous anticoagulation therapy, especially when the device is set at a 1:1 assist ratio.
- Currently, it is reasonable to use intravenous heparin with the goal of maintaining an activated partial thromboplastin time of 60 to 75 seconds in a patient without contraindications to anticoagulation and when IABP counterpulsation therapy is planned for longer than 24 hours or at lower assist ratios.
- Although no conclusive data exist in the literature, some authorities recommend gradual weaning of the balloon pump before it is finally removed.
- In patients in whom the IABP was placed to treat hemodynamic instability, a gradual reduction in the assist ratio from 1:1 to 1:2 and then to 1:3 over several hours is frequently employed.
- If hemodynamic stability is demonstrated at lesser assist ratios, the device can be removed safely.
- Complications arising from IABP counterpulsation therapy can be categorized into vascular and nonvascular events.
- In two studies of nearly 40,000 patients, death directly caused by an IABP or IABP placement was less than 0.05%.

TABLE 24.5 ▒ **Insertion and Removal of the Intraaortic Balloon Pump**

1. Anticoagulation should be stopped; confirm that the activated clotting time is less than 180 seconds or the activated partial thromboplastin time is less than 40 seconds.
2. Conscious patients should receive a low-dose narcotic and/or analgesic agent.
3. The securing sutures are cut.
4. The drive system console is turned off.
5. The intraaortic balloon is completely deflated by aspiration with a 20-mL syringe attached to the balloon inflation port.
6. The sheath and intraaortic balloon catheter are pulled as one unit.
7. Blood is allowed to flow from the arterial access site for a few seconds to remove any thrombi.
8. Manual pressure is applied above the puncture site for 30 minutes or longer if hemostasis is not obtained. A mechanical compression device can also be used to help apply pressure to promote hemostasis.
9. Distal arterial pulsations are palpated.
10. The patient should remain recumbent for a minimum of 6 hours to prevent any subsequent hemorrhage or vascular complications at the arterial access site.

■ Major complications—including major limb ischemia, severe bleeding, balloon leak, and death related directly to device insertion or to device failure—occurred in 2.6% of patients (see Table 24.3).
■ Vascular complications remain the most common serious complications to occur in patients with an IABP.
  ■ The most common types of vascular complications include limb ischemia, vascular laceration necessitating surgical repair, and major hemorrhage.
  ■ Arterial obstruction and limb ischemia can occur when the IABP is inadvertently placed into either the superficial or profunda femoral artery instead of the common femoral artery, because these arteries are usually too small to accommodate the IABP without compromising blood flow to the leg.
  ■ Prompt removal of the device and contralateral insertion (with avoidance of an excessively low needle puncture) is recommended.
  ■ Arterial dissection can occur with improper advancement of a guidewire with subsequent insertion of the IABP into a false lumen.
  ■ Less common vascular complications include spinal cord or visceral organ ischemia, cholesterol embolization, cerebrovascular accidents, sepsis, and balloon rupture.
  ■ The presence of PAD (including a history of limb claudication, femoral arterial bruit, or absent pulsations) has been the most consistent clinical predictor of complications.
  ■ These complications are more common in women (related to the size of the vessels) and patients with a history of diabetes mellitus and hypertension who are more likely to have PAD.
■ Because the helium gas used to inflate the balloon is insoluble in blood, helium embolization can cause prolonged ischemia or stroke.
■ These patients can be treated with hyperbaric oxygen to maintain tissue viability.

CLINICAL EFFICACY AND INDICATIONS

■ IABP counterpulsation therapy improves the hemodynamic and metabolic derangements that result from circulatory collapse.

- Historically, this modality has been used mainly in the setting of acute ischemic syndromes associated with hemodynamic decompensation.

Acute Myocardial Infarction

- Routine use of IABP counterpulsation in patients with acute myocardial infarction (MI), including ST segment elevation myocardial infarction (STEMI), is not indicated, although there may be patients who benefit from its use.
- A meta-analysis of IABP use in patients with acute MI in the absence of cardiogenic shock showed no mortality benefit.
- The routine use of IABP counterpulsation in patients with acute MI, including STEMI, is not indicated.

Cardiogenic Shock

- Early use of IABP in acute MI complicated by cardiogenic shock was based predominantly on small retrospective studies performed in the thrombolytic era that suggested improved outcomes.
- The Intraaortic Balloon Pump in Cardiogenic Shock II (IABP-SHOCK II) trial was one of the first large, multicenter randomized trials to compare IABP counterpulsation and standard medical therapy alone in patients with acute MI complicated by cardiogenic shock and treated with early revascularization.
- 600 patients were randomized to IABP or standard care.
- All patients underwent early revascularization (by PCI or coronary artery bypass graft) and received optimal medical therapy.
- At 30 days, 119 patients in the IABP group and 123 patients in the control group died (39.7% vs. 41.3%; $P = .69$).
- No significant differences were seen in secondary endpoints, including length of stay in the intensive care unit, duration of catecholamine therapy, and renal function.
- No difference was observed in 1-year mortality (52% vs. 51%; $P = .91$) between the groups.
- Based on clinical trials, routine use of IABP in patients with acute MI with cardiogenic shock is not indicated.

High-Risk Percutaneous Coronary Intervention

- An IABP is often used for mechanical circulatory support in patients undergoing high-risk PCI.
- These patients often have a higher risk of procedural morbidity and mortality owing to severe LV dysfunction, multivessel coronary artery disease, or uncontrolled angina.
- In this subset of patients, placement of an IABP before the intervention may be beneficial from the enhancement of coronary perfusion pressure and stabilization of hemodynamic parameters.
- The IABP may also allow them to better tolerate procedural complications, such as coronary artery dissection or the development of no-reflow.
- However, no data demonstrate a benefit of IABP placement as an adjunct to high-risk PCI.

Other Indications

- In patients with severe end-stage cardiomyopathy with refractory heart failure who are awaiting cardiac transplantation or LV assist device placement, IABP counterpulsation can be used as a bridging modality.
- IABP counterpulsation in this setting decreases aortic systolic pressure and impedance; thus, it can promote systolic unloading of the LV, leading to an increased stroke volume.

- The use of IABP counterpulsation has also been shown to improve right ventricular (RV) failure, as unloading the LV can increase performance of the RV and improve outcomes in carefully selected patients.
- Incessant ventricular tachyarrhythmias are occasionally treated with IABP counterpulsation to unload the LV or to improve perfusion to ischemic myocardium.

Left Ventricle to Aorta Support Devices

- The Impella (Abiomed, Inc.) is a miniature axial flow pump attached to a catheter (Fig. 24.4).
- Most commonly, devices are inserted percutaneously or surgically to position the pump across the aortic valve with the inflow in the LV and the outflow into the aorta (Fig. 24.5).
- The Impella now includes a family of devices that are used for cardiac support during high-risk percutaneous procedures, LV support in cardiogenic shock and, most recently, for circulatory assistance in the setting of RV failure.
- Current device models include the Impella 2.5, Impella CP, Impella 5.0, Impella 5.5 with SmartAssist, and Impella RP
- All devices, except the Impella RP, provide LV circulatory support.
- Impella RP provides RV circulatory support.

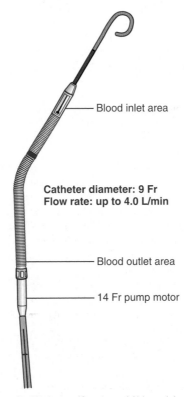

Blood inlet area

Catheter diameter: 9 Fr
Flow rate: up to 4.0 L/min

Blood outlet area

14 Fr pump motor

Fig. 24.4 Components of the Impella CP device. (Courtesy of Abiomed, Inc.)

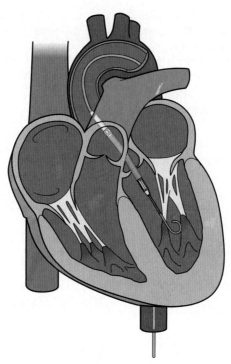

Fig. 24.5 Illustration of an Impella device positioned across the aortic valve. (From Thiele H, Smalling RW, Schuler GC. Percutaneous left ventricular assist devices in acute myocardial infarction complicated by cardiogenic shock. Eur Heart J. 2007;28:2057–2063.)

PHYSIOLOGY AND MONITORING

- The Impella devices contain a miniature pump with a rotating impeller based on the principle of the Archimedes Screw.
- The pump is mounted on a flexible catheter and inserted percutaneously or surgically through the arterial system and advanced to position the distal end of the pump in the LV apex with the proximal end in the ascending aorta.
- Blood is aspirated out of the LV and ejected into the aorta. The devices are most commonly inserted through the femoral artery, but alternative access sites, such as the subclavian and axillary arteries, have been described (see Table 24.1).
- Unlike the IABP, the Impella systems do not require timing, or a trigger based on the electrocardiogram or arterial pressure.
- By unloading the LV, the pump reduces myocardial oxygen consumption, improves mean arterial pressure, and reduces PCWP (see Table 24.2).
- Adequate RV function is necessary to maintain LV preload in cases of biventricular failure or unstable ventricular arrhythmias.
- The 12 Fr Impella 2.5, 14 Fr Impella CP, and 21 Fr Impella 5.0 and 19 Fr Impella 5.5 with SmartAssist provide a maximum flow rate of 2.5, 3 to 4, and 5 and 6 L/min, respectively.
- The pumps consist of inflow and outflow areas, a motor, and a pump pressure monitor.
- Heparin and glucose are continuously infused into the motor housing to prevent backflow of blood.

- The pump is attached to a flexible 9 Fr catheter that houses the motor power leads and lumens for pressure measurement and heparin infusions.
- The catheter's most proximal end contains a hub for attachment of a console cable and side arms for attachment of pressure measurement tubing.
- Impella devices are used with an automatic controller that can be run off a built-in rechargeable battery or from an electric power cord.
- The controller features a display with which users interact to determine pump positioning and the quality of pumping function.
- The degree of support for patients can be set by changing the revolutions per minute (rpm) in set levels designated as P1 to P9 on the controller.
- In addition to the use of radiography and echocardiography, appropriate Impella placement may be verified by the pressure waveform generated from the pressure sensor at the distal end of the pump.
- The placement signal is used to verify whether the Impella pump is correctly positioned in the LV or the aorta by evaluating the pressure differential on a pulsatile waveform.
- Appropriate placement can also be assessed on the display using the motor current waveform, which is a measure of the energy intake of the Impella pump.
- The energy used by the Impella varies with motor speed and the pressure difference between the inflow and outflow areas of the pump.
- When the Impella is positioned correctly with the inlet area in the LV and the output in the ascending aorta, the motor current should be pulsatile because of the pressure difference between the two areas.
- When the intake and output are on the same side of the aortic valve, the motor current will be dampened owing to the lack of a pressure differential.
- Once weaning is desired, the pump power can be reduced slowly over time to reduce the level of cardiac support.
- If the hemodynamics remain stable, the device can be pulled proximally into the aorta.
- If continued hemodynamic stability is observed, the device can then be removed entirely.

CONTRAINDICATIONS AND COMPLICATIONS

- Careful physical examination and imaging technology are necessary to assess the patient's vasculature and select an appropriate arterial access site.
- Traditional angiography, magnetic resonance angiography, or computed tomography angiography are often used for this purpose.
- Echocardiography is important to assess for LV thrombus, mechanical aortic valves, severe aortic stenosis, or aortic regurgitation.
- Insertion of a pulmonary artery catheter should also be considered to provide continuous hemodynamic monitoring of cardiac output, central venous pressures, and mixed venous oxygen saturation (SvO_2).
- Contraindications to the use of Impella devices include mechanical aortic valves or LV thrombus.
- The device should not be placed in patients with severe PAD owing to the risk of embolism during insertion.
- A minimum vessel diameter of 7 mm is required for the Impella 5.0 owing to the cannula size.
- Preexisting septal defects are considered a relative contraindication as, theoretically, the device could worsen right-to-left shunting.
- Severe aortic stenosis and regurgitation are considered relative indications, although Impella use in critical aortic stenosis has been reported.

- Anticoagulation is necessary to prevent thrombus formation on the pump housing and catheter.
- Therefore, the device should not be inserted in patients who cannot tolerate anticoagulation.
- The most common complications include limb ischemia, vascular injury, and bleeding (see Table 24.3).
  - Vascular complications include hematoma or pseudoaneurysm formation, arteriovenous fistula creation, and retroperitoneal hemorrhage.
  - Hemolysis is reported in up to 10% of patients with Impella devices. Obstruction to blood flow due to improper device placement is the most likely cause of hemolysis in the clinical setting.
  - Repositioning the device may reduce the degree of hemolysis.
  - Patients with persistent hemolysis associated with acute kidney injury should have the device removed.

CLINICAL EFFICACY AND INDICATIONS

- Although numerous case reports, case series, and observational studies of various Impella devices demonstrate improved hemodynamics and outcomes, few randomized controlled trials are available.

Cardiogenic Shock

- Only one randomized controlled trial evaluated the utility of an Impella device in cardiogenic shock.
  - In the Efficacy Study of LV Assist Device to Treat Patients With Cardiogenic Shock (ISAR-SHOCK), 26 patients with cardiogenic shock after acute MI were randomized to Impella 2.5 versus IABP.
  - The primary outcome was the change of cardiac index from baseline to 30 minutes after implantation.
  - Mortality at 30 days was a secondary outcome.
  - The trial demonstrated that the cardiac index was significantly higher in the Impella arm versus the IABP arm (Impella ΔCI: 0.49 ± 0.46 L/min/m^2; IABP ΔCI: 0.11 ± 0.31 L/min/m^2; $P = .02$), but there was no difference in mortality between the two groups.

High-Risk PCI

- Numerous observational studies have demonstrated the safety and efficacy of the Impella device in the setting of high-risk PCI, but only one randomized controlled trial exists that evaluates the utility of Impella in high-risk PCI.
  - In the Prospective, Multicenter, Randomized Controlled Trial of Impella 2.5 Versus Intra-aortic Balloon Pump in Patients Undergoing High-Risk Percutaneous Coronary Intervention (PROTECT II), patients with symptomatic, complex three-vessel coronary artery disease or unprotected left main coronary artery disease and severely depressed LV function undergoing nonemergent high-risk PCI were randomized to Impella 2.5 (n = 225) versus IABP (n = 223).
  - The primary endpoint was an adverse event during and after the PCI procedure at discharge or at 30-day follow up, whichever was longer.
  - Components of the primary outcome included all-cause mortality, MI, stroke or transient ischemic attack, repeat revascularization procedure, need for cardiac or vascular operation, acute renal insufficiency, severe intraprocedural hypotension requiring therapy, cardiopulmonary resuscitation, ventricular tachycardia requiring cardioversion, aortic insufficiency, or angiographic failure of PCI.

- The study demonstrated that, relative to IABP, Impella provided superior cardiac power output.
- However, no difference was observed in the primary outcome between the two groups at 30 days.

Left Atrium to Aorta Support Devices

- The TandemHeart percutaneous ventricular assist device (Cardiac Assist, Inc.) is the only commercially available left atrium to aorta assist device.
- This percutaneous device pumps blood extracorporeally from the left atrium via a transseptally inserted cannula to the ileofemoral arterial system, thereby bypassing the LV (see Table 24.1).

Physiology and Monitoring

- The TandemHeart has four components: a transseptal cannula, a centrifugal pump, a femoral arterial cannula, and a control console.
- A 21 Fr cannula is inserted into the right femoral vein, advanced to the right atrium, and finally into the left atrium via a transseptal puncture.
- The fenestrated cannula aspirates blood from the left atrium via a large end hole and 14 smaller side holes (Fig. 24.6).
- Blood flows to a 15 to 19 Fr arterial perfusion cannula inserted into the common femoral artery.
- The flow of blood is propelled by an extracorporeal centrifugal pump containing a spinning impeller.
- The pump has both a motor chamber and a blood chamber that are separated by a polymer membrane.
- An electromagnetic motor rotates the impeller between 3000 and 7500 rpm.
- The size of the arterial cannula determines the maximum flow rate.
- The 15 Fr arterial cannula can support flow rate up to 3.5 L/min, whereas the 19 Fr arterial cannula can achieve flow up to 5 L/min.
- Heparinized saline flows continuously into the lower chamber of the pump, providing lubrication and cooling, and preventing thrombus formation.
- An external controller controls the pump and contains a 60-minute backup battery in case of power failure.
- The hemodynamic effects of the TandemHeart are superior to the IABP (see Table 24.2).
- Similar to the Impella device and unlike the IABP, the TandemHeart does not require a trigger or timing based on the cardiac cycle.
- Because the TandemHeart device works in parallel with the LV, any intrinsic CO from the LV is additive to the support of the device.
- By virtue of unloading the LV, the TandemHeart results in increased CO, increased mean atrial pressure, decreased PCWP, and decreased central venous pressure.
- Both the LV and RV have decreased filling pressures, resulting in reduced ventricular workload and oxygen demand, and an increase in cardiac power index.
- However, owing to an increase in afterload and a decrease in preload, ventricular contraction may decrease.
- As a result, the LV often provides only a minimal contribution to CO, resulting in relatively nonpulsatile arterial pressure tracing.
- The amount of cardiac support provided by TandemHeart can be increased or decreased by changing the revolutions per minute on the centrifugal pump.

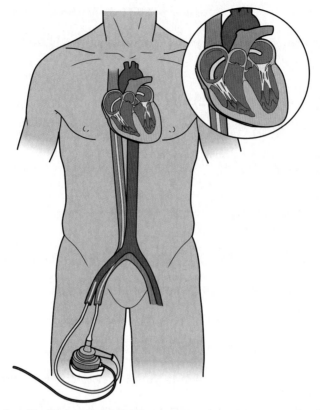

Fig. 24.6 Illustration of the TandemHeart device demonstrating an arterial catheter and a transseptal venous catheter connected to the centrifugal pump. The inset shows a close-up of the transseptally inserted fenestrated venous catheter. (From Thiele H, Smalling RW, Schuler GC. Percutaneous left ventricular assist devices in acute myocardial infarction complicated by cardiogenic shock. Eur Heart J. 2007;28:2057–2063.)

- Weaning is facilitated by monitoring hemodynamic stability while slowly reducing the revolutions per minute on the centrifugal pump.
- If hemodynamic stability is confirmed, the pump can be turned off and removed.

CONTRAINDICATIONS AND COMPLICATIONS

- Imaging modalities and physical examination are necessary to evaluate the patient's vasculature.
- Expertise with the transseptal puncture technique is required and is often a barrier to the use of TandemHeart given that proficiency with this technique is not universal.
- Upon insertion of the transseptal cannula, appropriate placement must be verified using a combination of echocardiography, pressure transduction, and blood gas analysis from the distal port.
- Contraindications for the use of TandemHeart include severe PAD, which may preclude the placement of the arterial cannula, contraindications to anticoagulation, and left atrial thrombus.

- Adequate RV function or support is necessary to maintain appropriate left atrial pressure for optimal device function.
- Complications include arterial dissection, groin hematoma, limb ischemia, hemolysis, and thromboembolism (see Table 24.3).
- Complications unique to the transseptal puncture technique, such as cardiac tamponade, may be increased in patients who are anticoagulated.
- Additionally, dislodgement of the left atrial cannula back into the right atrium will cause severe right-to-left shunting and associated hypoxemia.
- The cannula may also migrate into a pulmonary vein, which may cause device malfunction.

CLINICAL EFFICACY AND INDICATIONS

Cardiogenic Shock

- A 2006 randomized control trial of 42 patients across 12 centers compared patients with cardiogenic shock randomized to IABP ($n = 14$) or TandemHeart ($n = 19$).
- Patients treated with TandemHeart had improved hemodynamics compared with those treated with an IABP.
- However, survival did not differ between the two groups at 30 days; TandemHeart use was associated with more adverse events than the IABP.

High-Risk Percutaneous Coronary Intervention

- No randomized, controlled trials have compared TandemHeart with other devices or standard care.

Extracorporeal Membrane Oxygenation

- The two basic configurations of extracorporeal membrane oxygenation (ECMO) are venovenous (VV) ECMO and venoarterial (VA) ECMO.
- VV ECMO can be used to oxygenate blood and remove carbon dioxide in patients with respiratory failure.
- VA ECMO provides both hemodynamic and respiratory support.

Physiologic Principles of ECMO

- The ECMO circuit consists of a blood pump, membrane oxygenator, conduit tubing, and a heat exchanger (see Table 24.1).
- In VA ECMO, a drainage catheter is inserted into the venous circulation, which drains blood through an oxygenator and returns it to the arterial system using a pump (Fig. 24.7).
- VA ECMO is a supportive therapy with the goals of improving oxygen delivery and carbon dioxide removal while resting the heart and lungs to facilitate recovery.
- When recovery is not possible, VA ECMO may be used as a bridge to definitive therapy with a permanent ventricular assist device or cardiac transplant. The VA ECMO circuit can be set up in different ways.
- Although other vessels may be used, most commonly the femoral artery and vein are cannulated.
- Regardless of the setup, the drainage cannula is positioned in the vena cava or right atrium and the return cannula is positioned to deliver blood retrograde to the aorta.
- Blood flowing anterograde from the LV will meet resistance from blood flowing retrograde from the ECMO circuit.
- This nonphysiologic configuration has differing effects on the RV and LV.

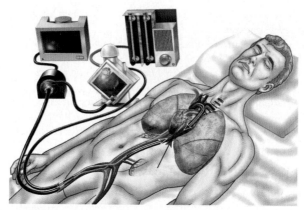

Fig. 24.7 Illustration of a patient with femoral venoarterial (VA) extracorporeal membrane oxygenation (ECMO). Deoxygenated venous blood from the femoral vein is infused through the ECMO circuit, and oxygenated blood is returned retrograde to the femoral artery. Poorly oxygenated blood flowing anterograde from the left ventricle will meet with resistance from the blood returned retrograde from the ECMO circuit. (From Abrams D, Combes A, Brodie D. Extracorporeal membrane oxygenation in cardiopulmonary disease in adults. J Am Coll Cardiol. 2014;63(25):2769–2778.)

- For the RV, drainage of blood from the venous system results in decreased preload, reduced RV output, and reduced pulmonary blood flow.
- For the LV, blood delivered retrograde into the arterial system results in increased mean arterial pressure and, consequently, increased afterload (see Table 24.2).
- The resultant increase in afterload often leads to reductions in LV stroke volume.
- The degree of reduction depends on residual LV function and the integrity of the aortic and mitral valves.
- Increasing hemodynamic support by increasing flow through the VA ECMO circuit further increases afterload.
- Concomitant increases in LV end-diastolic pressure may cause LV dilation, decreased coronary blood flow, and reduced subendocardial perfusion.
- The amount of support can be titrated by changing the flow rate on the blood pump.
- Although rates as high as 10 L/min can be accommodated with large-bore cannula, ECMO generally provides between 3 and 6 L/min of support.
- High flow also increases left atrial pressure and may precipitate pulmonary edema.
- Increases in afterload may be exacerbated further by the vasoconstrictive effects of vasopressor medications.
- Systemic hypertension is common; weaning of vasopressors and the addition of antihypertensive medications may be necessary to prevent complications.
  - Oxygenation and removal of carbon dioxide are facilitated by an oxygenator that uses a semipermeable membrane as an artificial lung to separate gas from blood.
  - In VA ECMO, deoxygenated blood is pulled from the venous system and oxygenated blood is returned to the arterial system.
  - Oxygenation is determined by the amount of blood flow through the ECMO circuit, gas flow through the oxygenator, and the contribution from the patient's own pulmonary function.
  - The rate of carbon dioxide removal is regulated by the flow of blood through the ECMO circuit and gas flow through the oxygenator, known as the sweep gas flow rate.

MONITORING OF ECMO

- Once cannulation has occurred and patients are connected to the ECMO circuit, flow through the circuit is slowly uptitrated to achieve appropriate respiratory and hemodynamic targets.
- Frequent adjustments may be necessary to achieve adequate arterial oxyhemoglobin saturation, mean arterial pressure, and venous oxygen saturation.
- Light sedation may be necessary to maintain patient comfort.
- Anticoagulation is essential during ECMO and is typically achieved with intravenous unfractionated heparin.
- Anticoagulation with the direct thrombin inhibitors argatroban and bivalirudin has been reported and is used in the case of heparin-induced thrombocytopenia.
- Anticoagulation is usually titrated based on activated clotting time (ACT).
- There is no universally agreed upon anticoagulation protocol; target ACT varies between institutions.
- The artificial material in the ECMO circuit results in activation of the coagulation, fibrinolytic, and complement pathways, which can result in both bleeding and thrombotic complications.
- Platelets are continuously consumed; current practice is to maintain platelet levels over 50,000/mL.
- Hemolysis, hemorrhage, and decreased bone marrow production owing to critical illness may result in a decreased hemoglobin concentration.
- Hemoglobin is often maintained between 12 and 14 mg/dL.
- For patients who are ventilated, ventilator settings should be minimized once adequate oxygenation and carbon dioxide removal is facilitated with the ECMO circuit to allow avoidance of ventilator-associated lung injury and oxygen toxicity.
- An ultraprotective lung strategy with target plateau pressures less than 20 cm H_2O and FiO_2 less than 0.5 is often used to improve outcomes.
- Reduction in ventilator settings decreases intrathoracic pressure, which may facilitate venous return and CO.
- Although near maximum flow rates are typically used for patients on VV ECMO, the flow rates used with patients on VA ECMO must be high enough to facilitate hemodynamic and oxygenation goals but low enough to allow for sufficient preload to maintain intrinsic CO.
- LV output must be monitored frequently owing to the risk of LV distention.
- Aggressive diuresis may be necessary.
- Ultrafiltration can also be added to the ECMO circuit to facilitate volume removal.
- LV output is assessed using the pulsatility on an arterial line waveform in combination with echocardiography.
- If LV output cannot be maintained, inotropes, an IABP, or Impella device may be inserted to improve forward flow.
- If cardiac output remains low despite these interventions, LV decompression may be necessary.
- Techniques include transatrial balloon septostomy or surgical insertion of an LV or right upper pulmonary vein drainage catheter.

CONTRAINDICATIONS TO THE USE OF ECMO

- ECMO should not be considered for patients who have preexisting conditions that are incompatible with recovery, such as severe neurologic injury and advanced malignancy.

INSERTION, REMOVAL, AND COMPLICATIONS

Insertion

- ECMO requires a multidisciplinary team, including a surgeon, anesthesiologist, perfusionist, cardiologist, pulmonologist, and intensivist. Once it has been decided that ECMO will be initiated, the patient is anticoagulated, and the cannula are inserted.
- The cannulas are inserted percutaneously using the Seldinger technique.
- The size of the cannulas chosen is determined based on the expected amount of circulatory support required for the patient based on residual LV function.
- For adults, inflow cannulas are available between 18 and 21 Fr and outflow cannulas are between 15 and 22 Fr.
- In VA ECMO, a venous cannula is typically placed in the femoral vein and advanced to the venocaval junction.
- The arterial cannula is typically placed in the common femoral artery.
- Given the large cannula sizes used in ECMO, ischemia to the limb ipsilateral to the arterial cannula is common.
- To compensate, a distal arterial cannula may be inserted into the posterior tibial artery to provide flow to perfuse the lower limb.
- If the femoral vessels are unsuitable for cannulation owing to severe PAD or prior arterial bypass, other arteries may be utilized, including the right carotid, right subclavian, and axillary arteries.

Removal

- The duration of ECMO support is typically 5 to 10 days, with a maximum implant time of 3 to 4 weeks.
- Once patients have recovered sufficiently to warrant consideration of weaning, weaning may be initiated as a series of trials where the support provided by the ECMO circuit is decreased incrementally while monitoring hemodynamic and respiratory stability.
- Because the VA ECMO also provides for gas exchange, the pump flow cannot be decreased without ensuring that respiratory support is adequate.
- Completely turning off the pump increases the risk of thrombus formation in the ECMO circuit, but short periods of reducing flow to 1 L/min can be performed.
- Because assessment of LV function may be compromised when the VA ECMO circuit is providing full support, cardiac monitoring during the weaning process with transthoracic or transesophageal echocardiography has been proposed.
- If weaning is successful and the decision is made to discontinue ECMO entirely, the cannulas are removed, and the venous and arterial access sites are compressed manually for at least 30 minutes to achieve hemostasis.

Complications

- Major complications include bleeding, thromboembolism, neurologic injury, and cannulation-related injury (see Table 24.3).
- Bleeding is the most common complication, occurring in 27% to 50% of patients, and may be severe enough to require intervention.
- Both anticoagulation and platelet dysfunction contribute to bleeding.
- Cannulation-related injury includes hemorrhage, dissection, distal ischemia, and compartment syndrome.
- Major bleeding from surgical wounds should prompt exploration. Thrombus may develop within the ECMO circuit or the patient's vasculature with an incidence of 8% to 16%.

- Routine inspection of all tubing and connectors for signs of clot formation is necessary.
- Changes in the pressure gradient across the oxygenator may reflect thrombus formation.
- Large clots necessitate immediate circuit exchange.
- If anticoagulation must be held or if there is heightened concern for thrombus development, circuits primed with anticoagulant may be kept at the bedside for urgent exchange.
- Intracardiac thrombosis may also develop if there is stasis owing to poor LV function.
- Neurologic injury occurs in up to 50% of patients with cardiac failure or those for whom ECMO is administered during cardiopulmonary resuscitation.
- Coma, encephalopathy, anoxic brain injury, stroke, brain death, and myoclonus have all been observed.
- Cerebral hypoxia is of particular concern for patients with femoral artery cannulation.
- Oxygenated blood returning from the circuit to the aorta will preferentially perfuse the abdominal viscera instead of the brain, heart, and upper extremities.
- To detect this complication, arterial oxyhemoglobin saturation should be monitored in the upper extremities.
- Other complications include pulmonary edema and pulmonary hemorrhage owing to elevated LV end-diastolic and left atrial pressures that may warrant LV or left atrial venting.
- Infection related to cannulation may result in prolonging the duration of ECMO or increased length of hospital stays.
- Heparin-induced thrombocytopenia may also develop and should prompt changing the anticoagulant to a direct thrombin inhibitor.
- Hemolysis, thrombocytopenia, acquired von Willebrand syndrome, disseminated intravascular coagulation, acute kidney injury, and air emboli have all been reported.

CLINICAL EFFICACY AND INDICATIONS

- Although randomized controlled trials exist demonstrating the utility of ECMO in respiratory failure and acute respiratory distress syndrome, there are no such trials for cardiac support or following cardiopulmonary arrest.
- In practice, ECMO is often used in cardiogenic shock or following cardiopulmonary arrest as a salvage therapy or a temporary bridge to definitive therapy with ventricular assist devices or cardiac transplant.

ACUTE RIGHT VENTRICULAR FAILURE

- Percutaneously delivered devices for right ventricular RV failure are relatively new and provide the opportunity for early intervention in RV failure without the need for surgery.
- Device options include venoarterial extracorporeal membrane oxygenation (VA-ECMO), the Protek Duo centrifugal-flow pump and the axial-flow Impella RP catheter (Fig. 24.1).
- These devices can be categorized according to their mechanism of action as either direct RV bypass or indirect RV bypass systems.
  - The Impella RP and the Protek Duo displace blood from the RA to PA, thereby directly bypassing the RV. VA-ECMO displaces and oxygenates blood from the RA to the femoral artery, thereby indirectly bypassing the RV.
  - Thus, these systems have distinct hemodynamic effects, depending on whether the patient has isolated RV failure or biventricular failure.

CHAPTER 25

Ventricular Assist Device Therapy in Advanced Heart Failure

Common Misconceptions

- Left ventricular recovery is common after placement of left ventricular assist devices (LVAD).
- Patients who are candidates for heart transplantation should never have an LVAD placed.
- Palliative care consultation is inappropriate for patients being considered for a destination therapy LVAD.

- The development of reliable left ventricular assist devices (LVADs) has revolutionized heart failure (HF) management.
- In the cardiac intensive care unit (CICU) context, LVADs are encountered in three situations:
  - Selection of the appropriate patient with heart failure for mechanical circulatory support (MCS) and preoperative evaluation
  - Treatment of these patients perioperatively
  - Treatment of complications and prevention of adverse events.

Technology of Left Ventricular Assist Devices

- The initial LVADs were volume displacement pumps known as pulsatile-flow devices.
- However, pumps had multiple moving parts, including bearings, valves, and pusher plates that were subject to failure.
- A paradigm shift in the field of assisted circulation occurred with the introduction of durable, implantable continuous-flow devices.
- The rationale for continuous flow was the observation that the initial pulsatile flow in the aorta is progressively dampened, transforming into continuous nonpulsatile flow at the level of the capillary (Fig. 25.1).
- Continuous-flow LVADs have only a single moving part and propel blood forward in a steady, continuous fashion with an axial or centrifugal rotor or an impeller.
- With this simplified design, the risk of mechanical failure has been greatly reduced.
- Currently, the HeartMate II (St. Jude Medical) and the HeartWare HVAD (HeartWare) are the only US Food and Drug Administration (FDA)–approved continuous-flow LVADs (Fig. 25.2).
- The HeartMate II is capable of providing up to 10 L/min of support and is surgically inserted into a preperitoneal pocket (See Fig. 25.2A).
- Blood is pulled out of the LV into the LV inflow cannula, accelerated by a rotor, and then ejected into the outflow graft, which is anastomosed to the ascending aorta.
- A percutaneous driveline exits in the upper abdomen and connects the device with a portable controller and two batteries for mobile operation, or to a power base unit and a wall outlet when a patient is stationary for several hours (e.g., while sleeping).

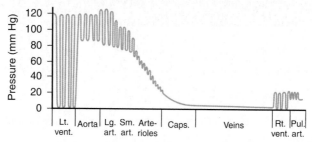

Fig. 25.1 Pressure and pulsatility distribution in the systemic circulation. *Caps.*, Capillaries; *Lg. art.*, large artery; *Lt. vent.*, left ventricle; *Pulm. art.*, pulmonary artery; *Rt. vent.*, right ventricle; *Sm. art.*, small artery.

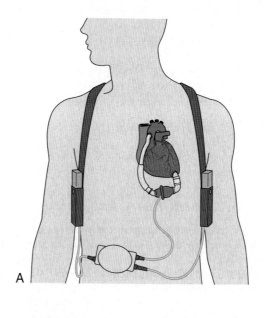

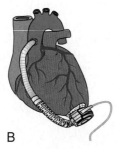

Fig. 25.2 Axial St. Jude HeartMate II (**A**) and centrifugal HeartWare HVAD (**B**) left ventricular assist devices.

- The device provides a constant flow of blood with one backup speed used in case of a sudden drop of preload.
- The typical operating speed range is 8600 to 9600 rpm.
- Despite antithrombotic coating with titanium microbeads, anticoagulation with a target international normalized ratio (INR) of 2.0 to 3.0 and aspirin are recommended.
- In distinction to the axial-flow HeartMate II, the HVAD is a miniaturized centrifugal pump (see Fig. 25.2B).
- The smaller size of this device allows implantation into the pericardial space and, often, a shorter operation.
- The housing contains an impeller suspended by magnets and the device is capable of providing 10 L/min of flow.
- The usual operating speed range is 2400 to 2800 rpm.
- The presence of a continuous-flow device does not necessarily eliminate the presence of a palpable pulse on physical examination.
- This has an important consequence when measuring a patient's blood pressure.
- In the absence of a palpable pulse, mean arterial pressure (MAP) is measured via Doppler.
  - The blood pressure cuff is inflated above where the Doppler tones are heard, and then the return of sounds auscultated via Doppler is taken as the MAP.
  - MAP measured by Doppler overestimates pressure in the presence of palpable pulse and should not be reported.
  - Instead, auscultation of the Korotkoff sounds should be performed.

BRIDGE TO TRANSPLANTATION (BTT) LVAD

- BTT refers to the implantation of a durable LVAD in a patient with end-stage HF with the intent of improving the hemodynamics and clinical course until a donor heart is available.
- As the donor shortage has worsened, the proportion of transplant recipients who required bridging with a durable LVAD increased from 26% in 2004 to more than 50% in 2014.
- Early studies in patients with a BTT have proven that prompt implantation of an LVAD is the only meaningful chance for survival available to the sickest patients.
- These studies also demonstrated a substantial reversibility of organ damage: that is, implantation of LVADs was followed by a significant improvement in biochemical markers of kidney and liver injury.

Destination Therapy LVAD

- Destination therapy (DT) refers to the implantation of an LVAD in a patient with end-stage HF who is not a candidate for heart transplant or who is unwilling to undergo a transplant.
- It is important to highlight that heart transplantation currently remains the "gold standard" for management of end-stage HF.
- As a result, patients who receive a DT LVAD are older and have more comorbid conditions than patients who undergo heart transplantation.
- In the landmark Randomized Evaluation of Mechanical Assistance for the Treatment of Congestive Heart Failure (REMATCH) trial, patients with end-stage HF were randomly assigned to undergo HeartMate I implantation or continued medical management.
  - The principal finding of REMATCH was a significantly better survival of patients randomized to the HeartMate I LVAD compared with those who were medically managed.
  - Estimates of survival at 1 and 2 years were 52% and 23% in the device group and 25% and 8% in the medical therapy group, respectively.

- Analysis of mortality revealed that sepsis and LVAD failure were the leading causes of death.
- In 2009, Slaughter and colleagues published outcomes of the first randomized trial comparing two LVADs for DT.
  - The patients were assigned to receive either a pulsatile-flow HeartMate I or a continuous-flow HeartMate II.
  - The primary study endpoint, "survival free from disabling stroke and reoperation to repair or replace the LVAD at two years" was achieved by 46% and 11% of patients in HeartMate II and HeartMate I groups, respectively.
  - The survival in the HeartMate II group was better than the survival in the HeartMate I group (58% vs. 24%).
  - Also, the HeartMate II LVAD had a lower hazard of adverse events compared with the HeartMate I LVAD: pump replacement hazard ratio (HR), 0.12 (95% confidence interval [CI], 0.06 to 0.26); right sided heart failure HR, 0.30 (95% CI, 0.16 to 0.57), sepsis HR, 0.35 (95% CI, 0.21 to 0.57), and cardiac arrhythmias HR, 0.53 (95% CI, 0.33 to 0.83).
- Quality of Life (QOL) improves after LVAD implantation.
  - In the HeartMate II DT trial, 80% of patients on a continuous-flow LVAD were in New York Heart Association (NYHA) class I or II 24 months after implantation with a remarkable improvement of their scores on The Minnesota Living with Heart Failure and The Kansas City Cardiomyopathy Questionnaires.
  - The improvement in exercise capacity, which is one of the components in QOL assessment, is often less than predicted owing to limitations related to a suboptimal increase in cardiac output (CO) during exercise and associated comorbidities.

Bridge to Recovery (BTR) LVAD

- A different approach for management of HF consists of a combination of MCS with aggressive medical therapy to promote LV recovery.
- If LV function normalizes, the device potentially could be explanted.
- Initial enthusiasm with BTR dropped off after the realization that only a small proportion (1% to 2%) of patients in large datasets could be weaned from MCS.
- Younger age, nonischemic etiology, and short duration of HF are associated with a greater likelihood of recovery.

PATIENT SELECTION AND EVALUATION

- A common clinical dilemma is whether to proceed with an LVAD implant or wait for cardiac transplantation.
- If the patient is a candidate for heart transplantation and if a prolonged wait time for a donor heart is anticipated, it might be reasonable to proceed with a durable LVAD if no contraindications exist to ensure hemodynamic and clinical stability while on the waiting list.
- Patients on LVADs are less likely to become deconditioned and lose muscle mass than those on chronic inotropic therapy.
- Conversely, in a stabilized patient with a favorable blood type and projected short wait time for a donor heart, the best decision might be to wait for a primary transplant without a bridging LVAD.
- In the United Network of Organ Sharing (UNOS) registry, overall posttransplant survival of patients requiring bridging with an LVAD is the same as patients who receive a transplant without having received an LVAD first, with the only exception being patients with increased transplant urgency status owing to device infection who possibly have decreased survival.

- For the purpose of prognostication and rapid assessment of patients with severe symptomatic HF, a staging system was developed known as the INTERMACS profiles.
  - INTERMACS profile I ("crash and burn") includes the sickest patients with cardiogenic shock who are hemodynamically unstable despite inotropes and/or intraaortic balloon pump counterpulsation.
    - Death is imminent without escalation of support for these patients.
    - A temporary MCS might be a good option in some of these patients while assessing potential reversibility of LV and end-organ damage.
    - If the LV damage is beyond recoverable (or is unlikely to recover without durable LVAD) and the need for assisted circulation persists, evaluation for a durable LVAD should be performed.
    - When an LVAD is implanted for patients with an INTERMACS profile I, survival to hospital discharge is only 70.4%.
    - As a result of this observation, fewer LVADs are now implanted for INTERMACS profile I (only 14.3% in 2014).
    - An appropriate strategy for these very sick patients has evolved to include temporary MCS to allow for reversal of end-organ damage and achievement of clinical stability prior to proceeding with a durable LVAD.
  - The majority (66%) of patients evaluated for LVAD are INTERMACS profile II ("sliding") and INTERMACS profile III ("stable on inotropes"); the benefit of LVAD is well proven in these patients.
  - Long-term therapy with inotropes is associated with poor survival and it is reasonable to proceed with an evaluation for durable LVAD as soon as the patient is declared inotrope dependent.
    - When an LVAD is implanted for patients who are INTERMACS profile II or III, survival to discharge is improved at 93.5% and 95.8%, respectively.
  - One fifth of LVADs are implanted into patients not receiving inotropes or temporary MCS (INTERMACS profiles IV to VII).
- A proposed algorithm for LVAD evaluation is presented in Fig. 25.3.

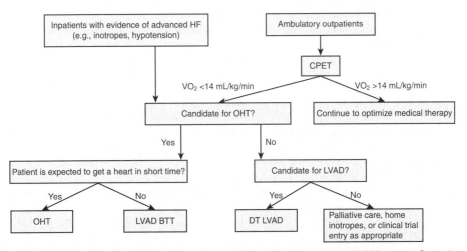

Fig. 25.3 A simplified algorithm of patient selection for left ventricular assist device (LVAD) support. Currently, only patients who are not candidates for OHT should be considered for DT LVAD. *BTT*, Bridge to transplantation; *CPET*, cardiopulmonary exercise test; *DT*, destination therapy; *LVAD*, left ventricular assist device; *OHT*, orthotopic heart transplantation.

ABSOLUTE CONTRAINDICATIONS TO LVAD IMPLANTATION

- Absolute contraindications for LVAD implantation are any irreversible end-stage organ damage that can limit survival after LVAD surgery.
    - This includes cirrhosis, permanent hemodialysis, dementia or severe stroke, severe chronic obstructive pulmonary disease, and malignancy with life expectancy less than 2 years.
    - In the CICU setting, important additions to this list include terminal multiorgan failure, ongoing bacteremia, incessant ventricular tachycardia, significant coagulation abnormalities, high bleeding risk, contraindications to anticoagulation with warfarin, severe RV dysfunction, and pregnancy.
- All contemporary LVADs require the patient's or caregiver's ability to comprehend and act on controller alarms, change batteries, and clean the driveline exit site.
    - Patients and caregivers who are unable to take care of the device owing to a medical or psychosocial issue cannot be considered for a durable LVAD.
- The decision about advanced cardiac therapies in patients with a history of cancer should be made in conjunction with an oncologist.

RELATIVE CONTRAINDICATIONS TO LVAD IMPLANTATION

- Relative contraindications to LVAD include severe peripheral vascular disease, poorly controlled diabetes with complications, severe malnutrition, frailty, and lack of a supportive caregiver.
- Chronic kidney dysfunction traditionally belongs to this group; however, the numeric value for a low glomerular filtration rate or an elevated creatinine level to set as a contraindication is a subject of ongoing debate.

ADVANTAGES OF LVADS OVER HEART TRANSPLANTATION

- Individuals with pulmonary vascular resistance greater than 5 Wood units can be supported by an LVAD in the absence of concomitant RV failure.
- So-called fixed pulmonary hypertension (pulmonary hypertension that does not improve despite medical therapy) does, in fact, improve post-LVAD implantation.
- Second, obesity with a body mass index greater than $35\,kg/m^2$ is only a relative contraindication for MCS.
- Improvement of hemodynamics and clinical state with an LVAD may allow a morbidly obese patient to undergo bariatric surgery and thus lose weight to become a heart transplant candidate.
- In patients who would be unable to tolerate immunosuppressive therapy owing to drug interactions or are otherwise unwilling to undergo a transplant for personal reasons, DT LVAD offers better survival than optimal medical therapy.

LVAD WORKUP

- A standard minimal workup should include evaluation by a heart failure specialist, social worker, psychiatrist, palliative care team, and a cardiothoracic surgeon.
- Palliative care consultation is now mandated by the Center for Medicare Services for DT implants.
- Because all contemporary FDA-approved LVADs require antithrombotic therapy, a history of bleeding diathesis must be investigated and documented.

- Individuals with a prior unprovoked deep venous thrombosis or pulmonary embolism should have a full hypercoagulable workup performed and be evaluated by a hematologist.
- For hospitalized decompensated patients, placement of a pulmonary artery catheter is required for optimization of right-sided pressures prior to the surgery (right atrial pressure below 15 mm Hg is a reasonable goal).
- For patients with a history of coronary artery bypass graft surgery, a chest computed tomographic (CT) scan is indicated to map bypass grafts and prevent trauma to the patient during the surgery.
- Cardiac anatomy and the presence of concomitant structural heart disease, including intracardiac thrombi, should be evaluated with an echocardiogram.
- Atrial septal defects, including patent foramen ovales, should be closed during cardiopulmonary bypass.
- Their absence should be confirmed by a bubble study in all patients, because their presence in the setting of an LVAD would turn a left-to-right shunt into a right-to-left shunt and lead to hypoxia.
- Because aortic regurgitation is likely to progress on a continuous-flow LVAD, in every patient with more than mild aortic insufficiency, the valve should be replaced with a bioprosthesis.
- Presence of a mechanical aortic valve is not a contraindication for an LVAD; however, the valve should be patch-closed or exchanged with a bioprosthesis to prevent left ventricular outflow tract and valve thrombosis.
- Patients with a bioprosthetic aortic valve or any prosthetic valve in the mitral position do not require any additional procedures.
- Severe mitral insufficiency does not necessarily require additional mitral valve procedures because it is likely to improve after LVAD implantation owing to normalization of LV filling pressures and reverse LV remodeling.
- Tricuspid valve insufficiency is extremely common in this population, but the approach to its management is a subject of controversy.
- Analysis of six studies addressing this issue suggested that tricuspid valve repair was associated with longer cardiopulmonary bypass time without any early mortality or morbidity benefits.

ADVERSE EVENTS

- Table 25.1 lists some of the adverse events post-LVAD placement.
- Of note, despite frequent hospitalizations for an adverse event, the majority of patients spend greater than 90% of their time out of the hospital.
- The two major perioperative complications are surgical bleeding and RV failure.
  - Early reports noticed an elevated risk of mediastinal bleeding post-LVAD compared with other open-heart procedures.
  - Importantly, bleeding requiring reoperation and the number of units transfused correlated with 1-year mortality in some studies.
  - Significant delayed bleeding requires interruption of anticoagulation and may predispose to pump thrombosis.
  - Before and during initiation of unfractionated heparin, chest tube output should be meticulously monitored.
  - Cardiac tamponade is suggested by a combination of elevated central venous pressure (CVP) and hypotension and mandates an emergent echocardiogram to look for pericardial effusion or pericardial hematoma in order to differentiate tamponade from RV failure (Fig. 25.4).

TABLE 25.1 ■ **Adverse Events Presented per Patient-Year in Individuals With HeartMate II (HM II) LVAD and HVAD**

Adverse Events	Hm II Event Rate	HVAD Event Rate
Bleeding requiring reoperation	0.09–0.23	0.19–0.26
Gastrointestinal bleeding	0.17–0.38	0.23–0.27
Drive-line infection	0.12–0.37	0.08–0.25
Sepsis	0.18–0.35	0.04–0.24
Right heart failure	0.16–0.36	0.04–0.33
Stroke	0.083–0.13	0.12–0.2
Ischemic stroke	0.031–0.06	0.09–0.11
Hemorrhagic stroke	0.052–0.07	0.08–0.09
Pump thrombosis	0.024–0.027	0.07–0.08
De novo aortic insufficiency	0.22–0.32	NR[a]

[a]One report suggests low incidence of *de novo* aortic insufficiency in HVADs equipped with Lavare cycle not available in the United States.

LVAD, Left ventricular assist device; *NR,* not recorded.

Modified from Slaughter MS, Rogers JG, Milano CA, et al. Advanced heart failure treated with continuous-flow left ventricular assist device. *N Engl J Med.* 2009;361(23):2241–2251; Jorde UP, Kushwaha SS, Tatooles AJ, et al. Results of the destination therapy post-Food and Drug Administration approval study with a continuous flow left ventricular assist device: a prospective study using the INTERMACS registry (Interagency Registry for Mechanically Assisted Circulatory Support). *J Am Coll Cardiol.* 2014;63(17):1751–1757; Jorde UP, Uriel N, Nahumi N, et al. Prevalence, significance, and management of aortic insufficiency in continuous flow left ventricular assist device recipients. *Circ Heart Fail.* 2014;7(2):310–319; and Soleimani B, Haouzi A, Manoskey A, et al. Development of aortic insufficiency in patients supported with continuous flow left ventricular assist devices. *ASAIO J.* 2012;58(4):326–329.

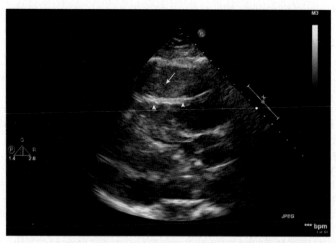

Fig. 25.4 A transthoracic echocardiogram from a patient with refractory hypotension shortly after left ventricular (*LV*) assist device implantation. Parasternal long-axis view shows a large anterior hematoma *(arrow)* and posterior pericardial effusion causing compression of the right ventricle free wall *(arrowheads)* and small LV cavity.

- Emergent drainage or hematoma evacuation is the only definitive treatment of cardiac tamponade.
- Approximately one in five patients develop some form of RV failure (need for a prolonged [> 14 days] course of inotropes or placement of a right ventricular assist device [RVAD]) after LVAD surgery.
- With a functioning LVAD in place, cardiac output is dependent on the ability of the RV to provide sufficient preload to the left side of the heart; however, increased RV preload may unmask preexisting RV failure.
- The presence of elevated CVP and significant RV dilation raises concerns that additional RV support may be required perioperatively.
- Patients with low pulmonary artery pressure in the setting of high CVP have, in fact, already developed RV failure.
- Patients with significant RV failure despite initial treatment, including inhaled nitric oxide, should not leave the operating room without an RVAD.
- The development of RV failure requiring an RVAD identifies patients with a poor prognosis.
- Patients who underwent an unplanned RVAD had only a 49% chance to be weaned from RVAD support and dismal 6-month survival (13%).
- The availability of the percutaneously placed Impella RP (Abiomed, Inc.) offers a new temporary mechanical support option for the failing RV with the ability to be removed at the bedside without requiring a repeat trip to the operating room to reopen the chest.
- Pharmacologic treatment of early and late RV failure consists of optimization of preload, augmentation of RV contractility, and reduction of pulmonary vascular resistance.
- If the patient is hypotensive and vasoplegic, the preferential vasoconstrictor is vasopressin, which does notincrease pulmonary vascular resistance as all other vasopressors do.
- LVAD speed must be optimized to avoid any left heart contribution to elevated pulmonary pressure.
- Care must be taken to optimize the speed to keep the interventricular septum midline and allow the RV to have a geometric shape conducive to contraction.
- Nitric oxide followed by sildenafil in combination with milrinone are used as pharmacologic agents to lower pulmonary artery pressures.
- With intermediate and long-term use, common LVAD complications are infection and gastrointestinal bleeding.
  - The relative immunosuppression of critical illness and the presence of large amounts of foreign material leave patients with an LVAD particularly susceptible to infectious complications.
  - Infections in patients with an LVAD can be classified into VAD-specific, VAD-related, and non-VAD infections.
  - LVAD-specific infections can occur in the device pocket or surrounding surgical area, along the percutaneous drive lines, and inside the device itself.
  - The majority of percutaneous site infections are bacterial (87.5%), with *Staphylococcus* and *Pseudomonas* the most common organisms.
  - Evaluation of patients with an LVAD with a suspected infection should include a complete blood count, blood cultures, and chest radiograph.
  - All patients with purulent drainage from a surgical site or driveline should have samples sent for Gram stain, potassium hydroxide test (for fungus), and routine bacterial and fungal cultures.
  - For patients with positive blood cultures with a pathogen known to cause endocarditis, an echocardiogram should be obtained.

- Management of device-related infections is challenging owing to the formation of an antibiotic-resistant biofilm on the surface of the device that is virtually resistant to penetration with antimicrobial agents.
- A prolonged course of culture-guided antibiotics is usually required.
- The most severe form of infection, VAD-related endocarditis, is rare.
- Urgent listing for transplantation or pump exchange once the blood cultures are sterile is required and suppressive antibiotics are necessary as long as the LVAD is still in place.

- Gastrointestinal (GI) bleeding in patients with an LVAD is common.
  - The observed higher GI bleeding rate in continuous-flow LVADs does not obviate the importance of antithrombotic management in thrombosis prevention.
  - The rate of GI bleeding following continuous-flow LVAD implantation ranges from 23 to 63 events per 100 patient-years and is disproportionately high compared with patients receiving warfarin for other indications (i.e., anticoagulation for mechanical valves, which carries a major bleeding risk of 1.2–2.6 events per 100 patient-years).
  - Formation of GI tract AVMs and acquired von Willebrand deficiency syndrome have been proposed as mechanisms responsible for this discrepancy.
  - In one study, de-escalation of double antithrombotic therapy to a single or even no agent still resulted in a subsequent major bleeding event in 43% of patients within 1 year.
  - This illustrates the intrinsic predisposition of continuous-flow LVAD recipients to bleeding complications even with minimal or no antithrombotic therapy.
  - Aspirin dose is an important factor that can potentially contribute to bleeding at high dose (325 mg) and thrombosis at low dose (81 mg).
  - Most LVAD GI bleeding events are managed therapeutically with blood transfusion and proton pump inhibitors.
  - Initial evaluation of GI bleeding should include endoscopy in an attempt to locate and manage the source of blood loss.
  - The upper GI tract is responsible for 40% to 50% of bleeding events from gastric erosions, ulcers, or arterio-venous malformations (AVMs).
  - Endoscopic maneuvers to stop bleeding are usually successful in the short term; however, in up to 50% of patients, rebleeding occurs.
  - Capsule endoscopy has limited diagnostic accuracy, but should be considered for recurrent and obscure bleeding events.
  - Octreotide should be considered for all patients with GI bleeding and angiodysplasias.

- Pump thrombosis is a potentially fatal complication of continuous-flow LVADs with a peak of pump thrombosis occurring within 3 months after insertion.
  - Pump-related factors are unique for each device and stem from abnormal flow and interactions between the blood components and LVAD surface.
  - Outflow graft kinking or impingement of the inflow cannula by the interventricular septum or LV free wall can also result in altered flow patterns and thrombosis (Fig. 25.5).
  - Patient-related factors include a preexisting or acquired hypercoagulable state, infection, sepsis, or dehydration.
  - Subtherapeutic INR is the most commonly encountered management-related factor.
  - Pump thrombosis has a diverse spectrum of clinical presentations.
  - Asymptomatic device alarms or hemolysis with darkening of the urine might be the only sign of pump thrombus.
  - On the other side of this spectrum are patients with thromboembolic events, new HF, and cardiogenic shock.
  - Understanding that elevation of plasma lactate dehydrogenase (LDH) level is related to pump thrombosis allows early diagnosis of this condition by routine measurement of LDH levels.

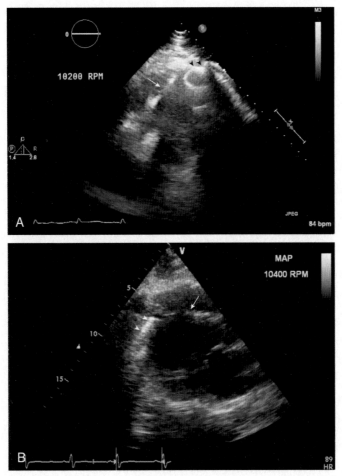

Fig. 25.5 In this patient with HeartMate II left ventricular assist device the inflow cannula *(arrowheads)* was malpositioned and the tip was occasionally impinged by interventricular septum *(arrows)*, causing symptoms. **(A)** Apical four-chamber view showing the circular-appearing left ventricular device inflow cannula abutting the interventricular septum. **(B)** Parasternal long-axis view showing the inflow cannula abutting the interventricular septum.

■ In addition to LDH level, all patients with a suspected pump thrombus should be admitted to the hospital, started on unfractionated heparin or bivalirudin, and should have a chest radiograph and echocardiogram.

■ Findings suggesting pump thrombus include poor LV uploading, worsening of mitral regurgitation, and one-to-one opening of a previously closed aortic valve (Fig. 25.6).

■ CT angiogram may be useful to evaluate the position of the inflow cannula and the outflow graft.

■ An echocardiographic ramp study has proven valuable for patients with a HeartMate II with an LV end-diastolic dimension slope absolute value of less than 0.16, which is highly suggestive of obstructive thrombus.

■ To evaluate patients with a HeartWare HVAD for possible thrombosis, the log files should be reviewed for presence of power spikes (Fig. 25.7).

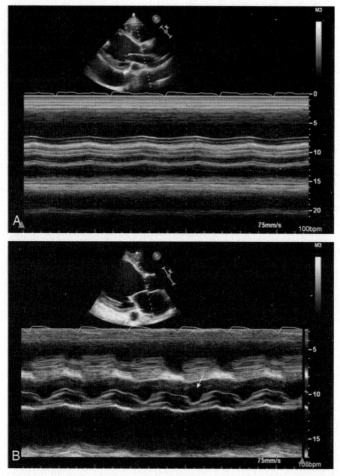

Fig. 25.6 M-mode echocardiograms from the same patient in Fig. 25.5 with a (**A**) normally functioning HeartMate II left ventricular assist device and (**B**) pump thrombosis. In **A**, the aortic valve is closed on each beat. In **B**, the left ventricle is now distended, and the aortic valve opens on every beat *(arrow)*. Pump thrombosis was confirmed during a device exchange.

- If the peak power is elevated less than 200% and growth rate of the power curve is less than 1.25, then thrombolysis might be helpful.
- Outcomes of thrombolysis for HeartMate II thrombosis are unsatisfactory, highlighting the importance of pump- and patient-specific treatment decisions.
- Emergent pump exchange or cardiac transplantation is the recommended treatment for HeartMate II and HVAD thrombosis with red alarms, pump stoppage, or shock.
- Patients with an LVAD with sustained ventricular tachycardia (VT) may tolerate the arrhythmia without hemodynamic collapse.
  - However, VT should be managed urgently to avoid deterioration of RV function.
  - The majority of VT occurs within the first 30 days of device implantation and might be caused by electrolyte abnormalities, β-blocker withdrawal, and the proarrhythmic effect of inotropes.

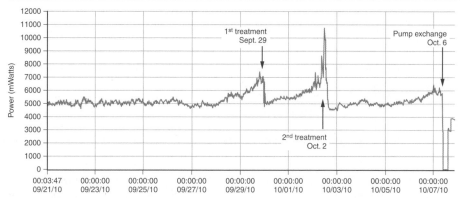

Fig. 27.7 HeartWare HVAD power consumption during pump thrombus and after multiple treatments. A device thrombus in which the patient received two unsuccessful doses of tissue plasminogen activator (on September 29 and October 2) before eventually requiring a pump exchange on October 6. (Modified from Jorde UP, Aaronson KA, Najjar SS, et al. Identification and management of pump thrombus in the HeartWare left ventricular assist device system: a novel approach using log file analysis. JACC Heart Fail. 2015;3(11):849–856.)

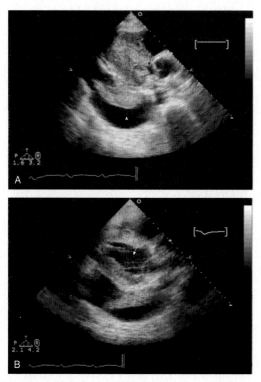

Fig. 25.8 A patient with a left ventricular assist device (LVAD) had recalcitrant ventricular tachycardia. (**A**) Parasternal long-axis view demonstrates almost complete obliteration of LV cavity *(arrow)*. A large pleural effusion was an incidental finding *(arrowhead)*. (**B**) The study was repeated after administration of intravenous fluids and LVAD speed decrease. LV cavity size has increased to 4 cm *(arrow)*. The patient was no longer in ventricular tachycardia after improvement in the LV chamber size.

- An LVAD-specific cause of VT is a suction event that occurs when the LV wall comes in contact with the inflow cannula in the setting of volume depletion or too high a pump speed.
- Rapid identification by echocardiogram is essential so that the speed can be decreased or volume given to correct this mechanical cause of VT (Fig. 25.8).
- Management of VT consists of discontinuing proarrhythmic drugs, correction of electrolyte abnormalities, appropriate use of β-blockers and antiarrhythmic drugs, and timely echocardiogram to rule out suction.
- In situations in which VT cannot be controlled, VT ablation can be attempted.
- Late aortic insufficiency (AI) has emerged as a complication of long-term therapy with continuous-flow devices.
  - The pathogenesis of AI relates to the loss of aortic valve opening followed by fusion of the leaflets.
  - At least moderate AI is expected to develop in 38% of patients after 3 years if an aortic valve opening strategy is not prospectively used.
  - Diagnostic evaluation is complicated by the fact that traditional echocardiographic methods of AI assessment underestimate its severity.
  - Although the best management approach is unknown, in severe symptomatic cases, use of transcatheter or surgical aortic valve replacement has been described.

Page numbers followed by '*f*' indicate figures, '*t*' indicate tables, '*b*' indicate boxes.